Third Edition

Clinical
ENT

Third Edition

Clinical ENT

Neha P Shah
MBBS, MS (ENT), DORL, FCPS, DNB
Consulting Ear, Nose and Throat Surgeon

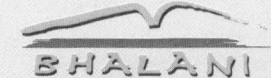

BHALANI PUBLISHERS
Mumbai

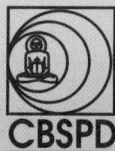

CBSPD

CBS Publishers & Distributors Pvt Ltd

New Delhi • Bengaluru • Chennai • Kochi • Kolkata • Lucknow • Mumbai
Hyderabad • Jharkhand • Nagpur • Patna • Pune • Uttarakhand

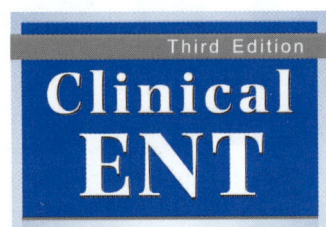

ISBN: 978-93-89688-86-3

© Bhalani Publishers

Third Edition: 2020

Reprint: 2025

First Edition: 2004

Second Edition: 2016

Published by Rajesh balani for

Bhalani Publishers, Mumbai
Mob: 09867214519   e-mail: bhalanipublishers@gmail.com

and

Published by Satish Kumar Jain and produced by Varun Jain for

CBS Publishers & Distributors Pvt Ltd

4819/XI Prahlad Street, 24 Ansari Road, Daryaganj, New Delhi 110 002, India
Ph: 011-23266838, 23289259   Website: www.cbspd.com
                                        e-mail: delhi@cbspd.com

Corporate Office: 204 FIE, Industrial Area, Patparganj, Delhi 110 092, India
Ph: 011-4934 4934   Fax: 011-4934 4935   e-mail: publishing@cbspd.com; publicity@cbspd.com

Branches

• **Bengaluru:** Seema House 2975, 17th Cross, K.R. Road, Banasankari 2nd Stage, Bengaluru 560 070, Karnataka, India
  Ph: +91-80-26771678/79   Fax: +91-80-26771680   e-mail: bangalore@cbspd.com

• **Chennai:** 18/8B, Subbarayan Street, Shenoy Nagar, Chennai 600 030, Tamil Nadu, India
  Ph: +91-44-42032115, 26681266   e-mail: chennai@cbspd.com

• **Kochi:** 42/1325, 1326, Power House Road, Opposite KSEB, Power House, Ernakulam 682018, Kochi, Kerala, India
  Ph: +91-484-4059061–65, 67   Fax: +91-484-4059065   e-mail: kochi@cbspd.com

• **Kolkata:** 147, Hind Ceramics Compound, 1st Floor, Nilgunj Road, Belghoria, Kolkata 700056, West Bengal, India
  Ph: +91-33-25633055/56

• **Lucknow:** Basement, Khushnuma Complex, 7 Meerabai Marg (behind Jawahar Bhawan), Lucknow 226001, UP, India
  Ph: +91-522-4000032   e-mail: tiwari.lucknow@cbspd.com

• **Mumbai:** PWD Shed, Gala No. 25/26, Ramchandra Bhatt Marg, Next to JJ Hospital, Gate No. 2, Opp. Union Bank of India, Noorbaug, Mumbai 400009, Maharashtra, India
  Ph: +91-22-66661880/89   e-mail: mumbai@cbspd.com

Representatives

• **Hyderabad**   0-9885175004   • **Jharkhand**   0-9811541605   • **Nagpur**   0-8692091830

• **Patna**   0-9334159340   • **Pune**   0-9664372571   • **Uttarakhand** 0-9716462459

Printed at: Goyal Offset Works Pvt. Ltd., Kundli, Haryana, India

Foreword

Dr Neha Shah was my student for her Masters course in TN Medical College and BYL Nair Ch Hospital. She studied under my guidance and secured a first place in her Masters and FCPS examinations. She was highly interested in academics and exuded sincerity in studies and practical work.

She is now in private practice but carries an urge to contribute to academics. I have known her for the last seven years and would say that she is an ideal candidate to write such a book. There are several books in ENT covering theoretical aspect of the subject but a book on practical knowledge was long required. This book attempts to bridge that gap. The book tries to put across the required data in a simple format with multiple charts, tables and illustrations. It is a very handy, comprehensive book for all students appearing for their final, diploma and masters examinations.

Simple presentations, multiple charts and an exhaustive coverage of practical examinations are the salient features of this book. Throughout the writing of the book, she was in touch with me and I have guided her for the same.

I hope, it will serve the purpose of every ENT student. I am extremely proud to say that she has lived up to the standards which I have tried to set for my students and I am equally pleased to forward her book *Clinical ENT* which will serve as a practical guide to help students through examinations.

Dr DS Grewal
Ex-Professor and Head
Department of ENT
TN Medical College and
BYL Nair Ch Hospital
Mumbai - 400 008

Preface

This book is dedicated to HIM. It was possible to complete this mammoth exercise only with His divine blessings and inspiration. At the time when this exercise was undertaken, the vast scope, complexity of the work and the limitations of resource availability were not fully comprehended and enthusiasm to author the book prevailed. It was the divine blessings, which guided me through this long and enriching journey.

The need for a good book, incorporating a compilation of numerous good notes, discussions and experience of professors and established doctors was felt very strongly by my colleagues and myself when we appeared for our Masters in Surgery practical examinations. This book is intended to help students, at all levels, to understand and comprehend the practical aspects of ENT examinations. It attempts to cover all such aspects.

Now, a brief description of the contents of this book. It includes six main sections which cover Case Presentation, Instruments, Operative Surgery, Surgical Pathology, Radiology in ENT and Anaesthesia in ENT.

In the section of Case Presentation, we have tried to follow a good format with related theory covered with each case. It tries to encompass all topics a student needs to know for practical exams. Contributions from many authors are included which not only ensures that all the topics are covered but also introduces to the case, a flair and flow pattern as distinct as the author. Another distinct feature of the Case Presentation section is the inclusion of numerous charts and blocks.

Contributions, help and support received from my professors, experienced and established doctors, my seniors and colleagues have been of immense value and thanks to all those who have made this effort possible: Dr DS Grewal, my guide, for his constant guidance and support, without which this publication would not have been possible. I am very grateful to Dr Kirtane and Dr Dabholkar for their encouragement and support. I am grateful to all my teachers, of the Nair Hospital ENT department for their immense help and guidance. I am thankful to Dr Divya Prabhat, Dr Bachi Hathiram, Dr Dinaz Irani, Dr Vijay Jagasia, Dr Rahul Mehta, Dr Ashwani Dwivedi, Dr Rohan Walvekar, Dr Meenal Shroff, Dr Yogesh Dabholkar, Dr Dilip Nair, Dr Sasz, Dr Kaushal Seth, Dr Ritu Agarwal, Dr Alok, Dr Chandrakant and Dr Sonali.

I am very thankful to all my teachers, who have written for this publication—Dr Vandana Lehiri, Dr Prerna Shroff, Late Dr Suren Kothari, Dr Jigna, Dr Behl, Dr Rajiv Joshi, Dr Uday Bhatt, Dr Shridhar Iyer, Mrs Geeta B Gore and Mrs Deepa A Valame.

• I am very thankful to Mr Rajesh Bhalani of M/s Bhalani Publishers for his publishing work and constant support for this book, Mr Chetan Sawant, for his excellent DTP work and Mrs Rayee Terdalkar for his simple and meticulously done diagrams.

• Special thanks to all my family members especially my son **Dev**, brother **Pratik**, my Mother and my spiritual teachers.

As I have already mentioned, this book is a reflection of the mammoth task to put an idea into practice. I present this compilation of knowledge in its current form knowing that even after numerous painstaking reviews, there is a tremendous scope for improvement and betterment of this book. God willing, I propose to incorporate this in the next edition.

I request your feedback and views to make the book more effective. We can incorporate these with due acknowledgement in the future editions. Please forward these suggestions by electronic mail at
Clinical ENT@yahoo.com

Dr Neha Shah

List of Contributors

Dr Vandana Lehiri
TN Medical College and BYL Nair Ch Hospital

Section: Anaesthesia

Dr Prerna Shroff
GS Medical College and KEM Hospital

Section: Anaesthesia

Dr Rajiv Joshi
TN Medical College and BYL Nair Ch Hospital

Section: Case Presentation – Thyroid Gland
Chapter: Ulcers of Tongue Operative Surgery -
Thyroidectomy

Late Dr Suren Kothari
Imaging Point, Hughes Road and
Professor, Department of Radiology
TN Medical College and BYL Nair Ch Hospital

Section: Radiology

Dr Jigna Rathod
Dr Uday Bhatt
TN Medical College and BYL Nair Ch Hospital

Section: Radiology
Section: Case Presentation – Cleft Lip and Palate
Operative Surgery - Rhinoplasty Instruments of Rhinoplasty

Mrs Geeta B Gore
Mrs Deepa A Valame
TN Medical College and BYL Nair Ch Hospital

Section: Audiology

Dr NK Behl
TN Medical College and BYL Nair Ch Hospital

Section: Surgical Pathology

Dr Shridhar Iyer
Tata Memorial Hospital

Section: Operative Surgery
– Commando Operation
– Radical Neck Dissection

Dr Kashmira P Chavan
Consultant ENT Surgeon
Dr LH Hiranandani Hospital
Powai, Mumbai 400076

Section: Tips for DNB Practicals

Dr Kashmira P Chavan
Consultant ENT Surgeon
Dr LH Hiranandani Hospital
Powai, Mumbai 400076

Chapter: Cochlear Implant
Chapter on "How to Read HRCT Temporal Bone"

Contents

Section II: Instruments

Section III: Operative Surgery

Section IV: Surgical Pathology

Section V: Radiology

Section VI: Anaesthesia

Section VII: Audiology

Section VIII: TIPS for DNB Practicals

Section IX: Additional Chapter

SECTION - I
CASE PRESENTATION

EAR

1. HISTORY AND EXAMINATION

HISTORY

Name, age, sex, religion, occupation, address.

Chief complaints:

- Discharge from the ear / Otorrhoea
- Decrease in hearing / Deafness
- Pain in the ear / Otalgia
- Giddiness / Vertigo
- Noise in the ear / Tinnitus
- Inability to close the eyes, mouth deviation etc. / Facial palsy.

(**Note:** It is preferable to present only two of the above complaints as chief complaints followed by their ODP i.e., Onset, Duration, Progress and then details of the rest of the complaints.)

ODP (Onset, Duration, Progress)

COMPLAINT	ODP (Onset, Duration, Progress)
Otorrhoea	• Unilateral / bilateral / state the side • Type - serous, serosanguinous, mucoid, mucopurulent, purulent, watery, blood • Foul smelling / not • Copious / moderate / scanty • Continuous / intermittent • Associated with pain / decrease in hearing / respiratory tract infection • Any aggravating / relieving factors - medications / ear drops, ear drops reaching the throat or not.
Deafness	• Unilateral / bilateral • Degree of hearing loss - cannot hear whispers / spoken speech / doorbell / loud sounds • Onset - sudden / gradual • Duration • Progress - rapid / slow • Fluctuant / constant • Associated with discharge / pain / tinnitus / fullness • Affecting routine work / not.

Otalgia	• Unilateral / bilateral
	• Type of pain-dull aching / throbbing
	• Intensity-mild / moderate / severe
	• Affecting routine work / sleep
	• Necessitates medication
	• Associated with upper respiratory tract infection
	• Relieving / aggravating factors
	  - Relieved with discharge
	  - Relieved with ear drops / medication

Vertigo	• Onset - sudden / gradual • Type-rotatory / swaying / tilting

COMPLAINT	ODP (Onset, Duration, Progress)
	• Positional element present or not • Gait disturbances present or not • Fluctuant / constant • Associated symptoms - Vomiting - Sweating - Hearing loss (Meniere's disease) - Tinnitus - Blackouts - Tullio's phenomenon (Meniere's disease) - Nystagmus. • Imbalance while walking - Precipitating factors - Sneezing - Change in position of head
Tinnitus	• Unilateral / bilateral • Onset • Duration • Type - Continuous / intermittent - Low pitched / high pitched - Fluctuant / constant - Rhythmic / pounding / roaring / dull / humming • Trigerring factors : mental or physical stress - Pregnancy / menstruation - Alcoholism - Exposure to excessive noise - Trauma - Associated with ear discharge / fullness in ear.
Facial Palsy	• Change in facial contour • Inability to close eye • Dribbling of saliva from one side • Difficulty in blowing cheeks and chewing food. • Inability to whistle. • Decreased / blurred vision • Redness / itching / watering of eyes • Characteristic of the palsy - Slow / sudden onset - Incomplete / complete palsy - H/o concurrent or preceeding upper respiratory tract infection with the palsy. - H/o pain or numbness around the ear - H/o surgical intervention / trauma to the nerve.

Positive / Negative history

• H/o post-aural swelling associated with fever or headache (mastoid abscess).

• H/o fever, vomiting, unconsciousness, headache, visual disturbances, speech problems (intra-cranial complications).

- H/o trauma, exposure to excessive noise, use of ototoxic drugs etc.
- H/o nasal blockage / recurrent attacks of rhinitis.
- H/o odynophagia, fever / recurrent upper respiratory tract infections
- H/o any other nose / throat complaints.
- H/o tuberculosis / tuberculous contact, blood pressure, diabetes.
- H/o asthma, allergy or sexually transmitted diseases.
- H/o otological / any major surgery / illness (meningitis) in the past.

Past history
- H/o any similar complaints in the past.
- H/o any major surgery or illness in the past.

Personal history
- Bowel / bladder habits
- T.B. / B.P. / D.M. / H.T.
- Socio-economic status.

Family history
- Similiar complaints in the family.
- Hearing loss
- Ear operations
- T.B. / B.P. / D.M.

GENERAL EXAMINATION
- Patient is conscious, co-operative and well oriented in time, space and person.
- General condition : - Built and nourishment
  - Afebrile or not
- Pallor
- Oedema
- Cyanosis
- Clubbing
- Jugular venous pressure
- Lymphadenopathy:
  - Cervical
  - Axillary
  - Inguinal

Respiratory System
- Air entry : - Bilaterally equal / not
  - Rales / rhonchi / foreign sounds.

Central Nervous System
- Consciousness, orientation in time, space and person.
- Cranial nerves I to XII.
- Muscle power
- Reflexes.

Cardiovascular System
- Heart sounds - first and second
- Apex beat

Gastrointestinal System

- Hepatosplenomegaly
- Ascites

LOCAL EXAMINATION

- Pre auricular region
- Pinna
- Post auricular region
- External auditory canal
- Tympanic membrane
- Mastoid region

Tuning fork tests

- Rinne's test with 256, 512 and 1024 Hz tuning fork
- Weber's test
- Absolute bone conduction test

Nystagmus

Fistula sign

Facial nerve

Tests for eustachian tube patency

Seigalization

Tests for balance

- Romberg's test
- Urtenburger's test

Examination of the eyes

- Inspection
- Nystagmus
- Corneal reflex

NOSE

External examination

External deviation, bridge of the nose, scars, sinuses etc.

Anterior rhinoscopy

- Septum   : Deviation, spurs, perforation
- Mucosa   : Congestion, atrophy, secretions.
- Turbinates : Hypertrophy, atrophy

Posterior rhinoscopy

- Secretions
- Adenoids
- Eustachian tube area
- Tenderness over paranasal sinuses.

THROAT

- Oral cavity : Teeth, tongue, buccal mucosa.

- Oropharynx : Tonsil, tonsillar pillars, posterior pharyngeal wall.
- Indirect laryngoscopy.

DIAGNOSIS

Right / left, inactive / active, chronic suppurative otitis media, with mild / moderate / severe conductive / mixed / sensorineural hearing loss with / without intracranial complications with nose / throat complaints, if any (e.g. with deviated nasal septum to the left and mild granular pharyngitis).

⟪ INITIAL PARTICULARS ⟫

PARTICULARS	IMPORTANCE	COMMENTS	COMMENTS
NAME (Full name with middle name and surname)	Gives identity to a person. It may help in identifying the unknown religion.		
AGE	Certain diseases are related to certain age groups.	Children ● Bilateral ear diseases ● Glue ear ● Tonsilloadenitis	Elderly ● Carcinomas ● Bone conduction decreases after the age of 50 years ● Sensorineural hearing loss is present in elderly ● Diabetes ● Hypertension
SEX	Certain diseases are common in a particular sex.	Males ● Meneire's disease. ● Carcinomas	Females ● Otosclerosis ● Goitre ● Postcricoid carcinoma ● Plummer Vinson syndrome ● Temporal arteritis During menstruation ● Increase in deafness can occur ● Tinnitus may occur. Pregnancy ● Deafness may occur following the pregnancy
RELIGION	Certain diseases are common in some races / religion.		
OCCUPATION	Occupational hazards	Noise Noise induced hearing loss / occupational deafness* is seen in : ● Boiler makers ● Black smiths ● Riveters. *Pathological effect is due to :	Hay / garden pollen can lead to : ● Allergic rhinitis ● Nasal polyposis Smoke / air pollution can cause : ● Asthma ● Carcinoma nasopharynx

PARTICULARS	IMPORTANCE	COMMENTS	COMMENTS
		• Constant vibrations • Loud and continuous noise Changes in air pressure : • Divers • Mountaineers.	Farmers can get : • Rhinosporidiosis.
ADDRESS	• Full postal address is necessary. • Essential for follow-up • Certain diseases are common in certain areas	Goitre is seen in : • Sahyadri range • Ratnagiri district	

OTORRHOEA

It means discharge from the ear.

TYPES	CHARACTERISTIC	CONDITIONS	COMMENTS
Serous	Like serum	Seborrhoeic otitis externa.	
Serosanguinous	Serum + blood tinged	Seborrhoeic otitis externa.	
Mucoid	Mucin threads seen on sucking the discharge through a suction cannula.	Secretory otitis media (with perforation). Otitis media • Acute • Chronic	Mucoid discharge is always from the middle ear as middle ear lining consists of goblet cells, which secrete mucin.
Mucopurulent	Mucoid discharge + pus	Otitis media • Acute • Chronic	
Purulent	Pus-like. A pus cell is a dead lymphocyte. It is yellow in colour and may have a foul smell.	Otitis media • Acute • Chronic : - Safe - Unsafe	Purulent non mucoid discharge is characteristic of chronic osteitis without cholesteatoma

Watery	Clear like water.	• CSF otorrhoea is seen in :
		  - Trauma
		  - Temporal bone fractures
		  - Intraoperative damage.
		• Eczematous otitis externa
			Confirmatory tests for CSF :
			1. Glucose estimation >30 mg/dl in the fluid
			2. Immunoelectrophoresis of the fluid : B2 transferrin band is present
			3. Halo sign : Halo around dried CSF on kerchief.

Blood	Actual blood.	• Trauma
		• Polyp
		  - External ear
		  - Middle ear
		• Glomus tumours
		• Acute otitis media
		• Foreign body	

TYPES	CHARACTERISTIC	CONDITIONS	COMMENTS
		• Tuberculosis • Granular myringitis • Malignant otitis externa. • Vascular anomalies	
Other characteristics • Foul smell	Fishy odour	Chronic suppurative otitis media-unsafe variety	Organisms responsible for the odour : • Anaerobes • Peptostreptococci • Bacteroides fusiformis • Bacteroides fragilis • Bacteroides melanogenicus • Saprophytic organisms.
• Copious quantity	RESERVOIR SIGN : Discharge filling the concha and reappearing on wiping it.	Reservoir sign is positive in : • Coalescent mastoiditis. • Operated radical mastoid cavity with secondary infection.	
• Scanty discharge		Chronic suppurative otitis media - unsafe variety	

Causes of otorrhoea:

EXTERNAL EAR	MIDDLE EAR	INNER EAR	MISCELLANEOUS
• Localised otitis externa (furunculosis) • Generalised otitis externa • Seborrhoeic otitis externa • Eczematous otitis externa • Bacterial / viral otitis externa • Otomycosis • Foreign body with secondary infection	• Acute otitis media • Chronic otitis media • Tumours	• Suppurative labyrinthitis	• Parotid abscess rupturing into ear • Temporomandibular joint abscess rupture

DEAFNESS

Definition

It is the term commonly used to indicate a change in hearing acuity.

Deafness   :   Total loss of hearing function

Hearing loss: Partial loss / partial hypoacusis

Types:

1. **Conductive deafness**   :   Defect in the conducting mechanism of the external and/or middle ear.
2. **Sensorineural deafness**   :   Due to lesions in the labyrinth, eighth nerve and the cochlea.
3. **Mixed deafness**   :   Both conductive and sensorineural components are present.

Difference between conductive and sensorineural deafness: (also on pg 10)

DEAFNESS	CONDUCTIVE	SENSORINEURAL
1. Site of lesion	External ear and middle ear	Inner ear, eighth nerve and central connections
2. Rinne test	Bone conduction better than air conduction	Air conduction better than bone conduction
3. Weber test	Lateralised to the worse ear.	Lateralised to the better ear.
4. Audiological tests	Bone conduction better than air conduction	Air conduction similar to bone conduction
5. Hearing loss	Not more than 60dB.	May be more than 60dB.
6. Speech	Speaks in a low voice.	Speaks loudly.
7. Speech discrimination	Good	Poor
8. Recruitment	Absent	Present in cochlear deafness.
9. Paracusis willisi	Present in otosclerosis	Absent

Causes of deafness

A. Conductive deafness

1. External ear:

   - Wax
   - Otomycosis
   - Otitis externa
   - Foreign body
   - Myringitis
   - Stenosis
   - Atresia
   - Tumours

2. Middle ear:

   - Congenital defects of the eardrum and ossicles.
   - Inflammatory:
     - Otitis media: acute / chronic
     - Secretory otitis media
     - Adhesive otitis media
     - Tuberculous otitis media
     - Syphilitic otitis media
   - Traumatic
     - Barotrauma
     - Rupture of eardrum
     - Haemotympanum
     - Ossicular discontinuity
     - Fracture of skull base
   - Others
     - Eustachian catarrh
     - Eustachian tube dysfunction.

B. Sensorineural deafness

   - Causes of sensorineural deafness:

UNILATERAL	BILATERAL	ASYMMETRICAL

1. Trauma
  - Head injury
  - Blast injury
  - Surgical damage
2. Vestibular schwannoma
3. Mumps
	1. Presbyacusis
	2. Noise
	3. Ototoxicity
	4. Heredity
	5. Bilateral acoustic neuromas
	6. Meneire's disease.
	7. Syphilis
		1. Weapon firing / explosion
		2. Head injury

C. Mixed hearing loss

- Chronic suppurative otitis media (toxins)
- Otosclerosis (abnormal mechanics of sound transmission)

D. Fluctuant hearing loss

Causes of fluctuant hearing loss

CONDUCTIVE	SENSORINEURAL
1. Upper respiratory tract infection	1. Syphilitic labyrinthitis
2. Eustachian tube dysfunction	2. Meneire's disease
3. Otitis media with effusion	3. Lermoyez's disease
	4. Perilymph fistula

Change in hearing loss associated with background noise is seen in patients on:

- Aminoglycosides
- Loop diuretics
- Quinine

E. Sudden deafness

Causes of sudden deafness:

- Vascular disease
- Viral disease / Mumps
- Perilymph fistula
- Meningitis
- Acoustic neuroma

F. Sudden and fluctuant deafness

Causes of sudden and fluctuant deafness:

COCHLEAR		RETROCOCHLEAR (VII) N AND CNS
Inflammatory	**Vascular**	• Meningitis
• Acute otitis media	• Hypertension	• Multiple sclerosis
• Typhoid	• Hypercoagulability	• Acoustic neuroma
• Syphilis	**Haematological**	• Alzheimer's disease
Viral	• Polycythaemia	
• Mumps	• Sickle cell disease	
• Measles	• Thalassaemia	
• Rubeola	**Autoimmune disease**	
• Infectious mononucleosis	• Systemic lupus erythematosus	
• HIV	• Wegener's granulomatosis	
Traumatic	**Metabolic disease**	
• Electricity	• Renal failure	
Iatrogenic	• Diabetes mellitus	
• Radiotherapy	• Hypothyroidism	
• Post operative	**Ototoxic drugs**	
	Idiopathic	

Common medical illnesses causing hearing loss :

- Meningitis
- Cerebral malaria
- Mumps
- Measles

Difference between conductive and sensorineural deafness:

	CONDUCTIVE	SENSORINEURAL
Site of pathology	External and middle ear	Inner ear, and VIII nerve
Tuning fork tests		
1. Rinne test	Normal	Reduced / nil
2. Weber test	Lateralised to worse ear	Lateralised to better ear
3. Absolute bone conduction test	Negative	Positive (not heard in severe cases)
Audiological tests		
1. Pure tone audiometry	Air-bone gap present	No air-bone gap
2. Impedance audiometry	Type 'A's curve in otosclerosis Type 'A' d curve in ossicular discontinuity Type B curve in otitis media with effusion	Both air and bone conduction are reduced
3. Bekesy audiometry	Type I	Type I – Cochlear deafness Type III / IV – Neural deafness
4. Recruitment	Absent	Present in cochlear deafness Absent in nerve deafness
5. SISI	Low score 0-20%	High score 0-60% in cochlear deafness 0-20% score in nerve deafness.

Important points:

- Conversation in a quiet environment is conducted at 40dB
- Telephonic conversation is at 40-70dB in the frequency range of 200- 1200Hz.
- Following decibels indicate the noise levels created by:

Automobiles-trains / buses	90dB
Aeroplanes	>90dB
Drills	85-115dB for patient
Music	Upto 120dB
Suction	140dB in EAC
Fire crackers	156dB
Guns	180dB

- Servicaeble hearing:

    Definition: An average loss of 40dB or better over the speech frequencies 500, 1000 and 2000Hz.

    Hearing reaches a serviceable level in

    80% - Type I and Type II ossicular reconstruction

    40% - Type III

    15% - Type IV

- Paracusis willisii   :   The phenomenon in which a person with a conductive hearing loss hears better in a noisy environment is termed as Paracusis willisii. It is seen in Otosclerosis. In sensorineural hearing loss, there is decreased discrimination of speech in background noise and it is not helped if the speaker raises the intensity of voice

    Reasons for this phenomenon:

    1. Reduction of masking effect of the background noise

    2. Increase in intensity of voice of the speaker

- Recruitment of loudness is a characteristic of cochlear hearing loss
- Poor-speech discrimination without recruitment suggests auditory nerve lesion
- Diplacusis is an apparent difference in the pitch of a tone between the two ears and is associated with conditions causing endolymphatic hydrops.
- Autophony: It is abnormal perception of one's own breadth and voice sounds and is associated with a permanently open or patulous eustachian tube
- Social noise trauma includes
  - Pop music
  - Rifle shooting
  - Motor racing

CONGENITAL DEAFNESS

Congenital deafness suggests deafness due to hereditary or genetic causes.

Classification:

Classification of genetic deafness / hereditary deafness

I. According to causes:
  1. Genetic
     a. Syndromic
     b. Non-syndromic
     c. Mitochondrial disorders
     d. Chromosomal disorders
  2. Non-genetic

II. According to type:
  1. Conductive
  2. Sensorineural
  3. Mixed
  4. Non-organic

CONDUCTIVE DEAFNESS

Causes of congenital conductive deafness:

AT BIRTH	APPEARING IN CHILDHOOD	PREDISPOSITION TO OTITIS MEDIA WITH EFFUSION	MISCELLANEOUS
• Down's syndrome • Crouzon's syndrome • Marfan's syndrome • Treacher Collin's syndrome	• Osteogenesis imperfecta • Otosclerosis	• Cystic fibrosis • Immotile cilia syndrome • Cleft palate • Immune deficiency states	• Isolated malformations • Congenital cholesteatoma • Rhabdomyosarcoma • Fibrous dysplasia

Isolated malformations: Marquet's classification into two types / Cremmer's, Oudenhoven and Marres into three types

TYPE I   :   Failure of canalization of external auditory canal
              Small external auditory canal, atretic laterally
              Normal / near normal auricle
              Small tympanic membrane

TYPE II   :   Largest group of ear deformities
              Rudimentary tag instead of an auricle
              Rudimentary tympanic membrane / partially / totally aplastic external auditory canal
              Fixed malleus and incus
              Abnormal course of VII nerve

TYPE IIA : Type II + partial bony stenosis of ear canal

TYPE IIB : Type II + complete bony stenosis of ear canal

Congenital Cholesteatoma:

Three criteria are set by Derlacki and Clemis

- Development behind an intact tympanic membrane
- No history of ear infections
- The lesion must arise from inclusion of squamous epithelium during embryonic development

Types

1. External auditory canal
2. Middle ear
3. Mastoid
4. Petrous apex
5. Cerebelllo pontine angle

    It behaves in the same way as an acquired cholesteatoma.

SENSORINEURAL DEAFNESS

Pathological abnormalities of the cochlea seen in these cases are of four patterns:

1. **Michel dysplasia**
    - Most severe
    - Total absence of labyrinth
    - Failure of otic capsule to separate from neural ridge
2. **Mondini deformity**
    - Affects cochlea and semicircular canal
    - Cochlear duct reduced to basal turn only
    - Absent / reduced organ of corti
3. **Bing - Siebenmann dysplasia**
    - Normal bony labyrinth
    - Decrease development of membranous part
4. **Scheibe (cochleosaccular) dysplasia**
    - Stria vascularis has alternate areas of aplasia and hyperplasia
    - Rudimentary organ of corti
    - Sparse / absent hair cells
    - Collapsed saccule

Genetic disorders with deafness present at birth

Syndrome:

1. Turner's syndrome
2. Usher's syndrome
3. Pendred's syndrome

Genetic disorders with deafness developing after birth

Syndrome:

1. Alport's syndrome
2. Renal tubular acidosis
3. Refsum's disease
4. Cogan's syndrome

Non genetic deafness

Causes of non-genetic deafness:

1. Intra-uterine disease

   a. Rubella

   b. Cytomegalovirus

   c. Syphilis

   d. Toxoplasmosis

2. Irradiation

3. Ultrasound

4. Maternal diabetes   :   Hypoplasia of IAC

                                    Fetal alcohol syndrome

5. Ototoxic drugs

   a. Aminoglycosides   :   Intrauterine cochlear damage

                                      Erythromycin, tobramycin

   b. Chemotherapeutic agents   :   Cisplatin

   c. Loop diuretics

Perinatal causes of SNHL

- Hypoxia: Decrease in cell no: of cochlear nucleii
- Hyperbilirubinaemia
- Low birth weight / Pre-term child

  It has immature metabolic function, more likely to suffer hypoxia. They may suffer from life threatening infections for which ototoxic drugs may have to be given
- Mumps   : Unilateral SNHL
- Measles : Degeneration of organ of corti, spiral ganglion, vestibular sensory cells
- Immunization: Tetanus injection: peripheral neuropathy
- Auto immune SNHL
- Meningitis: Bacterial labyrinthitis
- Trauma: Rupture of RW, OW
- Neoplastic disease: - Acoustic neuroma
  - Leukaemia of temporal bone
- Idiopathic: Vascular thrombosis, embolism

MIXED DEAFNESS

Causes of mixed deafness:

1. Earpits deafness syndrome
2. Osteopetrositis
3. Langerhans cell histiocytosis
4. Mucopolysaccharidosis

ASSESSMENT OF A CONGENITALLY HEARING IMPAIRED CHILD

Aims

- To determine if a hearing loss is present
- To decide the type and severity of hearing loss

- To determine the age of onset of the hearing loss

  (Prelingual hearing loss has more serious implications on the child)
- To look for other relevant handicaps

Assessment

1. History:

The parents are asked to state:

- Their main worry about the child
- About the child's hearing
- H/o of delivery / postnatal life
- ENT symptoms / family history
- Child failing to develop speech / screening tests

2. Audiological assessment:

1. Test for behavioural reflexes

AGE (IN MONTHS)	RESPONSES
First few weeks of life	• Loud sounds : startle reflex • Moro's reflex : change in heart rate and pattern of respiration and a backward head jerk and body movement on sound
Infant under 4 months of age	• Respond by stilling and listening • Smiles in a communicative way
4-6 months of age	• Turning the head towards the auditory stimulus
7-9 months of age	• Localizes sound accurately • Turns readily towards the sound source and searches for it • May also begin to copy sounds
10-12 months of age	• Localizes sound • Verbal comprehension of sound occurs
13-24 months of age	• Localizes sound, searches for sound start, therfore distraction may be necessary • Vocabulary increases, picks up toys on request
Over 2 years of age	• May carry out PTA also

2. Behavioural audiometry:

Behavioural responses seen on giving auditory stimulus

Pre requisites are:

- Appropriate test is chosen according to the developmental age of the child
- Auditory stimulus is given either live or through loud speakers in a sound free field

1. Distraction test of hearing:

It is for a child aged 9 months and above

Distraction is needed as such a child wanders or searches for sound.

2. Visual reinforcement audiometry

Similar to the above test but the response of the child is reinforced by a visual stimulus (flashing of light). This method is said to reduce the habituation to sound seen in children > 1yr. of age

3. Conditioning audiometry

The child is told to carry out a simple task (eg: putting a brick in a box) in response to sound

Difficult children are:

- Visually impaired children
- Mentally retarded children
- Cerebral palsy children
- Hyperactive children

Children which are difficult to handle and those below 3-4 months of age, in whom behavioural testing is not posible, objective methods of testing are used:

3. **Objective audiometry**

Electric response audiometry

- Auditory brain stem response
- Electrocochleography
- Period evoked potential
- Acoustic stapedial reflex

a) **Auditory brain stem response**

Brainstem responses measured in response to a click stimuli recorded in the 1-10ms.interval. The hearing threshold is determined by the lowest stimulus intensity at which the auditory evoked potential is detectable visually.

Principle:

When sound reaches the cochlea, it is converted into an electrical response which passes finally to the auditory cortex. Passage of the impulse through this pathway creates an electrical activity which can be monitored by placing a surface electrode on the scalp. Graphic recording of this electrical activity is done in a waveform, which is studied for any abnormality in the pathway.

b) **Electrocochleography**

The cochlear nerve action potential is an exogenous transient response recorded in the first 10ms. interval, from a number of sites around the ear.

c) **Period evoked potential**

It is a new technique, based on frequency following response, the frequency reflects auditory units in the brainstem

4. **Impedance audiometry**

The otoimpedance to the sound presented to the tested ear is measured. It gives an idea about middle ear impedance matching mechanism, the elasticity / compliance of the middle ear system

Results

INCREASED COMPLIANCE	DECREASED COMPLIANCE	NORMAL COMPLIANCE
• Ossicular chain discontinuity	• Otosclerosis • Adhesive / Secretory otitis media • Middle ear tumours like glomus tumours • Tympanosclerosis	• Eustachian tube obstruction

New related techniques

a) **TM displacement measurement**

Principle

Changes in hydrostatic pressure on the cochlear perilymph produces a minor variation in the movements of ossicles and tympanic membrane. The resulting tympanic membrane displacement is measured over time.

b) Acoustic reflectometry

It is a test performed as an impedance audiometry but instead, with the help of an acoustic otoscope

Advantages:

- Can be done on a crying child
- Does not require an air tight seal
- Useful in assessment of a difficult child

c) Otoacoustic emissions

The emissions are due to release of acoustic energy originating from outer hair cells of the cochlea. They are recorded in the external auditory canal and are evidence of a normally functioning cochlea.

d) Speech audiometry

- Speech detection
- Speech discrimination
- Speech perception

  This is done by, presentation of phonetically balanced words to the child with instructions to repeat the word heard.

Management of the hearing impaired child:

- Early detection:
  - By screening tests of hearing
  - High level of parental suspicion
  - Screening / testing children with undeveloped / poor speech
- Parental counselling
  - For future pregnancies
  - For rehabilitation and schooling of the deaf child
- Complete audiological assessment
- Other investigations

INVESTIGATION	REASON
Serological	• TORCH screening • Rubella specific IgG/IgM • Syphilis antibodies • Thyroxine levels
Urine	• Cytomegalovirus • Renal disease
X'ray skull	• Intracranial calcification in Toxoplasmosis
C.T. Scan / HRCT	• Structural abnormalities of middle ear, inner ear • For cochlear implantation
Ophthalmic checkup	• Rubella retinopathy
Paediatric / neurology opinion	• Head and neck abnormality • Syndromes • Mental retardation

MANAGEMENT

1. Appropriate hearing aid selection : - Hearing aid
   - Cochlear implant

2. Surgical correction of congenital malformations
3. Promotion of development of language / speech
4. Rehabilitation: education, schooling

1. Hearing aids

The hearing aid amplifies the presented sound stimulating the residual hair cells / sensory organ.

Indications

a) Children with SNHL

b) Congenital abnormality of external and middle ear not suitable for surgical correction

Types

1. Personal hearing aids
2. Body worn hearing aids
3. Behind the ear aids
4. In the ear / conchal aids
5. Bone conduction / bone anchored aids
6. Aids not entirely worn by the listener

The range of aids is such that a suitable aid can be found for most children. The behind the ear aids are too big for most children. The conchal hearing aid is most expensive and is reserved for children with deformities of the pinna. Bone conduction hearing aids are for children with deformed ears or severe recurrent ear infections which prohibit insertion of ear moulds.The bone anchored hearing aid is directly anchored to the mastoid bone with the help of screws without any intervening soft tissue and gives good results. It is used for uni / bilateral ear malformations with severe conductive losses. It is not suitable for children whose skull bones are not sufficiently thick to accept the osseointegrated screw.The greatest disadvantage of conventional hearing aid is their inability to distinguish between speech sounds and unwanted background noise. This is partly overcome by the following means (in school):

Aids not entirely worn by the listener

a) Speech trainer

In this, the microphone part of the hearing aid is kept close to the speaker (teacher's) mouth

b) Group hearing aids

Several children are connected to eachother and the teacher by amplifiers

c) Radio hearing aids

The teacher / parent wears a microphone transmitter and the child a receiver. FM (frequency modulation) radio systems are used

d) Infra red hearing aid system

The infrared signals pass from the teacher's transmitter to the child's receiver

e) Loop system

Input from the teacher's microphone is transmitted either directly around an electromagnetic loop installed on the classroom walls, or by means of a loop worn around the child's neck.

Cochlear Implants

Prerequisites

1. Profound sensorineural hearing loss with no conductive component
2. Proper developmental / mental / psychological age
3. No medical illness
4. Pre op. C.T.Scan
5. Good parental understanding / cooperation

Types

1. Intracochlear

   Simultaneous electrodes are implanted within the lumen of the cochlea in the scala tympani and which are typically multichannel

2. Extracochlear

   A single channel in which an active electrode is implanted in the region of the round window.

2. **Surgical management**

   Congenital aural atresia

   ● **Fenestration of the lateral canal**

      Disadvantages :   -   Creation of labyrinthine fistula

                        -   Wide exenteration of mastoid is required

   ● **Type III tympanoplasty**

      -   Direct contact between stapes and drum head

      -   Disadvantages: An open mastoid cavity with a constant risk of otorrhoea

   ● **Canalplasty technique**

      -   It is done in more severe cases with repair of microtia. In least severe cases, removal of atretic plate of the ear canal is carried out.

   ● **Plastic reconstruction of the pinna**

      -   It is carried out with surgery for hearing reconstruction

      -   Auricular prosthesis can also be used

3. **Rehabilitation / Education of the deaf**

a. Preschool children	● Teachers for the deaf ● Parental counselling : - Care of the hearing aid - To talk normally to the child etc.

b. School children	Sent to : - Ordinary classrooms using hearing aid
	              - Specialised teachers are appointed
	              - Speech and language units / hearing units
	              - School for profoundly deaf

4. **Communication methods**

   a) Auralism

      -   To use only speech and lip reading as a means of communication

      -   Signing is prevented

   b) Finger spelling

   c) Cued speech

      -   Uses 8 different hand shapes in 4 different positions to enable the child to discriminate lip movement

   d) Signing systems

      -   Signed English

      -   British sign language

   e) Total communication

      -   Use of all modes of communication eg. speech, gestures, writing etc.

OTALGIA

Otalgia: It means pain in the ear

Causes of otalgia

EXTERNAL EAR	MIDDLE EAR	INNER EAR
• Wax • Foreign body • Otomycosis • Otitis externa • Trauma • Herpes zoster • Exostosis • Keratosis obturans • Hypersensitivity to local eardrops	• Acute otitis media • CSOM with intracranial complications • Acute mastoiditis • Secretory otitis media • Traumatic perforation • Otitic barotrauma • Haemotympanum • Tumours / carcinoma	• Noise • Tinnitus - loud tinnitus is perceived as otalgia • Meniere's disease • Vestibular schwannoma - 30% of patients get pain in the ear

Character of pain

ACUTE OTITIS MEDIA	COALESCENT MASTOIDITIS	ACUTE OTITIS EXTERNA	AUDITORY TUBE DYSFUNCTION
• Acute • Deep seated • Violent / severe • Associated with continuous / paroxysmal pulsations • Increases in severity at night	Pain is behind the ear in coalescent mastoiditis and behind the eye in Petrous apex mastoiditis	• Diffuse pain generally • Severity of pain depends upon amount of oedema • Pain is aggravated by biting, chewing and pinna movements • Very severe pain is seen in furunculosis	Pain occurs within sometime on lying down

> **Conditions associated with severe pain :**
> • Herpes simplex oticus
> • Herpes zoster oticus
> • Bullous myringitis

Important points:

- As the skin is very closely applied to the meatal and auricular perichondrium, severe pain is associated with otitis externa
- Pain is not a feature of chronic otitis media unless associated with otitis externa or dural inflammation

Innervation of the ear

Cranial nerves V, VII, IX, X and C2, C3

ANATOMIC PARTS	INNERVATION
Pinna	• Greater auricular nerve C2, C3 • Lesser occipital nerve C3 • Auricular branch of vagus • Auriculotemporal nerve • Facial nerve
Tympanic membrane	• Tympanic branch of Glossopharyngeal nerve • Auricular branch of vagus nerve • Branches from facial nerve
Middle ear	• Glossopharyngeal nerve via tympanic plexus
Mastoid	• Meningeal branch of Trigeminal nerve

Referred pain

Pain is referred to the ear via the V, VII, IX, X, upper cervical and sympathetic nerves.

CAUSE OF REFERRED PAIN		NERVE CAUSING REFERRED PAIN IN EAR
Tonsil	Tonsillitis Peritonsillar abscess Post tonsillectomy Retropharyngeal abscess	Via Glossopharyngeal nerve
Parotid	Parotitis Mumps	Via Facial nerve Via Trigeminal nerve
Thyroid	Acute thyroiditis Subacute thyroiditis Hashimoto's thyroiditis	Via Vagus nerve
Larynx	Tuberculosis Carcinoma	Via Vagus nerve
Styloid process	Eagle's syndrome	Via Glossopharyngeal nerve
Oral cavity	Dental caries, Alveolar abscess Oral ulcers, Impacted molars	Via Trigeminal nerve
TM Joint	Trauma Infection Arthritis	Via Trigeminal nerve
Nervous origin	Herpes zoster Glossopharyngeal zoster	Via Trigeminal nerve Via Glossopharyngeal nerve
Spine	Cervical spine degeneration / tumours	Via Cervical nerves

Neoplasms (carcinoma) causing referred pain

- Pyriform fossa
- Glottis / supraglottis
- Post cricoid carcinoma
- Posterior pharyngeal wall
- Posterior ⅓ of tongue
- Parotid gland
- Nasopharynx

Common causes of referred pain
- Caries teeth
- Impacted molars
- Posterior tongue lesions
- Pharynx / tonsillar lesions

VERTIGO

DEFINITIONS

1. It is defined as an illusion of movement.
2. The disagreeable sensation of instability or disordered orientation in space
3. It is defined as a hallucination of movement.

ETIOLOGY

OTOLOGICAL	NEUROLOGICAL	VISUAL
• Chronic middle ear disease	• Cerebellopontine angle lesion	• Ocular pathology
• Meniere's disease	• Cerebellar lesions	• Retro-orbital lesion
• Benign paroxysmal positional vertigo	• Internal capsule / thalamic lesions	**TOXINS**
• Acoustic neuroma	• Epilepsy	• Ethanol
• Cholesteatoma	• Parkinsonism	• Carbon monoxide
• Otosclerosis	• Multiple sclerosis	**ENDOCRINE**
• Temporal bone lesions	• Hydrocephalus	• Hypothyroidism
• Labyrinthine contusion	• Meningitis	• Hypoglycaemia
• Syphilis	• Neurosyphilis	**SKELETAL**
• Viral labyrinthitis	• Subdural / extradural haematoma	• Osteoarthritis
• Tuberculosis	• Whiplash injury	• Paget's disease
		PSYCHOGENIC

CLASSIFICATION OF VERTIGO

I. a) **Rotational**
    1. Episodic
    2. Prolonged

   b) **Unsteadiness**
    1. Episodic
    2. Prolonged

II. a) **Central**

   b) **Peripheral**

   Difference between central and peripheral vertigo

CENTRAL VERTIGO	PERIPHERAL VERTIGO
Gradual	Sudden onset
Not an intense vertigo Increase disturbance of gait occurs instead	Intense vertigo
Not much affected by positional changes	Increases on head movements / positional changes
Swaying / tilting, more on one side	Rotatory in character
Due to lesion in the brain or its central connections	Due to lesion in the inner ear (labyrinth)

INVESTIGATIONS

- Complete blood count
- Blood sugar
- Cholesterol / Triglycerides

- Renal function test / Liver function test
- Blood pressure measurement
- X'ray cervical spine, internal auditory meatus, mastoid
- ECG
- CT scan / MRI

Subjective tests:

- Fistula test
- Rhomberg's test
- Urtenberger's test
- Caloric testing
- Hallpike manoeuvre

Objective tests:

- Pure tone audiometry / Impedance audiometry / BERA
- ENG, Craniocorpography, Posturography
- Acoustic reflex

MANAGEMENT

Medical treatment

1. Vestibular sedatives: These act by augmenting the "Cerebellar clamp"
   - Cinnarizine
   - Cyclizine
   - Prochlorperazine
   - Diazepam: labyrinthine sedative + anxiolytic properties

   Disadvantages
   - These drugs delay central compensation and can also make it incomplete
   - In vestibular inadequacy, these labyrinthine sedatives increase the unsteadiness
2. Mild tranquillizers
   - For suppression of emotional reaction
3. Cawthorne Cooksey exercises can accelerate the process of compensation.

Surgical treatment:

Indications:

1. Lack of response to adequate medical treatment
2. When symptoms are incapacitating, interfering with daily activity
3. In uncompensated vestibular disease

Surgical treatment for vertigo is grouped as:

1. Treatment of labyrithine fistula following chronic suppurative otitis media (unsafe type).
2. Surgical management of Meniere's disease
3. Surgery for acoustic neuroma
4. Surgery for benign paroxysmal positional vertigo.
5. Management of perilymph fistula

1. Treatment of labyrinthine fistula following CSOM

   A canal wall down mastoidectomy must be done, with the middle ear cleft disease to be cleared first and site of fistula last. Plugging the fistula with bone plate' or fat is done.

2. Surgical management of Meniere's disease

   i) Hearing conservative procedures:

   Indications

   1. When residual hearing is good
   2. Patient is young
   3. Disease is bilateral
   4. There is a possibility of disease developing in the other ear.

   Procedures

   a) Cervical sympathetectomy

   Rationale: - To correct the microcirculatory fault in stria vascularis

   Resection is done from C_3 to T_4 levels.

   b) Endolymphatic sac decompression

   Rationale   -   Decompression and drainage of endolymphatic fluid so that increased pressure directs itself away from the inner ear.

   Patients with positive SISI scores and positive Glycerol test, are said to benefit better with this surgery.

   c) Selective vestibular neurectomy: -

   Abnormal vestibular input is worse for vestibular compensation than absent input.

   Approaches i) Middle cranial fossa approach

   ii) Retro labyrinthine approach.

   iii) Retro sigmoid / Posterior cranial fossa approach.

   ii) Hearing destructive procedures:

   1. Labyrinthectomy - Removal of all nueroepithelial elements
   2. Chemical labyrinthectomy by transtympanic injection of streptomycin.

   Best result for Meniere's disease is that following labyrinthectomy with vestibular neurectomy.

3. Surgery for acoustic neuroma

   Approaches:

   a) Middle fossa approach
   b) Trans labyrinthine approach
   c) Posterior fossa approach

   Essentials of surgery are:

   1. Adequate exposure
   2. Facial nerve is to be identified and preserved
   3. Ability to control bleeding in posterior fossa with minimum trauma to brain stem and cerebellum

4. Surgical treatment of BPPV

   - Singular neurectomy
   - Posterior semicircular canal occlusion with bone dust
   - CO_2 laser neurectomy.

5. Surgical management of perilymph fistula

   Plugging of fistula with fat and covering with fascia.

TINNITUS

Definition:

The conscious experience of a sound that originates in an involuntary manner in a person, or may appear to him to do so.

Types:

1. Subjective / objective
2. Continuous / intermittent
3. Low pitched / high pitched
4. Physiological / pathophysiological / pathological / pseudotinnitus.
5. Fluctuant / constant

Source of Tinnitus:

- Cochlea
- Cerebral cortex
- Neural pathways.

Etiology

1. **Local**
   - Wax
   - Otitis media
   - Middle ear catarrh
2. **General**
   - Hypertension
   - Anaemia
   - Renal disease
   - Cardiac disease
   - Intracranial tumours
3. **Trauma**
   - Noise induced hearing loss
   - Ossicular discontinuity
   - Rupture oval / round window
   - Post-operative
4. **Drugs**
   - Salicylates
   - Streptomycin
   - Quinine
5. **Neoplasms**
   - Acoustic neuroma
   - Glomus jugulare
6. **Idiopathic**
7. **Psychogenic**
8. **Miscellaneous**
   - Palatal myoclonus
   - Aneurysms

Triggering factors for tinnitus:

1. Stress – Mental / Physical
2. Noise
3. Ototoxic drugs
4. Trauma
5. Pregnancy

Characteristics of tinnitus:

1. Dull / continuous - Conductive hearing loss
2. Rhythmic / pounding with pulse - Glomus tumours
3. Fluctuant tinnitus - Meniere's disease

Treatment of tinnitus:

- Reassurance
- Antidepressants
- Sedatives - Tab. Diazepam 5-10 mg Hs
- Vasodilators
- Anaesthetic drugs
- Injection Lidocaine HCl
  - Blocks multisynaptic channels
  - Short-term effect on tinnitus
- Tinnitus maskers
  - Electronic gadgets worn behind the ear to mask the patient's tinnitus.
- Psychotherapy
- Surgical treatment:
  - Stellate ganglion block
  - Cervical sympathetectomy
  - Tympanic neurectomy
  - Chordatympanic neurectomy
  - Labyrinthectomy

MANIFESTATIONS OF SYSTEMIC DISEASES IN E.N.T.

1. Syphilis

EAR	NOSE	THROAT / NECK
• Profound unilateral deafness (obliterative endarteritis) • Vertigo, tinnitus • Fusion of ossicles • Osteitis of temporal bone • Endolymphatic hydrops	• Syphilitic gummas • Septal perforations • Condylomatas • Syphilitic ulcers in oral cavity	• Cervical lymphadenopathy • Syphilitic laryngitis

2. Tuberculosis

EAR	NOSE	THROAT / NECK
• Tuberculous otitis media • Sensorineural hearing loss	• Lupus vulgaris • Nasal tuberculosis • Septal perforations	• Tuberculous laryngitis • Cervical lymphadenopathy / sinus / fistula • Cold abscess • Tuberculous ulcers in oral cavity

3. Diabetes mellitus

EAR	NOSE	THROAT / NECK
• Sensorineural hearing loss • Otomycosis	• Repeated furunculosis • Fungal sinusitis	• Oral thrush • Diabetic neuropathy / vocal cord palsy.

4. Hypertension

EAR	NOSE
• Sensorineural hearing loss	• Epistaxis • Increase bleeding at surgeries

2. GENERAL EXAMINATION

	DEFINITION	COMMENTS	CONDITIONS IN ENT
Pallor	Paleness of skin and mucous membrane due to decreased red blood cells or blood supply.	**Sites to look for pallor:** • Lower palpebral conjunctiva • Tongue • Soft palate • Palms and nails	**Conditions in ENT with pallor:** • Cases of dysphagia • Throat carcinomas • Nasopharyngeal angiofibroma. • Plummer-Vinson syndrome • Atrophic rhinitis.
Oedema	Collection of fluid in interstitial spaces or serous cavities	• Oedema occurs when 5-6 litres of water collects in the spaces. • Pitting on pressure occurs when circumfernce of the limb is increased by 10%.	**Conditions in ENT with oedema:** • Myxoedema • Angioneurotic oedema • Cachexia in malignancy • Liver metastatic carcinoma. • Metastatic lymph nodes pressing on lymphatics.
Cyanosis	Bluish discoloration of appendanges due to increased amount of reduced haemoglobin in the capillary blood (More than 5 gm %)	**Types** **1. Central:** Decreased arterial oxygen saturation seen on skin and mucous membranes (tongue, lips, cheek) **2. Peripheral:** Decreased blood flow to the part. seen on skin only.	**Conditions in ENT with cyanosis:** • Chronic obstructive lung disease • Foreign body bronchus with lung collapse
Clubbing	• Bulbous enlargement of soft parts of terminal phalanges • Interstitial oedema and dilatation of arterioles and capillaries • Curving of nails	**Grades** 1. Softening of nail bed 2. Obliteration of angle of nail bed 3. Parrot beak / drum stick appearance 4. Hypertrophic pulmonary osteo-arthropathy	**Conditions in ENT with clubbing:** • Bronchogenic carcinoma • Tuberculosis with secondary infection • Lung abscess • Myxoedema

Jugular venous pressure	The normal JVP consist of three positive pulse waves a, c and v and two negative pulse waves x and y.
	Normal = 3-4 cms.
		Elevated
		• Right ventricular failure
		• Hyper kinetic circulatory state
		• Increased blood volume
		• Pulmonary diseases
		  - Asthma
		  - Emphysema	

	DEFINITION	COMMENTS	CONDITIONS IN ENT
		Decreased • Shock • Dehydration	

Temperature
Fever is increase in temperature by more than 1^0C or any rise above maximal normal temperature.
	It reflects the temperature of the viscera and tissues of the body
	
	Sites: Oral
	       Axillary
	       Rectal
	
	Normal 98-99^{0}F
	Mild fever 99-100^{0}F
	Moderate fever 100-103^{0}F
	High fever 103-105^{0}F
	Hyperpyrexia upto 106^{0}F
		Types
		Continuous: Raised temperature, fluctuation not more than 1^0C over 24 hrs.
		Remittent: Fluctuation more than 1^0C over 24 hrs.
		Intermittent: Temperature only for some hours in a day.
			• Bacterial, viral, fungal infections
			• Thyrotoxicosis
			• Infectious mononucleosis
			• Specific infections like
			   - Diphtheria
			   - Tonsillitis
			   - Vincent's angina
			   - Herpes labialis
			• CSOM with intracranial complications.

Pulse	**Components of pulse** • Anacrotic wave. • Tidal / Percussion wave • Dicrotic notch • Dicrotic wave Normal rate = 60-100 / minute	**Types** • Anacrotic • Pulses Bisferiens • Dicrotic • Water hammer pulse etc.	**Conditions in E.N.T. with Tachycardia** • Anaemia • Thyrotoxicosis • Fever
Blood pressure	Systolic B.P. reflects: • Stroke volume of the heart • Stiffness of arterial vessels. Diastolic B.P. reflects: • Peripheral resistance **Normal Blood Pressure =** upto 120 / 80 mm of Hg	Hypertension is persistently elevated systolic or diastolic blood pressure.	**Hypertension:** • Thyrotoxicosis. • Raised intracranial tension. **Hypotension:** • Cachexia of malignancy • Tuberculosis • Anaemia • Functional

Lymphadenopathy	Enlargement of lymph nodes, inflammatory or non-inflammatory in origin.
	Neck nodes are examined by standing behind the patient with the patient's neck flexed. Nodes are examined from above downwards.

Neck nodes:

- Sub mental
- Sub mandibular
- Tonsillar
- Cervical
- Posterior auricular
- Occipital.

Tuberculous lymphadenitis:

- Affects deep cervical, axillary and mesenteric nodes
- Matted lymph nodes due to periadenitis
- Central caseation results in a cold abscess
- Bursting of the abscess results in a chronic non-healing sinus / ulcer.
- Constitutional symptoms are present.

Syphilitic lymphadenitis:

- Painless, firm, discrete and shotty glands.
- Epitrochlear and occipital nodes are involved in secondary syphilis.
- Generalised lymphadenopathy in secondary syphilis.

Lymphosarcoma:

- Affects cervical glands which are enlarged, firm and fixed
- Highly malignant tumour
- Overlying skin may show dilated blue veins under it.

Secondary carcinoma:

- Stony hard lymphnodes
- Enlarged, irregular and fixed nodes
- Primary growth may be there
- Constitutional symptoms are present.

Hodgkin's lymphoma:

- Affects young males
- Cervical glands are affected first
- Lymph nodes:
  - Elastic   - Discrete
  - Rubbery   - Mobile
- General signs:
  - Pel Ebstein fever
  - Hepatosplenomegaly
  - Anaemia
  - Weight loss by more than 10%
- Diagnosis:
  - Lymph node biopsy-
    - Reed Sternberg's cell
  - Peripheral smear-
    - Lymphocytosis
    - Eosinophilia

Non-Hodgkin's lymphoma:

- Waldeyer's ring and Supratrochlear nodes are affected.
- Less symptomatic than Hodgkin's lymphoma.
- Histological examination of the bone marrow confirms the diagnosis.

Cranial Nerves

CRANIAL NERVE	SENSATION	TESTS	INTERPRETATION
Olfactory	Smell	To smell non irritant substances like tea, coffee, clove oil, etc. Smelling irritating substances (eg. ammonia) leads to additional stimulation of Trigeminal nerve. Common bedside substances used are soap, scent, fruit etc. The patient can smell from smell bottles, UPSIT cards (a scratch on the card leads to eruption of smell) or an olfactometer	Anosmia: Abolition of sense of smell Hyposmia: Decrease sense of smell Parosmia: Perversion of sense of smell eg. offensive substance having a pleasant odour
Optic	Visual acuity Visual field	Bed side test - Finger counting at 1 meter. Distant vision test-Snellen's chart Near vision-Jaegger's chart	
Oculomotor	Eye movements	Test eye movements by confrontation method.	Squint
Trochlear	Eye movements	It supplies the superior oblique muscle	-
Abducens	Eye movements	It supplies the lateral rectus muscle	Lateral rectus palsy in VI nerve damage
Trigeminal (Ophthalmic, Maxillary, Mandibular)	**Ophthalmic:** Supplies the conjunctiva, lower lid, lacrimal gland, nose tip and skin, upper lids, forehead, scalp till the vertex **Maxillary:** Cheek, front of temple, side of nose, upper lip, upper teeth, roof of mouth, part of soft palate, tonsils **Mandibular:** Lower part of face, lower lip, ear, tongue and lower teeth. Parasympathetic fibres to the salivary gland. The motor root innervates the muscles of mastication. **Reflexes:** • Corneal • Conjunctival • Jaw jerk	The tactile sensibility includes light touch and pressure, tactile localisation and discrimination. Test sensations with cotton wisp / tip of index finger / pin. Test abnormal side first. **Corneal reflex:** Twist a light wisp of cotton into a fine hair and lightly touch the lateral edge of the cornea at its conjunctival margin with the wisp, having asked the patient to gaze into the distance or at the ceiling. The two sides should be compared. The cornea should not be wiped with cotton and the central part should not be touched in view of risk of corneal ulceration in cases of corneal anaesthesia. In a positive reflex, the patient blinks.	A lesion of the whole nerve leads to loss of sensation in the skin and mucous membrane of the face and nasopharynx. The salivary, buccal and lacrimal secretions may be diminished and trophic ulcers may develop in the mouth, nose and cornea. Weakness of muscles of mastication is also a feature.
Facial	The facial nerve is almost entirely a motor nerve. It	Ask the patient to close his eyes as tightly as he can. Affected eye	In facial paralysis, the affected side of face loses

CRANIAL NERVE	SENSATION	TESTS	INTERPRETATION
	supplies all the muscles of the face and scalp, except the levator palpebrae superioris. The chordatympani carries taste sensation from the anterior ⅔ of the tongue. There is a small area of cutaneous sensation in the auricle.	is barely closed or not closed at all. Test taste sensation on anterior ⅔ of tongue. To test the sense of taste, use strong solutions of sugar and common salt, and weak solution of citric acid and quinine, as tastes of sweet, salt, sour and bitter respectively. They are ideally applied with the help of a wooden rod on the surface of the protruded tongue.The patient is asked to indicate the perseverance of taste before withdrawing the tongue. After each sensation is tested, the mouth is rinsed. The quinine test is applied last as its effect is long lasting.	its expression. The nasolabial fold is less pronounced, the furrows of the brow are smoothened out, the eye is more widely open than on the normal side, and when the patient smiles, the mouth is drawn towards the normal side. The patient is unable to whistle and food is bound to collect between teeth and gums. Any fluid may escape from the angle of the mouth.
Vestibulocochlear	The nerve consists of two sets of fibres. One supplies the cochlea and subserves hearing, the other supplies the labyrinth and semicircular canals and maintains equilibrium, balance and bodily displacement.	All subjective and objective tests of hearing	
Glossopharyngeal	Afferent arm carries sensations from posterior part of tongue and oropharynx. It innervates the middle pharyngeal sphincter and the stylopharyngeus muscle. It contains taste fibres from posterior part of tongue.	Test taste sensation from posterior part of tongue Palatal reflex: Tickle the back of pharynx and note the reflex	
Vagus	Vagus is motor to soft palate (except tensor palati), pharynx and larynx. It is sensory and motor for respiratory passages, the heart and most of the abdominal viscera.	Ask the patient if he notices regurgitation of fluids through his nose on swallowing seen in total paralysis of the soft palate. Also patient may be unable to pronounce words requiring complete closure of nasopharynx. Unilateral paralysis doesn't cause these symptoms. For direct examination of the palate, ask the patient to say	Palatal reflex: The palate will get elevated and there will be generalised movement of the oro and hypopharynx Efferent - Vagus

CRANIAL NERVE	SENSATION	TESTS	INTERPRETATION
	The superior laryngeal branch of the vagus carries sensation above the vocal cords and also carries motor fibres that innervate the cricothyroid. The recurrent laryngeal nerve supplies sensation to the larynx below the vocal cord and to all muscles of larynx except the cricothyroid.	'ah' with an open mouth and depressed tongue. Watch for a motionless palate, bilateral paralysis, unilateral paralysis pulling the median raphe to the healthy side or a normal palate. Unilateral damage to superior laryngeal nerve does not produce any symptoms while bilateral damage leads to vocal cord relaxation resulting in a hoarse and deep voice in which high notes are difficult to pronounce. In recurrent laryngeal nerve affection, appearances of the vocal cord on laryngoscopy give an idea of the affection. The speech is characteristically blurred and the patient cannot cough clearly. Indirect laryngoscopy can help test vocal cord movements.	
Spinal accessory nerve	It is purely a motor nerve innervating the pharynx, larynx and supplies Sternocleidomastoid and Trapezius muscle	Each sternocleidomastoid is checked by turning the face / chin to the opposite side and applying resistance to it. Both sternocleidomastoids are checked by bending the face downwards and applying resistance. To check the trapezius, the patient is asked to shrug his shoulders while pressing the shoulders down.	
Hypoglossal	Motor supply to all muscles of the tongue except Palatoglossus	Examination of the tongue on its protrusion and movements	Unilateral hypoglossal affection: On tongue protrusion deviation of tongue occurs to affected side because of unopposed action of the contralateral genioglossus. Atrophy, fasciculations, fibrillations occur on the affected muscles. To assess fasciculation, keep the tongue relaxed in the mouth, not protruded. Bilateral hypoglossal affection : Dyspnoea, Dysarthria for 't' and 'd' phonemes occur

3. LOCAL EXAMINATION

It is ideal to begin examination with the normal ear as it decreases the chances of transferring infected debri from the pathological ear to the normal ear

PARTICULARS	RIGHT AND LEFT EAR - LOOK FOR
Preauricular region	Cysts, sinuses, scars, lymphadenitis
Pinna	Congenital deformities: anotia, microtia
	Acquired lesions: gouty tophi, carcinoma, perichondritis
Postauricular region	Scars-surgical / non surgical, keloid, erythema, tenderness, abscess
External auditory canal	Congestion, oedema, fungus, polyp, stenosis, osteoma, exostosis
	Inspect postero-superior region for erosion due to cholesteatoma or a mastoid cavity.

Tympanic membrane	1. **Normal appearance**
	   ● Glistening, light grey in colour (Pars tensa)
	   ● Dull red (Pars flaccida)
	   ● Cone of light in the anteroinferior quadrant
	2. **Retraction / Secretory otitis media**
	   ● Dull drum
	   ● Loss / distortion of light reflex
	   ● Flabby, bluish, thickened drum
	   ● Air bubbles / air fluid level seen
	   ● Foreshortened handle of malleus
	   ● Decreased mobility on seigalisation in adhesive otitis media
	3. **Perforation**
	   ● **Size**
	   ● **Type**
	     - Central / Marginal / Subtotal / Total / Attic
	   ● **Site**
	     - All / which quadrant
	     - Pars tensa / flaccida
	   ● **Rim of perforation**
	     - Thin / thick
	     - Red / pink / white
	     - Congested / fibrosed
	     - Oedematous / not
	     - Tympanosclerotic plaques +/-
	   ● **Middle ear mucosa** seen through the perforation
	     - Pale pink / pink / red / angry red
	     - Congested / not
	     - Granular / polypoidal / not
	     - Secretions / discharge, if any-serous / mucoid / purulent
	   ● **Ossicles** seen through the perforation
	     - Malleus
	     - Incudostapedial joint

PARTICULARS	RIGHT AND LEFT EAR - LOOK FOR

	• **Eustachian tube opening** seen / not
	   - Discharge at that site
	   - Inflamed mucosa +/-
	• **Round and oval window seen / not**
	• **Attic**
	   - Congestion / debri / flakes
	• **Retraction pocket**
	   - Site - quadrant
	   - Position - o'clock
	   - Fundus seen / not
	   - Flakes present within / not
	   - Neck wide / not
	   - Self emptying / not

Mastoid region	Erythema, induration, oedema, tenderness, abscess

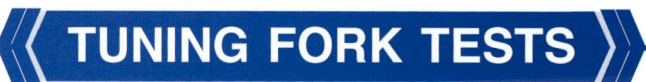

TUNING FORK TESTS

Simple and reliable tests

Tests are performed with 256, 512 and 1024 Hz frequency tuning forks.

RINNE'S TEST

It is a tuning fork test in which air and bone conduction of the test ear are confirmed.

METHODS

1. The tuning fork is struck gently on the elbow, knee cap or a rubber pad and then the vibrating prongs are held against the ear in line with the external canal at a distance of about 1 inch. This step tests the air conduction of the ear. The footpiece of the vibrating fork is then placed over the mastoid to test the bone conduction. The patient is asked to indicate the louder of the two sounds. Thus the test compares air conduction of sound to bone conduction. In normal / Rinne positive cases, the ear canal sound is better heard than that over the mastoid. i.e. air conduction is better than bone conduction

2. The foot of the vibrating fork is kept over the mastoid bone or the non-hair bearing skin posterosuperior to the external auditory meatus. When it is no more heard it is held infront of the ear.

   If it is still heard :   Rinne positive

   If it is not heard :   Rinne negative

   This is a better method as the ear has the property of adaptation and will not hear the sound if the fork is kept continuously over the mastoid.

RINNE TEST RESULTS

RESULT	INTERPRETATION	CONDITION
Rinne positive (R +)	Air conduction better than bone conduction (AC > BC)	• Normal individuals (AC: BC = 2:1) • Presbyacusis
Rinne negative (R -)	Bone conduction better than air conduction. The point at which Rinne turns negative is at an air-bone gap of 15-20 dB (18 dB)	Conductive deafness

RESULT	INTERPRETATION	CONDITION
Reduced rinne positive [R + (reduced)]	Air and bone conduction, both are reduced but air conduction is still better than bone conduction.(AC > BC both reduced)	Sensorineural deafness
False negative (R - False)	Bone conduction falsely better, with poor or no response to air conduction. This is because the patient is actually hearing the bone conducted sound across the skull through the normal ear. Masking (the normal ear) is done to avoid this false result. (BC > AC - False)	Severe unilateral sensorineural deafness
Rinne equivocal (R =)	Air conduction equals bone conduction (AC = BC)	Mild conductive deafness
Rinne infinite positive (R + infinite)	Air conduction is only heard. (AC only)	Severe sensorineural deafness
Rinne infinite negative (R - infinite)	Bone conduction only heard, untested ear is masked (BC only)	Severe conductive deafness

CORRELATION OF RINNE TEST RESULTS WITH DEGREE OF HEARING LOSS: -

RINNE TEST RESULTS			DEGREE OF HEARING LOSS	
TUNING FORK (HZ) FREQUENCY:			HEARING LOSS	dB
256	512	1024		
-	+	+	Mild	25-40
-	-	+	Moderate	40-55
-	-	-	Severe	> 55

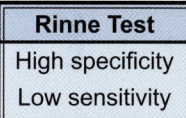

Rinne Test
High specificity
Low sensitivity

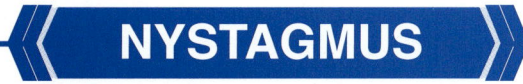

NYSTAGMUS

Definition:
1. Nystagmus is a disturbance of ocular posture characterised by a more or less rhythmical oscillatory movement of the eyes.
2. It is the term applied to a disturbance of ocular movement characterised by involuntary, conjugate and often rhythmical oscillation of the eyes.

Types:
1. According to the cause:
- **Central** with other signs of intracranial disease
- **Labyrinthine / vestibular** with signs of inner ear disease like vertigo, decrease hearing.
- **Ocular** with signs of ophthalmic disease

2. According to its origin:
- **Spontaneous** : nystagmus occurs on its own
- **Induced** : nystagmus is induced by caloric, rotational, galvanic, positional or optokinetic stimuli.

3. According to movement of the eyeball:
- **Horizontal**
- **Vertical**

- **Rotatory**
- **Pendular**

4. **According to its characteristic:**
   - **Phasic**
   - **Jerk**

Classification:

Nystagmus is classified into three degrees.

1. **First degree**   :   Nystagmus is present only when the patient looks in the direction of the quick component

2. **Second degree**   :   In addition, nystagmus is also present when the patient looks straight in front.

3. **Third degree**   :   Nystagmus is also present when the patient looks in the direction of the slow component. (in addition to the above two)

Mechanism of Nystagmus:

Labyrinthine   :   Normally the labyrinth of each ear tries to deviate eyes slowly to the opposite side because of its tonic activity. eg.: right labyrinth deviates the eyes to the left and vice-versa. The other ear also does the same and the effect gets neutralised and the eyes remain in the midline.

Abnormal state :   When one labyrinth gets stimulated either by disease or caloric / positional stimulus it moves the eyeball slowly to the opposite side-**slow component**. The cerebral cortex becomes aware of the situation and quickly corrects the deviation and brings the eyes to the original position. This quick deviation is the **fast component** of the nystagmus. The continuous slow and fast movement of the eyeball constitutes the two components of the nystagmus. The opposite occurs in case of hypoactive / dead labyrinth. The unaffected labyrinth becomes stronger and deviates the eye to the opposite ie; to the side of the affected eye, thus the slow component occurs on the affected side and fast on the unaffected side.

Central   :   This nystagmus occurs due to abnormalities in the central connections of the vestibular nerve.

Examination of nystagmus

The patient is placed in good light and the examiner faces the patient. The patient's head is kept steady and he is asked to follow the direction of the finger tip of the examiner.

The examiner's finger is then kept at a distance more than the focal length of the patient, at approximately 45 cms. Distance less than the focal length leads to convergence of the eyeball. The finger is then moved 30^0 laterally. Movement outside this field leads to physiological nystagmus caused by fatigue of ocular muscles. Nystagmus is tested by asking the patient to look at the three finger positions - centre, left lateral and right lateral. Observe the rate, amplitude and rhythm in each direction and whether or not nystagmus is sustained. The direction of the fast component is the direction of the nystagmus. Abolishment of nystagmus occurs by four weeks in labyrinthine destructive lesions.

Difference between labyrinthine and central nystagmus

LABYRINTHINE	CENTRAL
Unidirectional	Bidirectional
Associated with vertigo. The vertigo is always rotational, either the surrounding or the patient appears to move.	Not associated with vertigo. Vertigo, if present is like spinning movement in the head.
Not very long - lasting	Long-lasting

LABYRINTHINE	CENTRAL
Horizontal	Horizontal / Vertical / Oblique
Fine	Coarse / Sluggish / Violent jerk in cerebellar type
Lesion in semicircular canals	Involvement of central connections of the Vestibular nerve.
Nystagmus increases on visual fixation (eye closure, frenzel glasses, darkness)	Decreases on visual fixation
Increases in the direction of fast phase	Does not vary on gaze / eye movements
Falling and past pointing are present with third degree nystagmus	Falling and past pointing are often present but do not folllow the rules of direction.

Positional Nystagmus

WITH VERTIGO	WITHOUT VERTIGO
Nystagmus produced when head placed backwards and to one side	Nystagmus produced when head placed in any position.
Latent period present	No latent period (sudden nystagmus).
Giddiness present	Giddiness absent
Fatiguable	Unfatiguable
Above test can be repeated and is positive in peripheral disorders.	Above test can be repeated and is positive in central lesions.

Romberg's test

Falling test

Patient stands upright with the feet together and eye closed

RESULT	INFERENCE	LESION	
		LABYRINTHINE	CENTRAL
Positive	Patient falls	Patient falls towards the side of lesion,	Patient falls away from side of lesion,
	Tendency to fall	Towards the side of slow component	Towards the side of fast component.

Drugs causing nystagmus

1. Alcohol
2. Barbiturates
3. Tranquillizers
4. Anticonvulsants
5. Phenytoin
6. Benzodiazepines

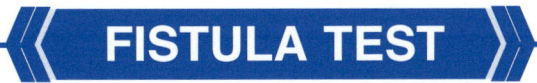

FISTULA TEST

This is the test performed to detect a fistula in the vestibule of the inner ear.

Principle:

Erosion of the bony part of the vestibule (usually the lateral semicircular canal) either by ear disease or trauma exposes the membranous labyrinth to external pressure changes. If the labyrinth is functioning, the pressure changes will lead to its stimulation and cause a subjective feeling of vertigo, vomiting and associated nystagmus.

In the test, external pressure changes are achieved by various methods and erosion / fistula is demonstrated by a subjective feeling of vertigo.

The external pressure can be altered by:

1. Alternatively, compressing and releasing the tragus against the external meatus, altering the pressure in the ear canal and stimulating the labyrinth.
2. Using a Siegle's speculum to increase and decrease the pressure in the ear canal.
3. Using the probe of an impedance audiometer to cause pressure changes.
4. By moving granulations / polyp in the ear by a cotton-tipped applicator.

Fistula test results:

INTERPRETATION	RESULT	CONDITION
Positive	Subjective feeling of giddiness, nausea, vomiting with or without nystagmus	Labyrinth is functioning and erosion is present
False positive	Subjective feeling of giddiness with no fistula in the labyrinth	Seen in congenital syphilis due to hypermobile stapes foot plate. It is called as **Hennebert's sign**. It is also seen after stapedectomy
False negative	Negative fistula test with the presence of a fistula in the labyrinth	Seen in a dead labyrinth which does not react to any stimulus.

SITE OF FISTULA	TYPE OF NYSTAGMUS
1. Lateral semicircular canal	• Nystagmus towards the normal side (If fistula is anterior to the ampulla, then nystagmus is towards the affected side)
2. Posterior canal	• Nystagmus in a vertical direction
3. Vestibule	• Rotatory horizontal nystagmus towards the abnormal ear
4. Superior semicircular canal	• Rotatory nystagmus towards normal ear.

EXAMINATION OF FACIAL NERVE

On Gross Examination:
- Facial asymmetry +/-
- One half / both halves affected
- UMN / LMN Facial Palsy
    - Same / opposite half of face affected
    - Fore head spared / not

On passive movements:
- Inability to close the eye
- Absence of wrinkling of forehead
- Loss of nasolabial fold
- Inability to blow cheek on one side

On active movements:
The above passive movements are tested with resistance to the particular action

Any associated movements:
- Synkinesis
- Facial twitching

- Hemifacial spasm
- Blepharospasm

Scars of any previous surgery

- Ear surgery - Postaural / Endaural scar
- Parotidectomy scar

Tests for facial nerve function

1. Schirmer's test / Lacrimation flow assessment (Topognostic test done at bedside)

   A small filter paper is placed on both the lower conjunctival fornices for 5 mins. and the amount of lacrimation is compared from side to side

   A reduction of lacrimation to 30% or less compared with total lacrimation of both eyes or bilateral reduction to 25mm. is considered significant

   It can be used as a potential for exposure keratitis. Reduction of lacrimation occurs when lesion is at point of origin of greater superficial petrosal nerve.

2. Stapedial relfex

   Contraction of stapedius muscle occurs on presenting loud sounds to the ear, as a protective mechanism. This reflex occurs only if the nerve to stapedius (branch of intact facial nerve) is functioning.

3. Electrodiagnostic tests
   - Electroneuronography
   - Electromyography.

TESTS FOR EUSTACHIAN TUBE PATENCY

TEST	METHOD	COMMENT
1. **Valsalva's manoeuvre**	It is based on the principle of forced expiration against a closed glottis. With the mouth tightly closed, the nose is pinched and air is blown out forcibly. This increases the pressure in the post-nasal space and air enters the middle ear causing the ear drum to bulge out, if the tube is patent and the drum is mobile.	Therapeutic uses of Valsalva's manoeuvre are for: • Retracted ear drum • Catarrhal otitis media • Aero otitis. Disadvantages of Valsalva's manoeuvre: • It can be performed only in expiratory phase of respiration • Pressure built up can be very high and can cause damage to middle ear / ear drum. • Patient has to learn the procedure. • Positive subglottic pressure can lead to hypoxia (rare) due to peripheral pooling of blood. • It can be negative in normal individuals.
2. **Politzerisation**	Politzer's bag is a rubber bag of 8 oz capacity. The bag is attached to a rubber tubing, the other end of which has a rubber / vulcanite nozzle. The tip of the nozzle is fitted into the nasal vestibule and the other nostril is pinched. The air in the bag is pressed while the patient is asked to either swallow	Bulging of the tympanic membrane is seen as the air gushes in.

TEST	METHOD	COMMENT
	with mouth closed or say the letter 'K' repeatedly. This manoeuvre opens up the tubes on swallowing and air gushes in the middle ear causing outward movement of the tympanic membrane. By swallowing or saying 'K' the soft palate touches the posterior pharyngeal wall and air is not allowed to leak into the pharynx and also nasopharyngeal pressure is maintained.	
3. **Eustachian catheterization.**	Eustachian catheters are malleable metallic catheters of varying sizes. A 8 oz rubber bag is used to blow air through the catheter. The ear canal is plugged with an auscultation tube, one end of which is placed in the examiner's ear and the other end in the patient's ear. The sound heard by the examiner indicates passage of air through the eustachian tube. Alternatively the movement of the tympanic membrane can be heard through the canal. Procedure: The nasal cavity is anaesthetized with 4% Xylocaine spray. The eustachian catheter with its tip facing down is passed along the floor of the nasal cavity without touching it till it reaches the posterior wall of the nasopharynx. The catheter is now brought forwards till the tip hooks against the posterior edge of the soft palate. The tip of the catheter (the direction of which is indicated by the ring at the proximal end) is rotated by 90° laterally. A politzer's bag is then attached to the proximal end and is squeezed to allow air to enter the tube. From this position if the catheter is rotated by 180° to the opposite tube, its patency can also be tested.	Interpretation: • Hollow sound: Normal • Wheeze: Narrow lumen stricture • Bubbling / Crepitations: Otitis media with middle ear effusion. Uses: • To test patency of tube. • To diagnose partial / complete obstruction of tube. • To dilate tubal strictures with bougies.

Seigalization

The Seigle's speculum consist of an aural speculum (of various sizes) with a 10 diopter lens.

The speculum is connected to a side tube which is attached to a rubber bulb. The rubber bulb can be pressed and released to alter pressure in the ear canal. The speculum should snugly fit into the earcanal to make the system air-tight. The pathology of the ear is examined by fitting the speculum in the earcanal and pressing the rubber bulb.

Functions:

The Seigle's speculum is helpful in the following ways:

1. To give a magnified view of the tympanic membrane
2. To give a magnified view of the pathology (eg.: perforation)
3. To assess mobility of the tympanic membrane
4. To elicit fistula sign by causing alteration in ear canal pressure
5. To instill medication or suck out discharge from the middle ear by varying pressure in the ear canal.

Examination of the eyes:

The eyes are inspected for nystagmus (refer page 35)

Corneal reflex:

This reflex is tested with a wisp of cotton wool applied to the cornea laterally which would result in brisk blinking or closure of the eyes. The afferent arm of the reflex is by the trigeminal nerve and the efferent is by the facial nerve. The reflex may be absent in lesions affecting the facial nerve.

4. INVESTIGATIONS

The following investigations may be done in a patient with chronic otitis media:

1. Ear microscopy
   - Confirmation of ear findings
   - Finding hidden cholesteatoma / squamous epithelium
   - Knowing ossicular chain status
   - Collection of discharge for smear, culture and antibiotic sensitivity testing
   - Suction and cleaning of ear
   - Probing of retraction pockets
2. Routine investigations
   - Haemogram
   - Blood sugar analysis
   - Urine examination
   - X'ray chest and electrocardiogram if required
3. Pure tone audiometry
   - To know the type and amount of hearing loss
   - To compare pre and post - operative results
   - For medico-legal purposes
4. X'ray mastoid - Schuller's view
   - For destruction of mastoid air cell system
   - To see cholesteatoma cavity
   - Boundaries / anatomy of mastoid region
   - To detect a low-lying dura or an anteriorly / posteriorly placed sinus plate
5. X'ray paranasal sinuses - Water and Caldwell's view to rule out sinus infection before surgery

5. CHRONIC SUPPURATIVE OTITIS MEDIA

DEFINITION

Chronic suppurative otitis media is a chronic inflammatory process involving the middle ear cleft and producing irreversible pathological changes. It is due to improper and inadequate treatment of acute suppurative otitis media.

Predisposing factors

- Poor general condition
- Improper diet / nutrition
- Chronic tonsilloadenitis
- Sinusitis
- Specific infections like
  - Measles
  - Scarlet fever
  - Diphtheria
  - Tuberculosis

Types:

It is basically of two types

1. **Tubotympanic type**
2. **Atticoantral type**

1. TUBOTYMPANIC TYPE

It is a benign type of chronic suppurative otitis media confined only to the middle ear cleft.

Types:

1. **Tubal** : The focus of infection lies in the nose, paranasal sinuses or nasopharynx and reaches the middle ear via the eustachian tube. It is usually seen in children of low socio-economic status.

2. **Tympanic** : In this type, the infection reaches the middle ear via a perforation in the tympanic membrane. This perforation is usually a large central perforation, persistent since a long-time and gives rise to recurrent infection by way of water entering the ear (Persistent perforation syndrome). It is usually seen in adults and involves one ear only.

Pathology:

1. **Persistent mucosal disease**

   Infection reaches the middle ear either via the eustachian tube or through a perforation in the tympanic membrane. Infection in middle ear leads to hyperplasia of middle ear mucosa. It can also lead to polyp formation by prolapse of oedematous mucosa. The mucosal proliferation leads to chronicity by trapping of infection.

2. **Cholesterol granuloma**

   Cholesterol granuloma like picture occurs when there is defective ventilation of the middle-ear cleft, leading to exudation of mucoid fluid with an inflammatory reaction. There is release of cholesterol crystals and blood pigments giving a blue tinge to the tympanic membrane. The mucous membrane of the middle ear cleft shows the typical histopathological picture of a cholesterol granuloma. It shows cholesterol crystals, foreign body giant cells, granulation tissue, haemosiderin and mucin granules.

Clinical features

1. Tubal type
   - Profuse bilateral mucopurulent discharge
   - Running nose
   - Bilateral anterior perforation in tympanic membrane
   - Nasal examination shows either a deviated septum or signs of sinusitis
   - Adenoids are usually present.
2. Tympanic type
   - Scanty discharge in one external auditory canal
   - Large (subtotal) central perforation seen, more often kidney shaped
   - Granulations and polypi may be seen in the middle ear
   - Pure tone audiometry reveals atleast moderate conductive hearing loss. These patients hear better when the external canal is full of pus as the thick pus seals off the defect in the tympanic membrane leading to better transmission of sound.

> **Types of tympanic membrane perforations:**
> - Central
> - Marginal
> - Attic
> - Subtotal
> - Total

PERFORATION	DEFINITION	PATHOLOGY
Central	It is a perforation situated in pars tensa and surrounded by tympanic membrane all around.	Tubotympanic disease confined to middle ear Sinusitis/adenotonsillitis may be present.
Marginal	It is a perforation in which bone forms any of the edge of the perforation	Bony necrosis associated with granulations and cholesteatoma.
Attic	It is a perforation, which occurs in the pars flaccida of tympanic membrane	Associated with cholesteatoma
Subtotal	It is a perforation, which is, surrounded by the annulus on all sides.	Tubotympanic disease
Total	It is a perforation in which there is complete loss of tympanic membrane and annulus.	Tubotympanic disease Associated exanthematous fever.

Stages of tubotympamic disease

1. Active
   - When there is active discharge from the ear
2. Quiescent
   - Discharge from the ear stops and becomes dry
   - A small perforation may heal in about 6 months
   - A big perforation remains open, needs repair
3. Inactive
   - No discharge
   - Disease is inactive
   - Ear has been dry for more than 6 months
   - When the ear stays in the quiescent stage for more than 6 months, it becomes inactive
   - Perforation needs to be closed by plastic repair

INVESTIGATIONS

1. Tuning fork tests
2. Pure tone audiometry
3. Smear, culture and antibiotic sensitivity test of the discharge
4. X'ray mastoid and paranasal sinuses may be needed in some cases.

TREATMENT

Aim:

1. To control infection
2. To treat underlying cause
3. To make the ear dry
4. To restore hearing.

Medical treatment

Aural Toilet

The external and middle ear is cleaned by

- Sterile dry cotton wool mops
- Syringing
- Suction

Cleaning is followed by instillation of eardrops in small perforations and powder insufflation in big perforations. The powder should be just enough to form a thin film and not a thick layer as it hinders drainage and causes irritation. Plugging the ear with nonabsorbent material like cotton vaseline should follow instillation of eardrops. With frequent aural toilet, the ear should become dry in 2-3 weeks. If the condition worsens, allergy to local drops or powder should be suspected.

Zinc Ionization

It is a line of treatment for safe chronic suppurative otitis media.

Principle: **Iontophoresis:** In which zinc ions are liberated which are germicidal and bactericidal. The inflammatory process subsides as soon as infecting organisms decrease in number.

Pre-requisites

- Central perforation, which is large.
- Infection confined to middle ear.
- No cholesteatoma, granulations or polyp.

Procedure

Supine position with affected ear up.

A vulcanite aural speculum is kept in the ear and the canal is filled with 2% zinc sulphate solution.

Positive electrode is attached to the speculum and negative electrode to a part of any limb wrapped in a moist cloth. The current is passed through the electrodes for about 20 minutes, increasing upto 3-4 mA and then decreasing to zero. It requires 3-4 applications to obtain a dry ear. Some patients may not improve and an aural swab culture may be required. Persistent perforation may have to be dealt by myringoplasty.

Surgical treatment

- Myringoplasty
- Tympanoplasty

Patch Test

- It is a test used to assess any gain in hearing following a myringoplasty in patients with a central perforation
- It helps in assessing whether myringoplasty will be helpful to a patient with a central perforation.

Procedure

A patch is made of cigarette paper or compressed gelatin sponge. It is then placed over the perforation. Tuning fork tests or audiological tests are done before and after application of the patch.

Interpretation

HEARING	INTERPRETATION	OPERATION
Gain	Intact ossicular chain	Myringoplasty suffices
No Gain	Ossicular discontinuity	Ossiculoplasty is needed
	Ossicular fixation	Stapedectomy is needed

2. ATTICO-ANTRAL TYPE

This is an unsafe type of chronic suppurative otitis media and is usually associated with cholesteatoma formation. It is a relatively dangerous type of disease because of its incidence of intracranial complications.

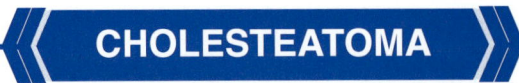

CHOLESTEATOMA

DEFINITION

Cholesteatoma has been defined as a three dimensional stratified squamous epithelial sac confirming to the anatomy of the middle ear cleft, containing keratin debri and having the capacity for progressive and independent growth at the expense of the underlying bone.

It is a misnomer as it is not a tumour nor does it contain cholesterol crystals or fat.

HISTORY

Johannes Muller - Cholesteatoma term

Schuknecht - Keratoma

ORIGIN OF CHOLESTEATOMA:

Toynbee	It arises from hair follicles / glands of external ear ("Molluscous tumour")
Habermann and Bezold	It arises from squamous epithelium of ear canal
Von Troeltsch	It arises from inspissated exudation of chronically inflamed mucosa
Politzer	Formation of epithelial lining in downgrowth of mucosa
Habermann	Role of embryonic remnant in development of attic cholesteatoma
Bezold	Role of eustachian tube in formation of cholesteatoma

PATHOGENESIS OF CHOLESTEATOMA

Cholesteatoma may be classified according to its etiology into:

1. **Congenital**
2. **Acquired**
   a) **Primary** b) **Secondary**

1. CONGENITAL CHOLESTEATOMA:

Definition: (Derlacki and Clemis)

Embryonic test of epithelial tissue in an ear without tympanic membrane perforation in a patient without a history of ear infection.

Criteria for definition

- White mass medial to a normal tympanic membrane
- Normal pars flaccida and pars tensa.
- No prior history of otorrhoea or perforation.
- No prior otologic procedures.
  (Canal atresia and intra membranous and giant cholesteatomas are excluded.
  Prior bouts of otitis media are not grounds for exclusion).

Incidence

- Sex - M:F = 3:1
- Mean age at presentation: 4.5 years
- Antero superior quadrant is affected more than the other quadrants

Pathogenesis of congenital cholesteatoma

A squamous cell rest - the epidermoid formation, identifiable from 10-33 weeks of gestation in the anterior superior lateral wall of the tympanic cavity has been held responsible for its origin

If the epidermoid formation failed to involute, its continued presence and later expansion could result in its eventual appearance medial to the tympanic membrane in the anterior superior quadrant of the middle ear as a congenital cholesteatoma. On further migration, the congenital cholesteatoma can occur in the posterior middle ear space.

2. ACQUIRED CHOLESTEATOMA

1. Primary acquired cholesteatoma
In this type, there has been no predisposing chronic otitis media and cholesteatoma occurs in the attic or in the posterior part of the tympanic cavity.

2. Secondary acquired cholesteatoma
In this type, cholesteatoma develops in ears which have suffered from active chronic disease with defects in the tympanic membrane.

THEORIES OF CHOLESTEATOMA

1. Implantation • Trauma	Penetrating or blast injury causes implantation of squamous epithelium into the pneumatized portions of the temporal bone.
• Iatrogenic	In ear surgery medial displacement of epithelium occurs during: i) burial of epilthelium under an onlay graft in tympanoplasty ii) during insertion of ventilation tubes iii) following removal of the ventilation tubes, retraction of the dimeric membrane can occur
2. Invasion - Mechanism **(Bezold)**	Invasion of squamous epilthelium inwards following perforation by acute otitis media
3. Metaplasia Mechanism I **(Reudi)**	Stimulation of basilar layer of squamous epilthelium of pars flaccida by inflammation ⇒ papillary ingrowth ⇒ expands ⇒ accumulation of keratin debri ⇒ cholesteatoma formation.
Mechanism II **(Sade)**	Residual mesenchymal tissue in epitympanum (pleuripotent) undergoes metaplasia due to inflammation ⇒ keratinizing epithelium capable of migration in both directions ⇒ cyst ⇒ bursts externally ⇒ cholesteatoma.
4. Negative middle ear pressure (Whitmacks)	Eustachian tube malfunction ⇓ Fluctuating positive and negative pressure ⇓ Marked excursions on the tympanic membrane, loss of elasticity and subsequent atelectasis ⇓ Attic and posterosuperior region ⇓ Retraction pocket formation ⇓ Grows inwards ⇓ Initially self cleansing ⇓ later ⇒ neck becomes narrow ⇓ accumulation of debris + foreign body inflammatory reaction ⇓ granulation tissue formation ⇓ destruction of bone ⇓ new areas into which squamous epithelium would penetrate

PATHOLOGIC ANATOMY OF CHOLESTEATOMA

Gross:

- Pearly grey or yellow, well defined structure
- Usually situated in the upper posterior part of the middle ear cleft
- May extend through the aditus into the mastoid antrum and mastoid air cells
- Ossicles and/or the scutum may be eroded
- Layer of granulation tissue is always present between the sac and underlying bone

Histopathology

1. **Perimatrix** :   Granulation tissue layer between the sac and the underlying bone.
2. **Matrix** :
   a) Corneal layer

   It is the pearly material of the cholesteatoma. It consists of dead, fully differentiated, anucleate keratin squames.

   b) Thin granular layer prior to the malphigian layer
   c) Malphigian layer of 5-6 rows of cells with intercellular prickles
   d) Basal layer made up of small cuboidal cells

   The deeper layers show downgrowths into the underlying connective tissue separating cholesteatoma into lobules.

Causes of bone erosion by cholesteatoma

1. **Pressure theory** :   Tumour causing pressure necrosis of the surrounding bone
2. **Pyogenic osteitis** :   Secondary bacterial infection causes pyogenic osteitis which causes necrosis and sclerosis of the surrounding bone
3. **Enzyme theory** :   In presence of the granulation layer, enzymes are released by the osteoclasts.

The enzymes are:

- Acid phosphatase
- Collagenase
- Proteolytic enzymes
- Epidermal growth factor (EGF)
- Transforming growth factor (TGF)
- Tumour necrotising factor (TNF)
- Interleukins
- Prostaglandins

SURGICAL ANATOMY OF CHOLESTEATOMA

A cholesteatoma can be a:

1. **Posterior epitympanic cholesteatoma:**

   Originating in the Prussak's space and passing via

   a) Superior incudal space into aditus and antrum
   b) Inferior incudal space by descending through the floor of Prussak's space into posterior pouch of von Troltsch into middle ear.

2. **Posterior mesotympanic cholesteatoma:**

   It is formed due to retraction of posterior portion of pars tensa and spreads to involve stapes, long process of incus, facial recess, sinus tympani or to mastoid via posterior tympanic isthmus. It passes medial to malleus head and incus while passing to mastoid in contrast to posterior epitympanic cholesteatoma which passes laterally to these structures.

3. **Anterior epitympanic cholesteatoma:**

   - It is formed from epitympanic retraction anterior to head of malleus.
   - It may involve geniculate ganglion, horizontal part of VII nerve causing facial nerve dysfunction
   - It reaches middle ear via anterior pouch of von Troltsch to involve the eustachian tube

Clinical Features

Symptoms

1. Otorrhoea
   - Purulent
   - Foul smelling
   - Scanty
   - Blood-stained
2. Deafness
   - Slow onset
   - Progressive
   - Associated with tinnitus
3. Onset of vertigo, vomiting, headache may signify intracranial complications.

Signs

1. Tympanic membrane defect
   a) Attic perforation: The perforation is present in the pars flaccida of the tympanic membrane. It is associated with cholesteatoma formation. The perforation may be covered by granulations or polypii.
   b) Posterosuperior marginal perforation: One of the edge of the perforation is formed by bone, rest by the tympanic membrane. It indicates bony necrosis associated with cholesteatoma and granulation. Cholesteatoma is seen as white shiny flakes present in the postero-superior region.
2. Fistula sign may be positive.

MANAGEMENT

History:

Bezold	Office management of cholesteatoma by irrigating with antral cannulas and a solution of 4% Boric acid + Salicylic acid at room temperature
Stacke (1893)	First radical mastoid surgery
Heath (1904)	Heath's modification of the above surgery.
Bondy (1910)	Modified radical mastoid surgery.
Tumarkin (1948)	Atticotomy.

History and assesment of the patient

- **Examination of the ear in detail**
   a) For character, colour, consistency of discharge
   b) In external auditory canal for:
      - Destruction of bone
      - Polyps, granulations
      - Flakes
      - Secondary otitis externa
      - Bulge in posterior canal wall
   c) Suction aspiration of the discharge

- **Fistula sign**
- **Examination under microscope**
   - Exact site of origin, posterior limit of cholesteatoma
   - Status of ossicles

- Status of tympanic membrane
- Swab for culture sensitivity

The culture usually reveals mixed group of organisms like -

- Bacillus proteus
- Pseudomonas aeruginosa
- Pseudomonas pyocyaneous
- Anaerobic bacteria, which are the cause for the secondary infection

INVESTIGATIONS

1. Pure tone audiometry
- For documentation
- It usually reveals conductive hearing loss unless the inner ear is involved.
- For comparing the pre operative and post operative hearing status
- For medicolegal purpose

2. X'ray mastoid (Schuller's view / Towne's / Law's view)
- Configuration of mastoid
- Anatomical landmarks
  - Sinus plate
  - Dural plate
  - Sinodural angle
- Extension of disease

  (seen as a lytic shadow with surrounding sclerosis)

> **Signs of cholesteatoma on x'ray**
> - Loss of normal osseous pattern of attic
> - Widened aditus
> - Antral enlargement
> - Radiolucent bone defect in the antral area surrounded by thin osteitic bone
> - Erosion of dural / sinus plate

3. C.T. scan of Temporal bone
The following features are looked for:
- Presence of soft tissue erosion and destruction of scutum
- Widened aditus
- Lateral displacement of ossicles with destruction
- Presence of fistula
- Erosion of facial canal
- Dehiscence of tegmen tympani
- Destruction of mastoid
- Dehiscence of sigmoid plate with or without sinus thrombosis
- Erosion and sagging of the EAC
- Atypical locations of cholesteatoma
  - EAC cholesteatoma
  - Petrous apex cholesteatoma

TREATMENT
Surgery is the treatment of choice for majority of the cases.

Aims and objectives of surgery:
- Complete eradication of the disease
- To provide the patient with a safe and dry ear
- To improve or preserve the hearing acuity
- To minimize the need for long-term care of the operated ear.

Approaches available:

1. Canal wall down (open) procedures

- Atticotomy
- Classical radical mastoidectomy
- Modified radical mastoidectomy
- Modern modified radical mastoidectomy (Tympanomastoidectomy)

2. Canal wall up procedures (closed)

- Combined approach tympanoplasty / Posterior tympanotomy

CANAL WALL DOWN	CANAL WALL UP
Easy to perform	Technically difficult
Good access	Relatively poor access
External auditory canal contour lost	Normal contour of external auditory canal is maintained
Shallow middle ear	Normal middle ear
Cavity problems are present • Discharge • Dizziness • Deafness • Disability • Doctor dependence	Absent cavity problems
Lesser recurrence rate	Higher rates for the same

RECIVIDISM

Residual cholesteatoma:

It can be defined as a disease that grows back from viable squamous epithelium that was not removed at the initial procedure

Recurrence:

It can be defined as a disease that grows back because of the inability of the eustachian tube to adequately aerate the middle ear, mastoid or both, resulting in retraction of the ear drum with keratin accumulation and bone resorption

Clinically it became difficult to differentiate between a residual and a recurrent cholesteatoma, so a new concept of RECIVIDISM was introduced, encompassing both the above types of disease.

Causes of residual cholesteatoma

1. Squamous epithelium left behind as in:
   a) Canal wall up surgery
   b) Inaccessible areas
   c) On purpose
      - To cover a lateral semicircular canal fistula.
      - To cover a facial nerve.
      - Over stapes foot plate.
2. Improper lowering of the facial ridge.
3. Improper drainage of the cavity
4. Inadequate meatoplasty.

Sites of residual cholesteatoma:

- Sinus tympani
- Anterior epitympanum and eustachian tube
- Medial to ossicular heads
- Sinodural angle
- Mastoid tip
- Peri labyrinthine region
- Over footplate of stapes

Management of residual cholesteatoma:

1. Small residual keratin pearls are excised

2. Revision mastoidectomy:
   - Canal wall up procedure is converted to canal wall down mastoidectomy
   - Adequate lowering of facial ridge is achieved
   - The affected sites are exposed and the matrix is removed
   - Good meatoplasty is made
3. Close follow up of the patient is essential

Difference between Safe and Unsafe ear

	SAFE EAR	UNSAFE EAR
Type of disease	Tubotympanic	Atticoantral
Perforation	Central	Attic/margnial
Discharge	Mucoid	Purulent, cheesy
	Copious	Scanty
	Non foul-smelling	Foul-smelling
	Intermittent	Continuous
Bleeding	Rare	Often
Granulation/polypi	Rare	Common
Squamous epithelium	Not present	Present
Focus of infection	Present in respiratory tract. Increase in discharge is seen during respiratory tract infection	Absent No change in discharge during respiratory infection
Ossicular chain	Less destruction	More destruction
Deafness	Mild to moderate	Moderate to severe
Audiogram	Conductive hearing loss	Mixed hearing loss
X'ray mastoid	Cellular/sclerotic	Sclerotic with a destruction cavity
Complications	Rare	Fatal complications can occur
Prognosis	Good	Not good because of complications

6. TUBERCULOUS OTITIS MEDIA

Tuberculous otitis media is quite common in India. It is almost always secondary to pulmonary tuberculosis.

ROUTES OF INFECTION

1. Eustachian tube : The tubercular bacilli are coughed out in the sputum from the infected lungs. This infected sputum reaches the eustachian tube while coughing and enters the middle ear via the tube.
2. Drinking unpasteurised milk of infected cows can cause the disease.
3. Blood borne infection in those suffering from pthisis (miliary tuberculosis)

   The infection can spread to the labyrinth through the round and oval window. It may spread to the mastoid via the haematogenous route.

CLINICAL FEATURES

1. Slow onset of disease
2. Painless condition
3. Thin, scanty and odourless discharge
4. Pale yellow colour of the tympanic membrane
5. Posterior part of tympanic membrane is bulging
6. Anterior part of tympanic membrane shows dilated blood vessels.
7. Multiple perforations of tympanic membrane. The perforations are caused by necrosis of the drum by the breakdown of multiple tubercles which are formed on the tympanic membrane.
8. The perforations may be associated with pale granulations, which recur after removal
9. Frequent involvement of the facial nerve occurs by the disease process.
10. Hearing loss is disproportionate to the ear findings.
11. Intraoperatively, lot of sequestra and bony granulations are seen.

DIAGNOSIS

Confirmation of disease is done by smear and culture of discharge or by biopsy of granulations.

TREATMENT

1. Antitubercular therapy consisting of four drug regime
   - Isoniazid
   - Rifampicin
   - Ethambutol
   - Pyrazinamide
2. Surgical treatment is indicated in tuberculous mastoiditis with caries and granulations
   - Removal of granulations
   - Removal of bony sequestra via a mastoidectomy approach.

7. TYMPANOSCLEROSIS

SYNONYMS

Chronic adhesive otitis media

Chronic adhesive catarrh

DEFINITION

It is an abnormal condition in which, local deposition of plaques of collagen along with calcerous deposits are seen in the submucosa of middle ear cavity. When it is confined to the tympanic membrane, it is called a **"Chalk patch."**

Sites :   It affects tympanic membrane, ossicular ligaments, interosseous joints, muscle tendons and submucosal spaces.

Common sites	**Other sites**	**Rare sites**
• Stapes-oval window area	• Long process of incus	• Hypotympanum
• Sub-fallopian groove	• Stapedius tendon	• Eustachian tube area
• Upper promontory	• Horizontal portion of fallopian canal.	• Round window niche
	• Epitympanum	
	• Malleus	

TYPES

1. Depending on the integrity of the tympanic membrane :
   - **Open**
   - **Closed**
2. Depending on the consistency :
   - **Soft**
   - **Dense / hard**
3. Depending on the histology :
   - **Sclerosing mucositis**

     It is a superficial non-invasive form in which surrounding mucosa and periosteum remain intact
   - **Osteoclastic mucoperiostitis**

     It is a deeper invasive form in which underlying bone is destructed.

PATHOLOGY

The main pathology is hyalinosis ie; hyaline degeneration of the collagen in which calcium is deposited. In the healing process of otitis media, the collagen in the fibrous tissue hyalinizes, loses its structure and becomes fused into a homogenous mass. Calcification then occurs followed by ossification. These deposits form in narrow spaces where inflammatory exudates accumulate during infection The reduction in ciliary activity and glandular secretion decreases the elimination of these exudates. They thus get organized to form tympanosclerotic plaques.

CLINICAL FEATURES

- Past history of otitis media
- Deafness
  - Stationary or progressive

- Mainly conductive, sometimes sensorineural
- Hearing loss of about 30 dB
- Tinnitus
- Signs
  - Signs of past attack of otitis media
  - Tympanic membrane will show white chalky patches
  - Drum may be mobile
  - Fibrosis and adhesions will be there between the drum, ossicles and promontory
  - Chalky patches over ossicles
  - Ossicular immobility
  - Fibrous tissue in round and oval window niches

DIAGNOSIS

- Past history of otitis media
- Deafness
- Chalky patches over drum
- Blocked eustachian tube

DIFFERENTIAL DIAGNOSIS

1. **Otosclerosis :** It is difficult to differentiate between the two especially if tympanosclerosis only involves the ossicles and tympanic membrane is normal. Past history of otitis media and a negative family history helps to differentiate the condition. Tympanotomy may be needed at times. Also the conductive deafness is usually nonprogressive and the mastoid is acellular.
2. **Cholesteatoma mass :** It lacks the glistening appearance of a tympanosclerotic plaque and is softer to touch.

TREATMENT

1. Prevent progress of disease
   - Tonsilloadenoidectomy
   - Treatment of sinusitis
   - Myringotomy / aspiration of effusion
2. No treatment for small plaques with no hearing loss
3. Surgical treatment (**only if eustachian tube is patent**)
   - Release of middle ear adhesions
   - Removal of plaques
   - Mobilization of ossicles
   - Stapedectomy (if the footplate is fixed)
   - Fenestration operation
4. Hearing aids are used for advanced cases.

8. OTOTOXICITY

The following drugs are ototoxic:

DRUG	SYMPTOMS	MECHANISM OF ACTION
1. **Antimalarials** • Quinine • Chloroquine	Decrease otoacoustic emissions	• Idiosyncratic reaction occurs with even small doses of Quinine • Decreases blood flow to cochlea / stria • Vasoconstriction of small vessels / ischaemic effect. • Degenerative changes in spiral ganglion.
2. **Diuretics** • Frusemide • Ethacrynic acid	Reversible hearing loss	Oedema and cystic changes in the stria vascularis
3. **Antiepileptics** • Phenytoin • Ethosuximide		Vestibulotoxic
4. **Antiheparinizing agents** • Hexadimethrine bromide	Deafness	Degeneration of organ of corti and stria vascularis.
5. **Antibiotics** • Vancomycin • Capromycin • Ampicillin • Chloramphenicol	Deafness	Ototoxic
6. **Topical Agents** • Chlorhexidine in alcohol • Ear drops containing Neomycin • Framycetin • Polymycin	Deafness	Absorption through round or oval window.
7. **Miscellaneous** • Mercury	Deafness	Eighth nerve neuritis
• Arsenic	Deafness	Herxheimer reaction
• Tobacco • Alcohol		Toxic neuritis

• B –Blockers
  - Propranolol
  - Oxyprenolol
  - Practolol
	Deafness	

• Nitrogen mustard		Cytotoxic changes in organ of corti.

MANAGEMENT

- Suspicion of ototoxicity if high pitched tinnitus and deafness occurs in a patient on drug therapy
- Stoppage of drug use.

- Multivitamins for nerve regeneration.
- Labyrinthine sedatives for vertigo
- Hearing aid for deafness.

NOSE

1. HISTORY AND EXAMINATION

HISTORY AND EXAMINATION

Name, Age, Sex, Religion, Occupation, Marital Status, Postal address.

Age:

Young   : - Nasopharyngeal angiofibroma
- Rhinosporidiosis

Elderly :   Carcinoma maxilla

Sex:

Males   : - Nasopharyngeal angiofibroma
- Rhinosporidiosis
- Carcinomas

Females : - Atrophic rhinitis

Address:

Rhinosporidiosis :   Along coastal areas in tropical countries like India, Bangladesh, Sri Lanka, Africa.

Rhinoscleroma   :   Rural areas of India, South Africa, Europe

Occupation:

Farmers   :   Rhinosporidiosis

Dusty environment: Vasomotor rhinitis.

> **Rhinosporidiosis:**
> Coastal areas of India
> Bangladesh
> Sri Lanka
> Africa

Chief Complaints:

- H/o Rhinorrhoea / nasal discharge
- H/o Nasal obstruction / blockage
- H/o Headache
- H/o Sneezing
- H/o Loss / decrease / change in sense of smell.
- H/o Epistaxis / bleeding from the nose.

  Each of the above complaint has to be described in detail with their onset, duration and progress.

Other Complaints:

- H/o fever with redness / swelling in association with nose or paranasal sinuses (acute vestibulitis, furunculosis, acute rhinitis / sinusitis, septal abscess, secondary infection of a nasal / paranasal mass, nasal fractures)
- H/o trauma / nose picking (cause of epistaxis, underlying nasal fracture.)
- H/o use of nasal packs (epistaxis, bleeding diasthesis, trauma, hypertension, spontaneous or induced bleeding due to surgical manipulation of a nasal mass, routine use of packs post-operatively in nasal surgeries).
- H/o lacrimation (nasal packing, nasal mass / polypii blocking nasolacrimal duct, orbital complication of sinusitis).
- H/o visual disturbances / diplopia (sinusitis with orbital complications, nasal masses with orbital invasion, malignancy).
- H/o earache (eustachian tube block by acute / chronic rhinosinusitis, nasal mass obstructing eustachian tube, malignancy.)

- H/o recurrent upper respiratory tract infection / cough (nasal mass / polypii / severe deviated nasal septum causing blockage of ostiomeatal complex and recurrent upper respiratory tract infection, secondary infection of nasal mass and chronic sinusitis causing post-nasal drip and cough.)
- H/o loss of sensations over front of cheek (infraorbital anaesthesia in carcinoma maxilla).
- H/o mouth breathing, snoring, (adenoid hypertrophy, nasal / nasopharyngeal mass, upper respiratory tract infection).
- H/o difficulty in speech / loss of nasal twang (huge nasal / nasopharyngeal mass hampering speech by its mechanical obstruction, absent / improper palatal movements and no nasal escape of air during speech).

Past History:

- H/o evening rise of temperature, loss of weight, appetite (Kochs / Koch's contact, tuberculosis of nose - nodular / ulcerative, lupus vulgaris).
- H/o blood pressure (Blood pressure - epistaxis, relative contraindication to surgery), Diabetes mellitus (fungal infections of nose), Asthma (associated nasal allergy), Allergy (allergic rhinitis, vasomotor rhinitis, ethmoidal polypii, asthma).
- H/o sexually transmitted diseases (syphilis gumma on septum, yaws - nodules in nose).
- H/o similar complaints in the past (recurrent ethmoidal polypii, recurrence of carcinoma).
- H/o any medical / surgical treatment in the past.

Personal History:

- H/o smoking, alcoholism, drug / snuff addiction (septal perforation in addicts.)
- H/o excessive use of nasal decongestants, hypotensive drugs (rhinitis medicamentosa, chronic nasal obstruction)

Family History:

- H/o similar complaints in the family (Allergy, Asthma, Polypii).
- H/o Bleeding disorders / hypertension / diabetes mellitus

GENERAL EXAMINATION
Pallor is seen in:
- Nasopharyngeal angiofibroma
- Repeated epistaxis.

LOCAL EXAMINATION
- External examination
- Intranasal examination
- Examination of paranasal sinuses.

EXTERNAL EXAMINATION:

Inspection	:	For obvious deformities of nasal form.
Nasal bridge deformities	:	Saddle - nose
		Hump deformity
		Crooked nose
		Bridge deviation

Obvious scars, sinuses, cysts, ulcers, growth (Rodent ulcer, lupus vulgaris on skin of nose.)

Broadening of nose. (Large polyps, malignancy)

Swelling, redness of skin over nose, surrounding area (Vestibulitis, furunculosis, rhinophyma)

Saddle nose deformity is seen in:
- Congenital Syphilis
- Tertiary Syphilis
- Post-traumatic
- Post-operative
- Septoplasty
- Nasal surgeries
- Septal abscess / haematoma
- Sarcoidosis
- Wegener's granulomatosis.

Examination of the shape of the nose, columella and position of caudal septum with respect to the columella can be done by asking the patient to raise the chin and looking from the front and the sides.

Simple elevation of the tip of the nose allows assessment of the membranous septum, the valve region and the floor.

Palpation:

- Palpation of cyst, sinuses, growth, ulcers etc.
- Palpation of the bridge for assessment of deformity, fractures, crepitus, oedema,.
- Look for woody feel in rhinoscleroma.
- Palpation of the bony and cartilaginous vault with special emphasis on the areas around the inner canthus of the eye and the alar base.
- Patient can be told to take a heavy breath and alar collapse can be looked for during inspiration.

Anterior Rhinoscopy

It is the examination of the anterior nares and nasal cavity using a nasal speculum. Usually a Thudicum's nasal speculum is used. The speculum is held at the junction of the two prongs by the thumb and index finger in the left hand with the blades facing the patient. The spring action of the prongs is controlled by the ring and middle finger. It is introduced with the blades closed which gently open up when the spring action is released in the nasal cavity.

Structures seen on anterior rhinoscopy:

STRUCTURES SEEN	LOOK FOR / COMMENTS
1. **Nasal septum**	Normally mildly deviated or in the midline. Look for: Deviated nasal septum 1. 'C' or 'S' shaped 2. Anterior / posterior 3. Presence of spurs, if any. Septal perforation: • Anterior / Posterior • Small / Medium / Large • Edges can be probed to rule out bleeding / irregularity.
2. **Nasal mucosa**	Normal mucosa is pinkish red in colour • Bright red: Acute inflammation • Pinkish white: Anaemia • Pale white: Allergy Topical vasoconstrictor solution can be used to decongest a congested mucosa.
3. **Nasal floor**	Normally seen as a concave tunnel. Look for foreign bodies, rhinoliths etc.
4. **Lateral wall**	The anterior ends of the inferior and middle turbinates are seen with their respective meatuses. **Causes of hypertrophied turbinates:** • On opposite side of DNS • Allergic rhinitis • Vasomotor rhinitis. Vasoconstrictor drops are used to differentiate between hypertrophied turbinates and polypii. A hypertrophied turbinate shrinks on vasoconstriction while a polyp does not. **Meatus:** • Purulent secretions are seen in chronic sinusitis

STRUCTURES SEEN	LOOK FOR / COMMENTS
5. Cavity	Both cavities ideally should be almost equal on both sides. A wide cavity is one through which one can get the view of the postnasal space. Causes of a roomy cavity: Unilateral: Secondary atrophic rhinitis, Deviated nasal septum Bilateral: Primary atrophic rhinitis The cavity is inspected for: ● Secretions ● Foreign body / maggots ● Tumours ● Polypii ● Adhesions
6. Lesion	Note: ● Surface ● Colour ● Ulceration ● Consistency ● Tenderness ● Sensitivity to touch ● Bleeding on touch
7. Secretions	● Discharge from middle meatus indicates inflammation of one of the anterior group of sinuses ie; frontal, maxillary or anterior ethmoidal cells
8. Inferior meatus	● It is the first meatus to be identified ● Collection of mucus or pus may be seen, beneath which a foreign body may be present.
9. Middle meatus	● Middle meatus is pear shaped and appears as a dark cleft. ● Repeated suction and decongestant drops helps to locate source of pus or polypii. ● Frontal sinusitis: Discharge, swelling, redness and oedema is seen high up and forward. ● Ethmoiditis: Generalised swelling of outer wall of middle meatus.
10. Superior meatus	● It is difficult to see ● It can be seen in Atrophic rhinitis and only after repeated decongestion

Posterior Rhinoscopy:

It is the visualisation of the posterior nares / choana with the help of a mirror. The size of the mirror ranges from 8-15 mm in diameter. A 10 mm diameter mirror is adequate. The instrument has a bayonet shaped handle and is used with the mirror facing upwards.

Method:

The mirror is first warmed to prevent condensation of vapour on it by:

● Dipping the mirror in warm water.

● Warming the mirror in the flame of a spirit lamp.

● Rubbing the mirror surface on the buccal mucosa and generating minimal heat by friction.

● Dipping the mirror in commercially available demisting / defogging solutions like cetavlon.

The warmth is tested on the flexor aspect of the wrist before putting it in the mouth.

The tongue is then depressed with a tongue depressor and the mirror is passed behind the soft palate without touching the uvula and surrounding structures to prevent gagging.

Patient must breathe through the nose and mouth to relax the soft palate. (Smiling often relaxes the soft palate)

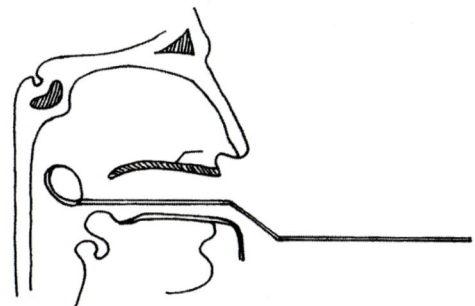

METHOD OF PERFORMING POSTERIOR RHINOSCOPY

Structures Seen:

Anteriorly:
- Posterior end of nasal septum. (It is vertical and the first structure to be identified)
- Posterior end of middle and inferior turbinate.
- Posterior end of superior turbinate (Superior turbinate is small and the highest landmark)
- Posterior part of superior and middle meatus.
- Nasal surface of the soft palate and the uvula on tilting the mirror further anteriorly.

Laterally:
- Eustachian tube openings on either side with the tubal elevations seen behind the posterior end of inferior turbinate.
- Fossa of Rosenmuller behind the eustachian tube orifice (difficult to examine).

Superiorly:
- Roof of nasopharynx
- Superior part of posterior pharyngeal wall.

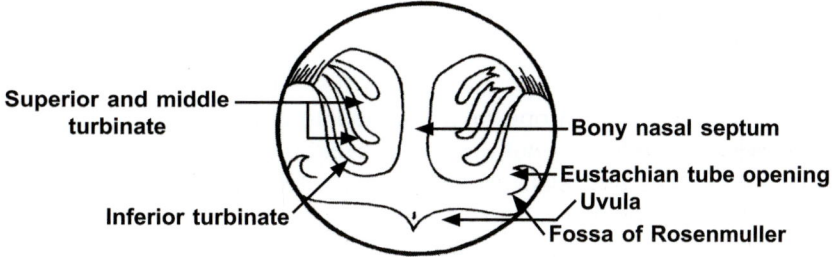

STRUCTURES SEEN ON POSTERIOR RHINOSCOPY

Abnormalities to be looked for:
- Polyps
- Cysts
- Secretions
- Foreign bodies
- Ulcers
- Tumours

Difficulties encountered:

- Difficult to perform in children and mentally retarded patients, due to lack of cooperation.
- Gag reflex: It can be prevented by proper method of examination and using 4% local anaesthetic / Xylocaine spray on the posterior pharyngeal wall.
- Recurrent fogging of the mirror surface of the instrument.

Methods for examination of Nasopharynx:

- Posterior rhinoscopy.
- Digital examination of the nasopharynx
- Rigid Yankauer's nasopharyngoscope under general anaesthesia.
- Lifting of soft palate with the help of retractors or rubber catheters passed through the nose into the mouth under general anaesthesia.
- Digital palpation of nasopharynx under general anaesthesia.
- Use of 90° / 120° nasal endoscope through the nose.
- Fibreoptic flexible nasopharyngoscope.
- Radiological examination of nasopharynx.
    - X-ray lateral view nasopharynx
    - Xeroradiogram soft tissues nasopharynx.
    - C.T. Scan / MRI nasopharynx.

Digital examination of nasopharynx:

It is useful in children when the postnasal space cannot be inspected. It is always felt through the soft palate and never behind it except under general anaesthesia. The child is held and the examiner stands on the right side. The child is asked to open his mouth and the left cheek is pressed between the teeth. The examiner passes his index finger of the right hand along the hard palate and presses it up into the postnasal space at the edge.

Tests for Nasal Obstruction:

1. **Spatula Test:** The air blast from both the nostrils is compared by asking the patient to exhale through the nostrils on the tongue depressor or a metal spatula. The area of fogging on the tongue depressor allows an assessment of the degree of nasal obstruction.

2. **Cotton-wool Test:** A wisp of cotton-wool is held under each nostril and the degree of its movement gives an idea about the air blast.

Probe Test:

Nasal masses can be probed with a probe or a eustachian catheter to find their site of origin and / or attachment. Vascular masses are preferably not probed to avoid bleeding. A mass can gently be touched with a probe to test its sensitivity. Polyps are relatively asensitive to touch, because of the dearth and splaying of nerve endings in their submucosal plane.

EXAMINATION OF PARANASAL SINUSES

Inspection:

Look for signs of inflammation - swelling, redness, oedema over the skin of the sinuses caused by under-lying sinusitis, osteomyelitis. There may be ulceration or a fungating growth encroaching the skin in cases of sinus tumours, especially carcinoma maxilla. Also look for scars, sinuses, fistula, pigmentation over the sinus area. Asymmetry of the face / sinuses.

Palpation:

To confirm inspectory findings and elicit tenderness in sinusitis.

SINUS	SITE TO ELICIT TENDERNESS
1. **Maxillary sinus**	Canine fossa or anterolateral wall of maxilla (thinnest wall)
2. **Frontal sinus**	Above the inner canthus of the eye - this area corresponds to the floor of the sinus which is the thinnest part, the anterior wall comprising of 2 layers of bone.
3. **Anterior ethmoidal cells**	Side of the nose midway between inner canthus and nasion, against the orbital plate of ethmoid.
4. **Posterior ethmoidal cells**	Deep in the skull, not amicable to palpation.
5. **Sphenoid sinus**	Deep in the skull, not amicable to palpation. A probe can be passed over its anterior surface and patient feels pain in occiput or temporal region.

Each sinus has to be palpated on both sides simultaneously with moderate pressure after steadying the head.

Posture Test:

This test differentiates between frontal and maxillary sinusitis. The nose is cleared of its discharge and the patient is made to sit. If the discharge appears in the middle meatus in the sitting position, it is said to be coming from the vertically draining frontal sinus. If it does not appear, the patient is made to lie down on the unaffected side (for drainage of the possibly affected maxillary sinus). If the discharge reappears in the middle meatus, it is said to be coming from the maxillary sinus. Thus by variation in posture, the pathological sinus is identified.

Transillumination Test:

This test is performed in a dark room after removal of any oral cavity denture / prosthesis. Maxillary sinus: Light is shun with the help of a torch placed in the oral cavity facing upwards and an infraorbital glow / crescent and retinal illumination is looked for. It appears if the sinus is clear, or if there is a cyst with clear fluid within which is able to transmit the light. The glow and retinal reflex do not appear in a sinus filled with pus or neoplasm.

Light is also pressed against the floor of the frontal sinus. Presence of illumination indicates a normal sinus but its absence is not necessarily pathological since the sinus may not have got developed.

Other Relevant Examination

Oral cavity:

- Teeth : Tooth involvement by tumour
  Loosening of teeth
  Dental caries
- Palate: Bulge due to tumour
  Perforation
  Movements
- Tumour extension to gingivo-buccal sulcus.

Eyes:

- Unilateral / bilateral proptosis

Cranial nerves:

- Involvement of cranial nerves V, VI, IX, X in nasopharyngeal carcinoma / masses.

Regional lymph nodes:

Involved in nasopharyngeal carcinoma.

INVESTIGATIONS

1. **Routine and specific blood investigations:**
   - Hb / CBC
   - ESR
   - Peripheral smear if lymphoma is suspected.
   - Blood sugar / RFT: if fungal infection is suspected
   - VDRL
   - HIV

2. **Bacterial / Fungal Culture** of Nasal Swab

3. **Radiography:**
   - X-ray Para nasal sinuses   : - Occipito mental (Water's) view
                                        - Occipito frontal (Caldwell's) view
   - X-ray Skull   :   Anteroposterior and lateral views
   - X-ray Nasopharynx
   - Orthopantomogram
   - X-ray Chest

4. **High Resolution CT Scan of Nose and PNS:**
   - Extent of involvement by any neoplasm or any pathology can be known
   - Invasion into brain, orbit, palate can be assessed
   - Good image of ostiomeatal complex
   - Details of bony invasion, calcification
   - It can't differentiate between soft tissue and cystic lesions

5. **MRI**
   - Good soft tissue differentiation
   - Poor bone - soft tissue differentiation
   - Superior to CT scan in assessing invasion of ossified hyaline cartilage.
   - Advantageous in nasal / nasopharyngeal tumours with intracranial extension.

6. **Diagnostic endoscopy**

7. **FNAC**
   - FNAC of the swelling and secondary lymphnode can be performed.
   - FNAC of vascular tumours may cause a lot of bleeding
   - Ultrasound / CT guided FNAC is valuable in posterior nasal space lesions.

8. **Biopsy**

   It is necessary if malignancy is suspected.

9. **Allergic test**

10. **Tests for olfaction**
   - Pure olfactory stimulants are used eg: asafoetida, clove, coffee (Ammonia is not used as it is an irritant and it stimulates trigeminal nerve in addition). Commercial kits are also available.
   - Evoked response olfactometry

MUCOCILIARY / CILIARY FUNCTION TESTS

SACCHARIN TEST: 0.5 mm diameter crystal of saccharin is kept 0.5 mm behind the anterior end of the inferior turbinate and the time taken to taste sweetness in pharynx is noted. Normal time taken is 20 minutes.

A time of more than 60 minutes indicates abnormal mucociliary clearance as seen in:

- Kartagener's syndrome
- Young's syndrome
- Cystic fibrosis

These conditions are associated with nasal polyps

RHINORRHOEA

It is the term used to denote discharge from the nose.

Types

- Watery
- Mucoid / Mucopurulent
- Purulent
- Blood-stained.

Etiology

TYPE	CONDITION
1. Watery	Allergic rhinitis
	Vasomotor rhinitis
	Viral rhinitis
	Rhinitis medicamentosa
	CSF rhinorrhoea
	Ethmoidal polypii
2. Purulent	Bacterial rhinitis: acute or chronic
	Sinusitis: acute or chronic
	Tuberculosis
	Syphilis
	Long standing foreign body
	Nasal granulomas
	Atrophic rhinitis
	Choanal atresia
	Nasal mass with secondary infection
	Foreign body
	Rhinitis sicca
	Furuncle
	Vestibulitis
	Leprosy
3. Blood-stained	Rhinosporidiosis
	Nasopharyngeal angiofibroma
	Atrophic rhinitis
	Carcinoma with sloughing
	Nasal granulomas
	Inverted papilloma
	Nasal diphtheria
	Acute / chronic rhinosinusitis
	Sarcoma

Causes of Unilateral Nasal Discharge
- Foreign body
- Rhinolith
- Antrochoanal polyp
- Unilateral choanal atresia
- Nasal tumours on one side
- Secondary atrophic rhinitis (Unilateral).

NASAL OBSTRUCTION

ETIOLOGY

1. **Congenital**
   - Choanal atresia
   - Congenital tumours

2. **Inflammatory**
   - Acute/chronic rhinitis
   - Acute/chronic sinusitis
   - Allergic rhinitis
   - Vasomotor rhinitis
   - Atrophic rhinitis

3. **Neoplastic / Swellings**
   - Nasopharyngeal angiofibroma
   - Rhinosporidiosis
   - Inverted papilloma
   - Carcinoma of nose/paranasal sinuses
   - Nasal polypii
   - Adenoids
   - Turbinate hypertrophy
   - Haemangiomas

4. **Granulomatous diseases**
   - Rhinoscleroma
   - Wegener's granuloma
   - Sarcoidosis
   - Tuberculosis
   - Midline granulomas
   - Foreign body granulomas

5. **Traumatic**
   - Fracture nasal bone
   - Facio maxillary injuries
   - Septal haematoma
   - Septal abscess

6. **Mechanical obstruction**
   - Deviated nasal septum
   - Synechiae
   - Modified Young's operation

7. **Miscellaneous**
   - Foreign body
   - Hypotensive drugs
   - Hypothyroidism
   - Smoking
   - Alcoholism
   - Drug addiction
   - Rhinitis medicamentosa

Causes of Unilateral nasal obstruction
- Deviated nasal septum
- Unilateral choanal atresia
- Foreign body
- Hypertrophied turbinate
- Antrochoanal polyp
- Rhinosporidiosis
- Inverted papilloma
- Synechiae
- Modified Young's operation on one side
- Tumours in one nostril

Causes of nasal obstruction in children:
- Foreign body
- Adenoids
- Rhinitis
- Choanal atresia
- Nasal diphtheria

HEADACHE

Causes of headache:

NOSE	PARANASAL SINUSES

• Deviated nasal septum
• Rhinitis
• Atrophic rhinitis
• Nasal masses / granulomas / polyp
• Rhinolith
• Malignancy
	• Sinusitis
	• Ostial block: vacuum headache
	• Complications of sinusitis
	  - Pyocoele
	  - Cavernous sinus thrombosis
	  - Orbital complications
	  - Intracranial abscess
	  - Aural complications

EPISTAXIS

Epistaxis means bleeding from the nose.

TYPES

TYPE	SITE	SEEN IN
1. **Anterior**	Little's area	Children and young persons
2. **Posterior**	Woodruff's plexus	Elderly

Epistaxis digitorum
- Epistaxis in children due to nose picking
- Commonest cause of epistaxis in children.

SOURCE OF BLEEDING

1. **Little's area (Locus valsalvae) (James Little in 1879)**	Anastomosis of nasopalatine, greater palatine, anterior ethmoidal arteries (Arterial bleed) - Commonest site of bleeding
2. **Woodruff's plexus (Nasal-Nasopharyngeal plexus)**	Collection of large blood vessels Situated in the lateral wall of inferior meatus posteriorly Venous bleed.
3. **Septal turbinate**	Engorged vascular nasal mucosa on the septum Can cause severe epistaxis Submucous resection helps to cure.
4. **Haemorrhagic nodules**	Aneurysmal dilatation of an unusually placed muscular artery with hypertensive changes in its walls.
5. **Venous bleed**	From retrocolumellar vein, common in young persons.

ETIOLOGY

Local:

1. **Inflammatory**	**Non-Specific:** • Rhinitis • Sinusitis • Atrophic rhinitis

	• Bacterial / viral infections
	• Adenoid infection
	Specific:
	• Granulomatous diseases
	- Syphilis
	- Tuberculosis
	- Rhinoscleroma
	- Sarcoidosis
	- Rhinosporidiosis
	• Leprosy
	• Fungal infections
	• Nasal Diphtheria
2. Neoplastic	**Benign tumours**
	• Angioma
	• Angiofibroma
	• Inverted papilloma
	• Haemangioma
	Malignant tumours
	• Nasopharyngeal carcinoma
	• Carcinoma maxilla
	• Malignancy of nose
	• Squamous cell carcinoma
	• Adenocarcinoma
	• Adenoidcystic carcinoma
3. Traumatic	**Injuries to the nose**
	• Nose picking
	• Surgical / Iatrogenic
	- Reactionary haemorrhage
	- Secondary haemorrhage
4. Drugs / Inhalants	**Topical decongestants**
	• Cocaine
	• Tobacco
	• Cannabis
	• Heroin
	• Wood dust
	• Phosphorus
5. Miscellaneous	**Foreign bodies**
	• Inanimate
	- Buttons
	- Batteries
	- Peas
	- Nuts
	• Animate
	- Maggots
	• Rhinolith

General:

1. Congenital	• Rendu-Osler-Weber syndrome
	   - Epistaxis
	   - Multiple mucosal telangiectasia
	   - Cutaneous telangiectasia
	• Meningocoele
	• Von-Willebrand's disease
	• Hereditary telangiectasia of Little's area
	• Unilateral choanal atresia
	• Glioma

2. Cardiovascular	• Hypertension • Atherosclerosis • Congestive cardiac failure • Mitral stenosis • Secondary hypertension due to nephritis
3. Haemopoietic	• Blood dyscrasias • Haemophilia • Leukaemia • Thrombocytopenia • Coagulopathies
4. Endocrinal	• Puberty • Vicarious menstruation • Pregnancy • Granuloma gravidarum • Hypothyroidism
5. Hepatic	• Cirrhosis of liver • Portal hypertension • Vitamin K deficiency.
6. Drugs	• Aspirin • Anticoagulants • Methotrexate • Immunosuppressants • Alcohol • Chloramphenicol
7. Exanthematous fevers	• Measles • Chicken pox
8. Miscellaneous	• High altitude • Extremes of temperature • Head injuries • HIV • Barotrauma
9. Idiopathic	

Common causes of epistaxis in E.N.T.

CHILDREN	ADULTS
Nose picking	Hypertension
Trauma	Angiofibroma
Acute rhinitis	Malignancy
Foreign body	Rhinosporidiosis
Exanthematous fever	Head injury
Diphtheria	Idiopathic
Blood dyscrasias	
Idiopathic	

Pathology: (In elderly)

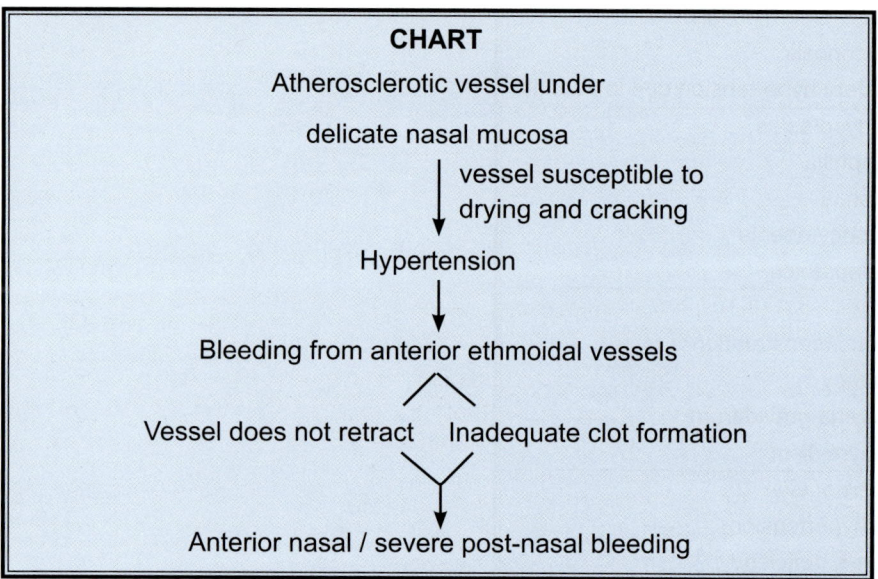

CHART

Atherosclerotic vessel under

delicate nasal mucosa

↓ vessel susceptible to drying and cracking

Hypertension

↓

Bleeding from anterior ethmoidal vessels

Vessel does not retract   Inadequate clot formation

↓

Anterior nasal / severe post-nasal bleeding

INVESTIGATIONS

1. Detail history of epistaxis

   Epistaxis

   - Quantity
   - Frequency
   - Duration
   - Previous episodes
   - Unilateral / bilateral
   - Clots / frank blood
   - Onset
   - Anterior / post-nasal blood
   - Haemoptysis / haematemesis

2. History

   - Trauma
   - Exanthematous fevers
   - Foreign body
   - Bleeding disorders
   - Hypertension
   - Drug intake

3. Examination of nose and sinuses

4. Systemic examination
   - Blood pressure
   - Pulse
   - Temperature
5. Blood Investigations
   - Bleeding time
   - Clotting time
   - Prothrombin time
6. Radiology
   - X'ray nasal bones for trauma
   - C.T. scan for nasal mass
7. Biopsy for non-vascular masses
8. Endoscopy of nose and sinuses

TREATMENT

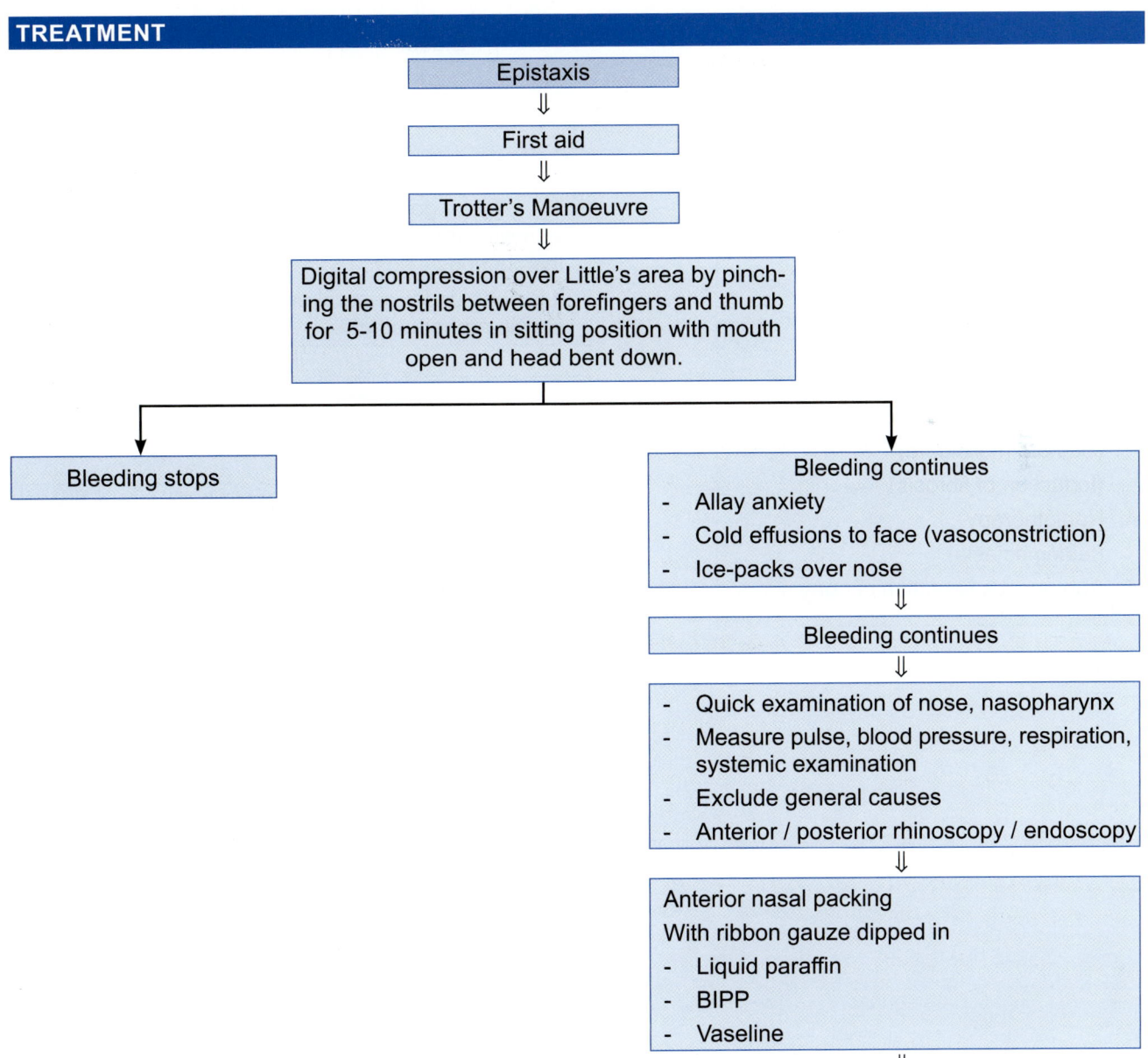

Epistaxis
⇓
First aid
⇓
Trotter's Manoeuvre
⇓
Digital compression over Little's area by pinching the nostrils between forefingers and thumb for 5-10 minutes in sitting position with mouth open and head bent down.

Bleeding stops

Bleeding continues
- Allay anxiety
- Cold effusions to face (vasoconstriction)
- Ice-packs over nose
⇓
Bleeding continues
⇓
- Quick examination of nose, nasopharynx
- Measure pulse, blood pressure, respiration, systemic examination
- Exclude general causes
- Anterior / posterior rhinoscopy / endoscopy
⇓
Anterior nasal packing
With ribbon gauze dipped in
- Liquid paraffin
- BIPP
- Vaseline
⇓

(Adrenaline pack is not used in hypertension.)

- It is done in a layered fashion starting from below. This method of packing gives uniform gentle pressure and prevents loosening of pack in oropharynx.
- It is removed by 48 hrs.
- Now a days synthetic sponge nasal tampons are available.
- Send blood for
  - Haemoglobin
  - Blood counts
  - Bleeding and clotting time
  - Platelet count
  - Prothrombin time (Extrinsic clotting system)
  - Partial prothrombin time
  - Blood grouping / cross-matching if required

⇓

Bleeding

⇓

Stops

Repeat episode of bleeding

1. Cauterization of Little's area with
   - Silver nitrate,
   - Trichloroacetic acid
   - Diathermy
2. Cryosurgery
3. Local sclerosing injections
   (Sodium morrhuate)
   (Induction of fibrosis)
4. Radiotherapy
   (telangiectasia)
5. Submucous resection of bony spurs

Continues

- A 4 x 4 inch gauze rolled to 1 inch diameter, secured with silk threads or umbilical cord tapes is placed in the post nasal space
- It is done under general anaesthesia with the help of simple rubber catheters

⇓

Bleeding continues

Repacking or Foley's catheter placement

⇓

Catheter passed transnasally till balloon reaches behind the uvula

15 ml air is injected into the balloon which should snugly fit into the post-nasal space

The catheter is pulled anteriorly to place the balloon against the posterior nares

⇓

Intractable cases

⇓

-   Blood transfusion
-   Ligation of
    - External carotid artery
    - Internal carotid artery
    - Maxillary artery
    - Common carotid artery
-   Angiography with embolization

SURGICAL LIGATION

ARTERY	METHOD
1. Internal maxillary artery	Sublabial incision Posterior wall of antrum is pierced Ligation is done in pterygopalatine fossa
2. External carotid artery	Division is done close to sphenopalatine foramen Curved incision over the neck at the upper border of thyroid cartilage is taken. Incision is centred over the bifurcation of common carotid artery. External carotid artery is identified by its branches and ligated in continuity with 3/0 silk or linen thread.
3. Anterior ethmoidal artery	External ethmoidectomy incision Artery is identified at junction of medial and superior walls of orbit Posterior ethmoidal artery located 1 cm. behind anterior ethmoidal artery.

2. DEVIATED NASAL SEPTUM

Deviated nasal septum is a very common condition found in adults. Nasal septum is usually never central.

Types of deviations:

I. 1. Cartilagenous
    2. Bony
    3. Combined
II. 1. 'C' shaped
    2. 'S' shaped
    3. Caudal deviation.

Etiology

1. **Birth Moulding Theory:** The intrauterine position of the foetus and that during labour influences the deviation of the septum
2. **Trauma** during birth and further on
3. **Hereditary**
4. **Racial:** Common in white races
5. **High arched palate**

Pathology in deviated nasal septum

1. **Deviations**	1. More or less a generalized bulge 2. Bony or cartilagenous deviation 3. 'C' or 'S' shaped.
2. **Spurs**	A spur is a sharp angulation that occurs at the junction of the vomer below with the septal cartilage and / or ethmoid above.
3. **Dislocations**	Lower border of septal cartilage gets displaced from its medial position into one of the nostrils.
4. **Lateral nasal wall**	Compensatory hypertrophy of turbinates occurs.

Cottle's classification

The septal lesion is classified into three types.

TYPES	PATHOLOGY	VASOCONSTRICTION	TREATMENT
1. **Simple deviation**	1. Mild deviation of the septum 2. Does not cause obstruction	- -	No treatment is required
2. **Obstruction**	1. More severe deviation 2. Septum touches lateral wall	Obstruction is relieved by shrinkage of the turbinates	Medical decongestants Surgery may be required
3. **Impaction**	1. Marked angulation of the septum 2. Spur lies in contact with the lateral nasal wall.	No relief occurs on vasocons - triction	Surgery is essential

Clinical features

Symptoms

1. **Nasal obstruction**
   - Unilateral, mostly on the side of the convexity
   - Bilateral due to compensatory hypertrophy of the turbinate, on the opposite side.
   - Snoring may be present.

2. **Headache**

   Causes of headache in a case of deviated nasal septum are:
   1. Sinusitis
   2. Obstruction of the frontonasal duct
   3. Pressure over anterior ethmoidal nerve by the middle turbinate **(Sluder's neuralgia) (Anterior ethmoidal nerve syndrome)**
   4. Severe deviation of the septum can cause pressure on the lateral nasal wall causing referred trigeminal pain.

3. **Anosmia**

   In acute deviation, blast of air does not adequately reach the olfactory nerves.

4. **Epistaxis**

   It occurs due to stretching of vessels over the bony spur.

Paradoxical Nasal Obstruction

It is seen in patients complaining of unilateral nasal obstruction but anterior rhinoscopy reveals deviation of the septum on the opposite side. These patients have a long-standing fixed nasal obstruction to which they have become accustomed to and are now unaware of it. Mucosal swelling occurring on the opposite side associated with the nasal cycle causes intermittent obstruction, which the patient appreciates as the main symptom.

Signs

1. 'C' or 'S' shaped deviation
2. Spurs
3. Caudal deviation may be present
4. Compensatory hypertrophy of turbinate occurs on the opposite side
5. Mucosa around the deviation may be oedematous (Bernoulli's phenomenon).

'C' shaped deviation

Displacement of the upper bony septum and pyramid to one side and the whole of the cartilagenous septum and vomer to the opposite.

'S' shaped deviation

Deviation of the middle third (upper cartilagenous vault and associated septum) is in the opposite direction to that of the upper and lower third.

Treatment

1. **Medical**
   - Decongestants
   - Analgesics for pain relief
   - Antibiotics for concomitant sinusitis.

2. **Surgical**
   - Submucous resection
   - Septoplasty

3. SEPTAL PERFORATION

It is a condition in which a perforation is present in the nasal septum. Septal perforations are important in children since if not treated they can hamper the growth of the nose and mid-third of the face.

ETIOLOGY

I Congenital

II Acquired

1. Trauma
- Septal haematoma
- Septal abscess
- Nose picking

2. Surgical trauma
- Submucous resection of the septum
- Submucous cauterization
- Rhinoplasty

3. Inflammation
- Syphilis
- Tuberculosis
- Leprosy
- Diphtheria

4. Granulomatous disease
- Sarcoidosis
- Wegener's granulomatosis

5. Malignant tumours of the nose

6. Drugs
- Addiction to cocaine
- Topical corticosteroids

7. Occupational / Industrial
- Chromium
- Arsenic
- Mercury

8. Idiopathic

PATHOLOGY

Chart I

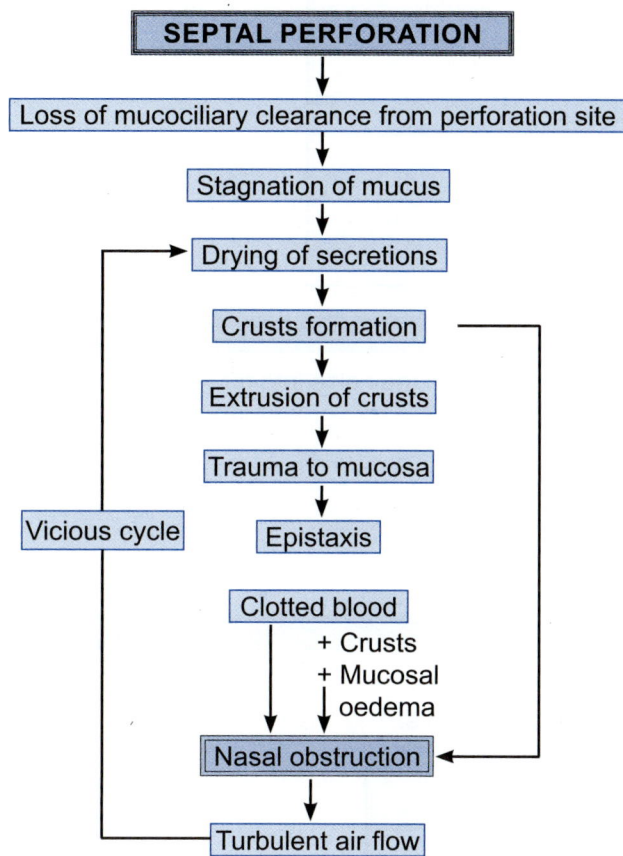

Chart II

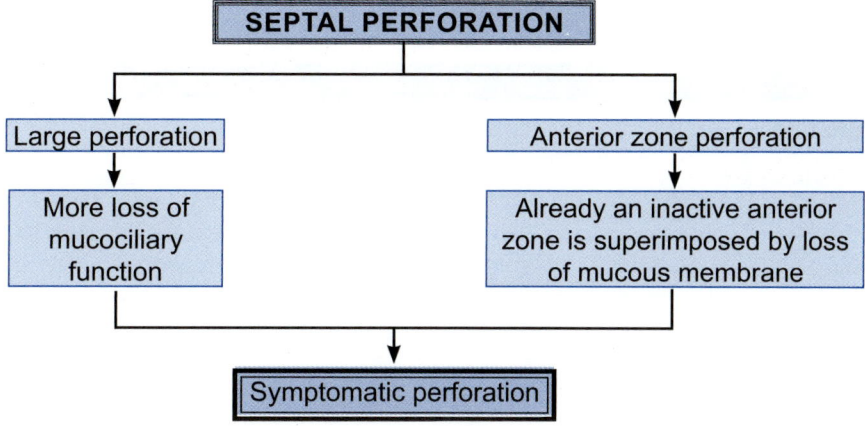

STAGES OF SEPTAL PERFORATION

The following are the stages of development of a septal perforation

STAGE	FEATURES
I	Redness and congestion of mucosa Irritation and rhinorrhoea
II	Blanched and anaemic mucosa
III	Development of crusts over the area Necrosis of the area starts
IV	Crusts extend into the substance of the cartilage Septal perforation

CLASSIFICATION OF SEPTAL PERFORATION

Septal perforations are classified according to their size into three types:

PERFORATION	DIAMETER
Small	Up to 1 cm
Medium	1-2 cm
Large	>2 cm

CLINICAL FEATURES

Small septal perforations may be asymptomatic

A perforation may have the following symptoms:

SMALL PERFORATION	LARGE PERFORATION
Whistling sound at respiration	Dryness Crusting Epistaxis Nasal obstruction Disturbed phonation

Septal perforations are usually preceded by ulceration.

DIAGNOSIS

History and examination
- Crusting
- Epistaxis
- Trauma
- Occupation

Biopsy
- When edge of perforation is raised
- In Wegener's granulomatosis

Serological tests for Syphilis

Erythrocyte sedimentation rate for Wegener's granulomatosis

C.T. Scan / MRI

- It is rarely required
- The size of the perforation can be determined
- Bone erosion can be determined

TREATMENT

Principles:

Asymptomatic perforations require no treatment

- Perforations usually do not heal spontaneously
- It is difficult to close perforations >2cm surgically
- Avoidance of nose picking, blowing
- Clearance of occupational hazards
- Treatment of underlying disease

Medical treatment

- Local application of
  - Petroleum jelly
  - 25% Glucose glycerol
  - Cicatrin cream
- Nasal douching to remove crusts

Closure of perforation by prosthesis

- Obturators made of Acrylic / silastic
- Prefabricated silastic buttons.

Advantages of using a prosthesis

- Simple, safe method
- Reliable method
- Better insertion and retention occurs with silastic obturators
- Closure of defect can be achieved

Disadvantages of prosthesis

- Prosthesis do not replace lost septal mucosa
- Replacement is needed for a loose prosthesis
- Retention of silastic buttons is poor
- Displacement of obturators occur
- Acrylic obturators are rigid for insertion

Surgical treatment

Surgical closure can be achieved by the following approaches:

APPROACH	PERFORATION SITE ON SEPTUM
External rhinoplasty	High
Alar facial crease incision	Low (Upper limit of such a perforation is 2 cm or less from nasal floor)

Closure

After selecting a proper approach, depending on the site of the perforation, the perforation is closed by either grafts or flaps raised from the surrounding structures.

GRAFTS	FLAPS

• Temporalis fascia
• Free grafts from turbinates
• Three layered composite graft from pinna
• Fascia lata
	• Mucosal flaps
	  - Septal
	  - Upper lip
	  - Buccal mucosa
	  - Labial flap
	• Lateral nasal wall
	• Cartilage flap
	• Bipedicled flap based on
	  - Sphenopalatine artery
	  - Superior labial artery

Disadvantage • Amount of tissue available from turbinate grafts is limited	**Disadvantage** • Limited width of buccal flap (2 cm) • Thinness of buccal flap

4. ATROPHIC RHINITIS

It is a chronic nasal disease characterized by progressive atrophy of mucosa and underlying bone with formation of crusts and characteristic foul smell called ozaena emanating from the nose.

TYPES

I. It is classified into primary and secondary atrophic rhinitis
1. **Primary:** It is usually bilateral
2. **Secondary**: It is secondary to
   - Deviated nasal septum: atrophic changes occur on the concave side
   - Specific infections which cause atrophic changes in the nasal mucosa
     - Syphilis
     - Leprosy
     - Tuberculosis
     - Lupus vulgaris
     - Atrophic stage of rhinoscleroma
   - Chronic sinusitis
   - Irradiation
   - Radical surgery of nose
     - Over correction of deviated nasal septum
     - Extensive rhinoplastic procedures
     - Turbinectomy
     - Rhinosporidiosis removal
     - Nasopharyngeal angiofibroma removal
     - Removal of nasal polypi.

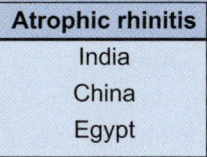

Atrophic rhinitis
India
China
Egypt

II. Histopathologically, it is divided into type I and type II

TYPE	PATHOLOGY	ESTROGEN THERAPY
I	Endarteritis Periarteritis	Benefits
II	Vasodilatation of capillaries	Worsens

ETIOLOGY

1. Zaufal's mechanical theory: anatomical abnormalities like deviated nasal septum cause unilateral atrophic rhinitis.
2. Endocrine / hormonal dysfunction: estrogen deficiency. It affects females more and worsens during menarche, menopause and pregnancy.
3. Deficiency of fat-soluble vitamins, especially vitamin A.
4. Hypoproteinaemia
5. Malnutrition and poor general condition
6. Autonomic dysfunction.

7. Reflex sympathetic dystrophy syndrome.
8. Bacterial infection caused by:
   - Coccobacillus foetidus ozaena (Perez)
   - Klebsiella ozaena
   - Diphtheroids
   - Bacillus mucosus
   - Coccobacillus
9. Autoimmune disorder
10. Heredity: racial preponderance
11. Familial: occurs in members of the same family.
12. Environmental: common in tropical countries.
13. Exanthematous disease in childhood predisposes to atrophic rhinitis due to altered immunity
14. It is seen in blood groups O and B.

PATHOLOGY

The following pathological changes occur in atrophic rhinitis:
1. Atrophy of mucosa
2. Metaplasia of epithelium to stratified or cuboidal type
3. Atrophy of cilia and secretory glands
4. Drying of secretions to form crusts
5. Secondary infection leading to foul smell (ozaena) from the nose
6. Atrophy of turbinates leading to roomy nasal cavity
7. Periarteritis and endarteritis of blood vessels leading to ischaemia and atrophy of mucosa.
8. Atrophy of sensory nerves and olfactory nerve endings.

CHART

Pathological changes in Atrophic rhinitis:

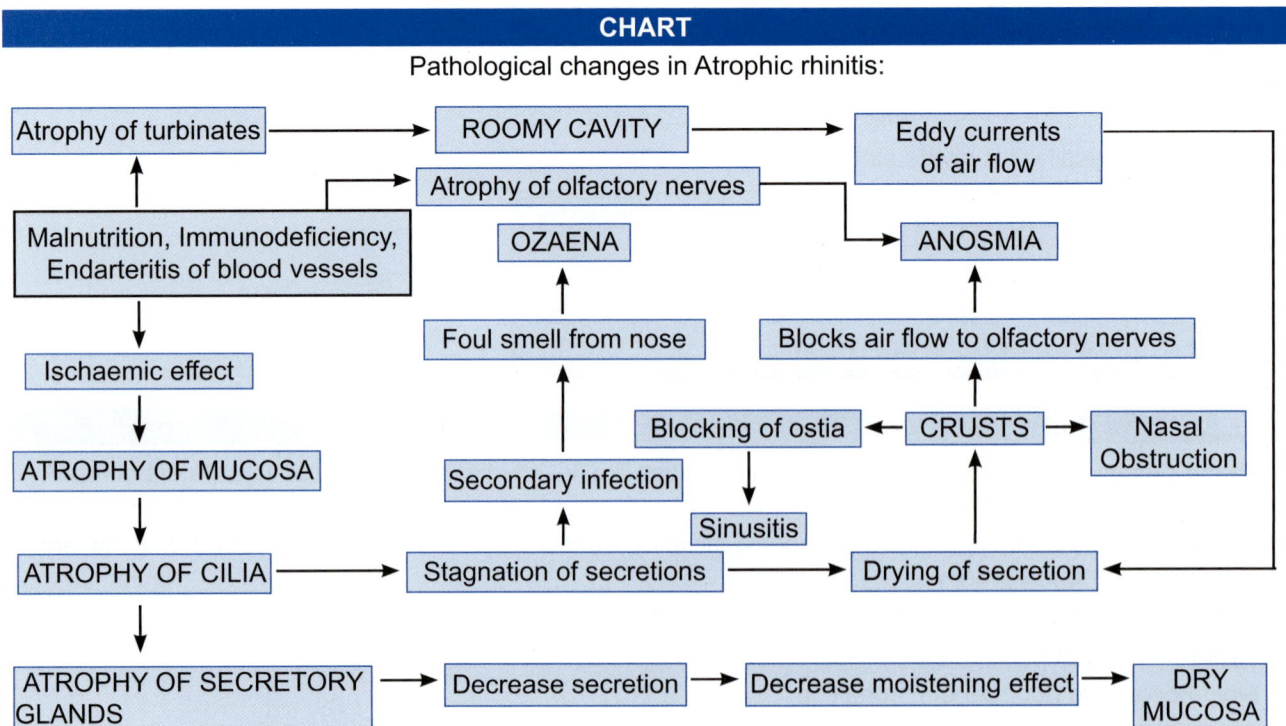

CLINICAL FEATURES

Symptoms

SYMPTOMS	COMMENTS
Foul odour	• Perceived by neighbours, relatives • Patient unable to perceive because of atrophy of olfactory epithelium • Called as **"Merciful anosmia"**.
Nasal obstruction	Causes of nasal obstruction: • Crusts in nasal cavity • Atrophy of sensory nerves giving false sense of obstruction, as patient cannot feel the air flow
Purulent discharge	Causes of purulent discharge • Secondary infection of the crusts • Sinusitis
Headache	Causes of headache: • Associated sinusitis as crusts block the ostia • Change in "eddy currents" in the nose due to widening of nostrils
Anosmia	Causes of anosmia: • Atrophy of olfactory nerve endings • Obstruction of airflow to the nerve endings by crusts
Dry cough	Causes of dry cough: • Drying of pharyngeal mucosa • Crusts extending downwards from choanae • Pharyngitis sicca
Dyspepsia	It is due to ingestion of septic material.
Epistaxis	It is caused by removal of crusts by the patient
Psychiatric disturbances	They are due to • Foul-smell emanating from the nose • Social out-casting

Signs

Primary
• Bilateral atrophy of nasal mucosa.

Secondary
• Unilateral atrophy
• Deviated nasal septum
• Signs of the causative factor

Common features

External examination
• Bridge of nose may be depressed due to atrophy of nasal bones and the septum.

Anterior rhinoscopy
• Roomy nasal cavities
• Pale, atrophied dry mucosa
• Atrophied and shrivelled turbinates
• Yellowish green crusts in the cavity
• Meatus may be seen
• Posterior nares and nasopharynx may be seen
• Loss of anatomical landmarks
• Crusts on posterior pharyngeal wall

Posterior rhinoscopy

It is relatively easy to perform as atrophy of sensory nerves causes diminished sensations. It shows atrophied mucosa and crusts.

Differential Diagnosis

- **Syphilis:** Atrophy of mucosa and systemic signs of the disease are present like chancre, gumma etc.
- **Tuberculosis:** Atrophy of mucosa, anaemia, cachexia, cough, cervical lymphadenopathy etc.
- **Leprosy:** Atrophy of mucosa and systemic signs like skin lesions, nerve palsies are present
- **Atrophic stage of rhinoscleroma:** Mucosa is pink and the turbinates are not affected.
- **Rhinitis sicca:** Crusting is present only in anterior part of nose and there is no foul smell

Investigations

(Clinical diagnosis usually suffices)

- X'ray paranasal sinuses:
    - Sinusitis
    - Walls of the sinus may be thickened
- X'ray chest: for Tuberculosis
- Nasal smear: for Leprosy, Tuberculosis
- VDRL test: for Syphilis
- Dermatological tests for Leprosy
- Biopsy to rule out rhinoscleroma.

Complications

- Sinusitis
- Pharyngitis
- Laryngitis
- Nasal myiasis
- Middle ear infection
- External nasal deformity
- Psychiatric problems

Treatment

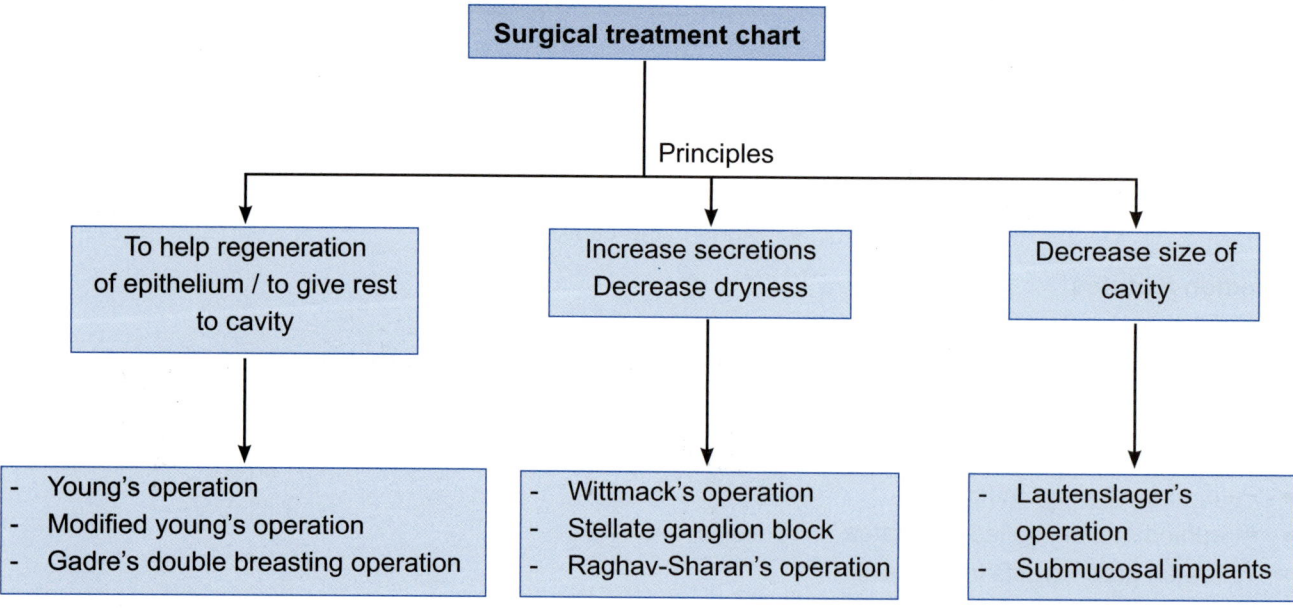

PRINCIPLE	OPERATION		\DIAGRAM\
• Regeneration of epithelium • Rest to cavity • Avoidance of turbulent air currents	Young's operation (1967)	Closure of anterior nares Folds of skin are raised from within the nostril and then sutured. The closure is maintained for 9 months – 1 yr, followed by opening after healthy mucosa and absence of crusts is confirmed by posterior rhinoscopy. The nasal mucosa is given rest and helped to regenerate in the closed nostrils. The high CO_2 concentration in the expired air collecting in the closed nostrils helps to regenerate mucosa and goblet cell growth. Patient has to breathe through the mouth leading to halitosis, snoring	**Closed anterior nares**
	Modified YOUNG'S operation	A 3mm. opening is left during closure of anterior nares. A 3mm. size opening is just about adequate to allow rest and maintain minimal respiration. Advantages of the opening: • Allows minimal respiration • Opening allows visualization of regeneration of mucosa, if any with an endoscope / otoscope	**Opening**
	GADRE'S double breasting	Similar to Young's operation but two folds are raised within the nostril Double layered closure is done	
• Increase secretion • Decrease dryness.	Wittmack's operation	Transplantation of parotid duct (Stenson's duct) into maxillary sinus It moistens nasal mucosa. Disadvantage: Profuse rhinorrhoea occurs while eating food	
	• Stellate ganglion block • Cervical sympathectomy / blockade	By abolishing sympathetic supply, parasympathetic predominates causing an increase in blood supply. It thereby makes the nasal mucosa more supple, increases secretions and also helps it to regenerate.	
	Raghav Sharan's operation	Transplantation of antral mucosa into nasal cavity.	
• Decrease in size of cavity	Lautenslager's operation	Medialization of the lateral nasal wall. The lateral wall is displaced by the intranasal route.	

	Submucosal implants	The width of the septum is increased by the following submucosal implants:
		• Bone (autogenous medullary bone graft)
		• Cartilage
		• Injection of
		  - Teflon
		  - Paraffin
		  - Dermofat
		  - Acrylic resin.
		• Placental extracts
		• Gold
		• Ivory	

MEDICAL TREATMENT

Aim:

-   To reduce crusts
-   To prevent foul smell
-   Nasal hygiene / toilet

-   Adequate nutrition / high protein diet
-   Administration of vitamin A and dilute hydrochloric acid to improve appetite.
-   Injection of placental extracts intramuscularly (biogenic stimulator)
-   Injection Streptomycin (against gram negative ozaena bacilli).
-   Potassium iodide orally to increase nasal secretions
-   Mandl's paint applied to nasal mucosa increases nasal secretions
-   Massage of turbinates to stimulate the glands.

-   **Nasal drops:**

    i)   25% glucose in glycerine nasal drops or tampoons put three times a day.
         (glucose – 8 gms, glycerine – 30 cc)

         Action:

         -   Saccharolytic organisms break up the glucose and lactic acid is produced
             This inhibits growth of proteolytic organisms
         -   Glycerine helps to moisten the crusts and mucosa and prevents drying.

    ii) Ethylene oestradiol in Arachis oil (1:10,000)

    iii) Chloramphenicol / Streptomycin nasal drops

    iv) Liquid paraffin nasal drops to soften the crusts.

-   **Nasal Toilet**

    i)   Alkaline Nasal Douche

Sodium bicarbonate	28.4 gms	Creates an alkaline medium, necessary to dissolve the crusts.
Sodium diborate	28.4 gms	Antiseptic
Sodium chloride	56.7 gms	Maintains isotonicity

One teaspoonful of the above powder is added to half pint of water (280 ml). The resulting solution is used for nasal washing twice a day. A simple rubber catheter with a 20 cc plastic / glass / Higginson's syringe can be used for nasal toilet

    ii) Hydrogen peroxide

         Hydrogen peroxide is used to dissolve the crusts before douching. Oestrogen in arachis oil / coconut oil is then applied to improve vascularity of the musoca. (Edinburgh school treatment)

    iii) Kemicitin   Antiozaena solution:

         Each ml contains

         Chloramphenicol   90mg
         Oestradiol dipropionate   0.64 mg
         Vit. D_2 900 IU
         Propylene glycol   Base

    iv) Removal of crusts after application of oestradiol in arachis oil.

-   Autogenous vaccines
-   Tissue therapy with systemic human placental extracts (Sinha, Sardana, Rajvanshi)
-   Rifampicin 600 mg orally once a day for 12 weeks.

5. DIFFERENTIAL DIAGNOSIS OF A NASAL MASS

NASAL POLYPS

A nasal polyp is prolapsed, pedunculated, oedematous and hypertrophied mucosa of the nose and sinuses. Antrochoanal polyps are common in children while ethmoidal polyps are common in adults

TYPES

1. Antrochoanal polyp
2. Ethmoidal polyp

ETIOLOGY

1. Infection: Antrochoanal polyps are of infective origin.
2. Allergy: Ethmoidal polyps are of allergic origin.
3. Vasomotor imbalance: Imbalance of sympathetic and parasympathetic system
4. Bernoulli's phenomenon: Air passage through a narrow constriction results in fall of air-pressure in the vicinity of the constriction. As regards to the paranasal sinuses, the ostium is considered as a constriction, a fall in pressure results in prolapse of mucosa around the constriction and subsequent blockage.
5. Polysaccharide changes: In the ground substance of the mucosa, predispose to polyp formation.
6. Mast cell reactions in the mucosa
7. Immunoglobulin changes predispose to polyp formation.

PATHOLOGY

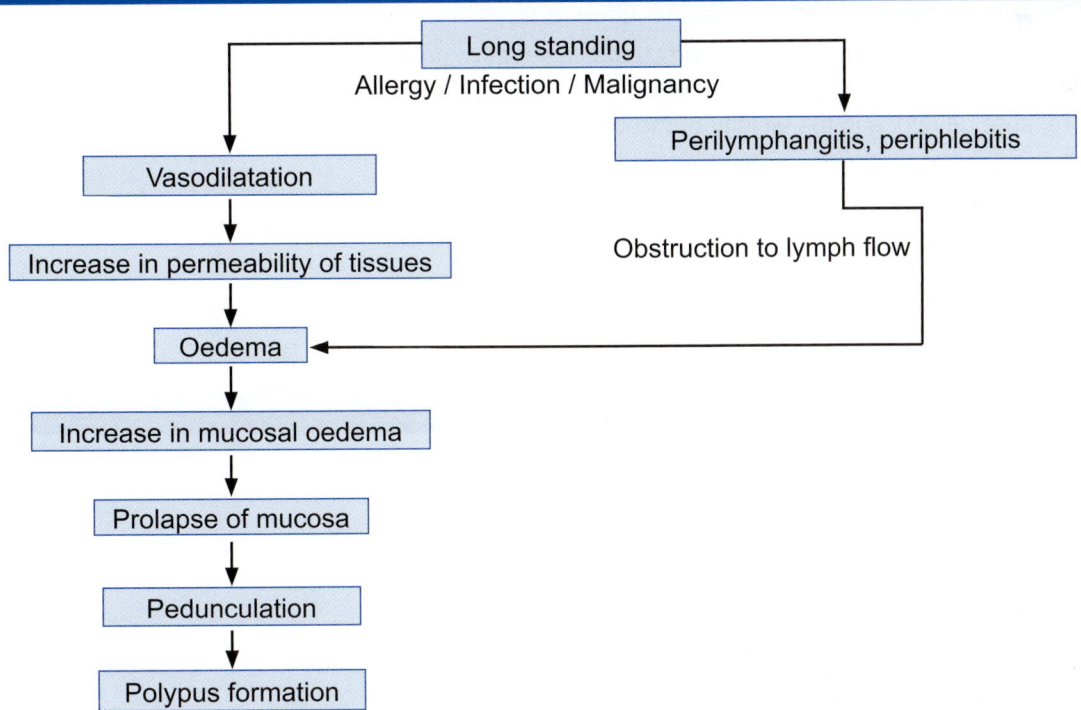

91

COMPLICATIONS

- Secondary sinusitis
- Epistaxis due to inflammation / infection
- Metaplastic changes due to trauma
- Mucocoele and pyocoele formation
- Deviation of septum to opposite side
- Broadening of nasal bridge
- Hypertelorism.

DIFFERENTIAL DIAGNOSIS

- Hypertrophied turbinates
- Rhinosporidiosis
- Inverted papilloma
- Malignancy
- Angiofibroma
- Rhinoscleroma
- Rhinolith
- Nasal granulomas

1. ANTROCHOANAL POLYP

It arises from the mucosa of the maxillary antrum, passes through its ostium and enters the nasal cavity. It then passes backwards to the posterior choana, nasopharynx and throat hanging behind the palate. Sometimes it may project anteriorly into the nasal cavity.

PATHOLOGY

Gross:

It is ideally trifoliate in shape and consists of three parts

Antral : It is the first part to form and it fills the maxillary antrum.

Nasal : It is the smallest part present in the nasal cavity. Its exposed part may show metaplastic changes.

Choanal : It is the part seen in the posterior nares and nasopharynx. It grows backwards because:

- Ciliary movement is towards posterior choana.
- Inspiratory blast is more powerful and creates a negative pressure which pulls the polyp backwards.
- Bernoulli's phenomenon: When gases or fluids pass through a constricted area, a negative pressure develops in the vicinity of the constriction with resultant oedema.
- Floor of nasal cavity slopes backwards
- Direction and opening of maxillary sinus is downwards and backwards.

Microscopy

Polyp is lined by columnar ciliated epithelium with subepithelial oedema and plenty of round cells, due to infective origin.

CLINICAL FEATURES

Symptoms

- Unilateral nasal obstruction (bilateral if nasopharynx is obstructed).
- Nasal discharge.
- Hyponasality
- Sneezing
- Mouth breathing
- Headache
- Deafness

Signs:

- Trifoliate shaped
- Soft, smooth mass
- Greyish / pearly white in colour
- Probe test:
    - Soft, mobile and insensitive to touch.
    - Probe can be passed all around.
    - Does not bleed on probing (relatively avascular mass)
- Posterior rhinoscopy
    - Globular smooth mass in the choana.

X'ray Sinuses

- Thickening of mucosa in the antrum
- Opacification in the antrum
- Lateral view nasopharynx: Crescent sign positive. (Soft tissue mass with radiolucent curvilinear zone between it and the roof of nasopharynx).

DIFFERENTIAL DIAGNOSIS

- Ethmoidal polypii
- Nasopharyngeal fibroma
- Adenoids
- Rhinosporidiosis
- Hypertrophied turbinate
- Malignant tumours

PROGNOSIS

Prognosis is good since it rarely undergoes malignant change. Recurrence is not very common if Caldwell-Luc surgery is performed. Nowadays FESS with canine puncture is done to remove the entire polyp.

TREATMENT

- Surgical removal of the polyp.

    Nasal polypectomy with the help of a nasal snare and avulsion technique so that the polyp is removed from its root-the antrum. If polyp has extended to the throat, it can be removed by the oral route in tonsillectomy position.

    Polyp if recurs, is removed by Caldwell-Luc operation.

    Nowadays Functional Endoscopic Sinus Surgery is performed with a pre-operative C.T. scan of the sinuses.
- Medical treatment of the underlying infection.

ETHMOIDAL POLYP

These are polyps arising from ethmoidal air cells.

They are common in adults, rare in children.

PATHOLOGY

Gross:

They are multiple, bilateral, soft, greyish / pearly white masses. They are multiple because the ethmoid cells are multiple. They appear like a bunch of grapes. They arise from ethmoid cells present in middle concha, hiatus semilunaris and rarely the roof.

Polyps are common in the ethmoids because:
- Laxity of tunica propria
- Narrowness of roof
- Erect posture
- Gravity.

Microscopy:

A polyp has ciliated columnar epithelium with subepithelial oedema with plenty of eosinophils. Immunoglobulin IgE is high in polyps of allergic origin.

CLINICAL FEATURES

SYMPTOMS

- Bilateral nasal obstruction
- Nasal discharge
- Frontal headache
- Anosmia
- Sneezing

SIGNS

- Big polypii cause broadening and frog-face deformity
- Anterior rhinoscopy: multiple greyish white masses like bunch of grapes bilaterally.
- Soft, mobile, insensitive and do not bleed on touch.
- Posterior rhinoscopy: no abnormality.
- X'ray sinuses:
  - Haziness of ethmoidal air cells
- Blood examination: eosinophilia
- Cytology of nasal secretion: eosinophilia

TREATMENT

Treatment of allergy

- Prolonged therapy with antihistaminics prevents recurrence
- Local steroid sprays pre and post-operatively prevent recurrence
  - Budesonide
  - Beclomethasone

SURGICAL TREATMENT

Intranasal polypectomy with Luc's / Citelli's forceps under local / general anaesthesia.

A piece of the underlying bone is removed as it undergoes osteitis. If the polyps recur, intranasal ethmoidectomy is performed.

Nowadays Functional Endoscopic Sinus Surgery is performed with a pre-and post-operative C.T. scan of the sinuses.

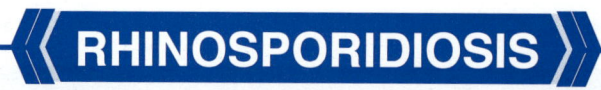

RHINOSPORIDIOSIS

A chronic fungal disease of the nose caused by fungal - parasite Rhinosporidium seeberi (Rhinosporidium Kinealy). Australia is the only continent from which this disease has not been reported. It is endemic in India and Sri Lanka. In India, the incidence is highest in Tamilnadu and Kerala followed by Madhya Pradesh, Orissa and West Bengal. Hyperendemic areas in Tamilnadu are the districts of Madurai and Ramnand. Young males are commonly affected.

Hyperendemic areas in Tamilnadu:	Rhinosporidium seeberi:
• Madurai	• Described by Seeber and also by Kinealy
• Ramnand	• The fungus does not satisfy koch's postulates - cannot be cultured

> **Endemic regions:**
> **India:**
> - Tamilnadu
> - Kerala
> - Madhya Pradesh
> - Orissa
> - West Bengal
>
> **Sri Lanka - Ceylon**
> **Not reported from Australia**

It is acquired by:
- Swimming in water contaminated by cow dung.
- Inhaling dust of dried dung.

Common site: Nose
- Septum
- Lateral wall of nose
- Inferior turbinate
- Middle turbinate

Sites of affection:
- Nose
- Nasopharynx
- Lacrimal apparatus
- Conjunctiva
- Palate
- Genitalia
- Middle ear
- Maxillary antrum

Clinical features:
Symptoms:
- Epistaxis - chief symptom
- Mucoid / blood stained nasal discharge
- Itching
- Sneezing

Signs:
- A bleeding polypus is the commonest lesion.
- Friable, red, polypoidal strawberry like mass.
- Studded with sporangia, showing as minute white spots on undersurface
- Pedunculated / sessile mass
- Polypoid / nodular / granular mass
- Broad nose if the mass is big.

Nasal secretion:
- Viscid

- Spores present
- Hyperaemic nasal mucosa

Spread:
- To surrounding regions by autoinnoculation by finger nails
- Lymphatic: widespread cutaneous and subcutaneous rhinosporidiosis.
- Haematogenous: visceral rhinosporidiosis

HISTOPATHOLOGY

- Papillomatous hyperplasia of mucosa lined by ciliated columnar epithelium
- Fibro-myxomatus stroma
- High vascularity in stroma
- Sporangia in various stages of development

Stains used to study rhinosporidiosis include:
- Conventional Eosin and Haematoxylin stains
- Sudan black, stains the wall of the spherule deeply and the body of the spherule lightly
- Methyl green stains the centre of the spherule deeply.
- Toludine blue and Bismarck brown are also used.

Sporangia:
- Mature sporangium is 300-400 μ in size.
- Has a double layered wall.
- Outer wall is thick chitin.
- Numerous spores are released from mature sporangia through pores covered by an operculum.
- Sporulation occurs and the spores spread through the lymphatics, the trophic stage is then seen.
- Size of spore is that of RBC i.e. 7.2 μ.

Diagnosis:
- Characteristic clinical appearance.
- Microscopic examination of the nasal discharge for spores
- Histopathological examination of the biopsy specimen
- High tendency to recur

Differential Diagnosis
- Papilloma
- Rhinoscleroma
- Malignant tumours

Treatment:
Surgery: Excision of growth with cauterization of base.
        It is mandatory to cross match and reserve at least 1 bottle of blood pre-operatively.
- Recurrences are common if inadequately excised.
- Recurrences are prevented by:
    - Cauterization of base
    - Dapsone 100 mg tds with Iron and multivitamins
    - Local application of 2% acqueous solution of Antimony tartarate to the nose and conjunctival lesions.
- I / V Amphotericin
- Local injection of steroids

RHINOSPORIDIOSIS

- Chronic fungal infection
- Rhinosporidium seeberi
- Endemic: India, Sri Lanka
- Swimming in dung contaminated water
- Inhalation of dried dust dung
- Strawberry-like bleeding polypus
- Undersurface: Sporangia
- Affects septum, lateral nasal wall
- Surgical excision with cauterization of base
- High tendency to recur

RHINOSCLEROMA

Synonym: Scleroma

It was first described by Hebrew in 1878.

It is a chronic granulomatous disease of the nose caused by Gram negative bacilli, Kleibsiella Rhinoscleromatis or Diplobacillus of Frisch characterized by sclerosis and stenosis of the nasal cavities. It initially affects the nose and then extends into the nasopharynx, oropharynx, sub glottis, trachea and bronchi.

It affects both the sexes, is contagious and is mainly seen in poor unhygienic conditions associated with low socio-economic status. It is common in Central and Northern India.

Rhinoscleroma
Central and Northern India
Eastern Europe
Middle East
Africa
Indonesia
South America

CLINICAL STAGES

STAGES	FEATURES	PATHOLOGICAL DIAGNOSIS
1. **Atrophic stage**	Atrophy of mucosa Crusting and painless foul smelling discharge Pink nasal mucosa	• Diagnosis only by complement fixation test
2. **Nodular stage/ stage of granulations**	Nodules • India-rubber consistency • Bluish-red • Non-ulcerated External deformity • Hebra nose	• Predominant cells are plasma cells • Difficult to demonstrate the organism
3. **Cicatrisation/ stage of sclerosis / fibrosis/stenosis**	Scarring occurs all over the nose Tapir nose-coarsening of external nose Fibrosis starts anteriorly and progresses posteriorly.	• Typical histological picture

Histology:

Granulomatous tissue infiltrates submucosa. The predominant cells are plasma cells with hyaline bodies-Russel bodies (fuschinophil degeneration). Other cells are fibroblasts, endothelial cells, lymphocytes and eosinophils. The characteristic cell is the Mikulicz cell

Mikulicz cell:

- Large mononuclear cell
- 30-40um in size
- Foamy / vacuolated cytoplasm
- Nucleus is irregular, central or compressed to one side
- Cytoplasm contains clusters of capsulated Frisch bacillus.

    There is a high content of mucopolysaccharides around the walls of the organism (Klebsiella), thus protecting it from antibiotics and antibodies.

CLINICAL FEATURES

- Atrophic changes in nasal mucosa in the initial stages
- Slow progressively increasing nasal obstruction
- Hard, non-tender, non-ulcerated swelling
- Swelling initially anteriorly below the nostril and lips
- Stenosis of the nose
- Cough, hoarseness and stridor due to subglottic stenosis

Indirect laryngoscopy:

- Atrophy of vocal cords
- Subglottic stenosis
- Lymph node involvement is rare as fibrous tissue deposition blocks the lymphatics.

DIAGNOSIS

- History
- Clinical features
- Smear examination for bacilli
- Biopsy shows typical histological picture.

DIFFERENTIAL DIAGNOSIS

- Atrophic rhinitis
- Syphilis (tertiary stage)
- Tuberculosis
- Leprosy
- Rhinosporidiosis

TREATMENT

STAGE	TREATMENT
1. **Atrophy / Granulations**	Antibiotics: • Streptomycin • Chloromycetin • Tetracycline • Ampicillin with Trimethoprim Local Application: • Rifampicin • Acriflavin 2% (2% Acriflavine is very effective. 5% causes vestibulitis, epistaxis, septal perforation. 1% produces no effect.) Kailash Rai regime: Local injection of carbolic acid with glacial acetic acid in glycerine mixture
2. **Cicatrization**	• Laser excision of stenosis with polyethylene tube insertion for 8 weeks • Electrocautery • Cryosurgery • Plastic reconstructive surgery • Tracheostomy for stridor • Local steroid injection • Radio therapy-3000-3500 CGY over three weeks destroys scleroma organisms • Surgical removal of stenosis and dilatation therapy

RHINOSCLEROMA
- Chronic granulomatous disease.
- Klebseilla rhinoscleromatis
- **3 stages:**
  - Atrophic
  - Granulomatous / nodular
  - Cicatrization / fibrosis
- Features:
  - Hard nodules which do not ulcerate
  - Hebra nose
  - Tapir nose
- Pathology:
  - Mikulicz cells
  - Russell bodies
- Treatment:
  - Local acriflavin / rifampicin
  - Antibiotics, streptomycin, tetracycline
  - Excision of stenotic tissue

INVERTED PAPILLOMA

- **Synonyms:**
  - Ringertz tumour
  - Transitional cell tumour
- It arises from lateral wall of nose and sinuses
- 1-4% of all nasal neoplasms
- Males: Females = 5 : 1, seen in old men.
- Soft, pinkish-red, friable vascular mass
- They are often single.
- Clinical features
  - Nasal obstruction
  - Bleeding
  - Nasal discharge
  - Deformity of nose
- **Histology:**
  - Inversion of epithelium beneath the stroma
  - Basement is intact
  - The surface is covered with alternating layers of squamous as well as columnar epithelium. It is also called transitional cell papilloma.
  - Malignant change can occur

Treatment:
- Wide excision by lateral rhinotomy.
- Recurrence is common.

MIDDLE TURBINATE HYPERTROPHY

- Less common
- Could lead to chronic sinus disease
- Pneumatised middle turbinate - Concha bullosa.

Treatment:
- Decongestants
- Reduction with punch forceps
- Submucous diathermy
- Removal at Functional Endoscopic Sinus Surgery
- Complete excision by Lateral rhinotomy

INFERIOR TURBINATE HYPERTROPHY

- Usually due to submucosal oedema
- Bony hypertrophy is rare
- Dilatation of the submucosal venous sinusoids occurs
- Venous sinusoids are under sympathetic control

- Agonist drugs cause vasoconstriction and mucosal decongestion

Clinical features:

- Soft sensitive mass arising from the lateral wall.
- Associated with symptoms of intrinsic rhinitis

Treatment:

- Systemic and local decongestants (No response if submucous fibrosis has occurred)
- Submucous cautery (diathermy, laser)
- Partial or total turbinectomy

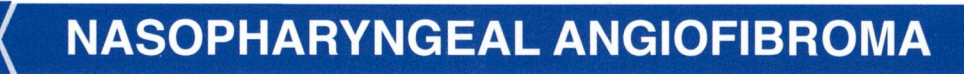

NASOPHARYNGEAL ANGIOFIBROMA

Synonym

- Juvenile Angiofibroma
- Nasopharyngeal fibroma

It is a vascular swelling arising in the nasopharynx of prepubertal and adolescent males and having a strong tendency to bleed.

SITES OF ORIGIN

- Vault of nasopharynx
- Choana
- Sphenopalatine foramen

THEORIES OF DEVELOPMENT OF ANGIOFIBROMA

Ringertz	Arose from periosteum of nasopharyngeal vault
Som and Neffson	Inequality in the growth of bones forming skull base resulting in hypertrophy of underlying periosteum
Bensch and Ewing	Tumour arose from embryonic fibrocartilage between basiocciput and basisphenoid
Brunner	Tumour originates from conjoined pharyngobasillar and buccopharyngeal fascia
Osborn	Hamartomatous theory: • Hamartomas • Residual erectile tissue subject to hormonal influence
Girgis and Fahmy	Paragangliomas are forerunners of this tumour
Hormonal theory	Arose from vestiges of atrophied stapedial artery Androgen and oestrogen imbalance

PATHOLOGY

Gross

- Pink, smooth mass
- Firm, hard to touch
- Bleeds on touch
- Broad based/small base
- Pedunculated
- Covered with mucous membrane
- Ulceration is rare

- Tendency to spontaneous regression
- Can be bilobed, dumb-bell swelling with one portion in nasopharynx, other in pterygopalatine and infratemporal fossa, stalk in the sphenopalatine foramen.

Microscopic

- Tumour is made up of plenty of young fibroblasts, blood vessels, and collagen.
- Tumour has no capsule, hence it has to be removed from its attachments without breaking into the growth.
- Surface epithelium is columnar ciliated.
- Blood vessels are more in the centre than the periphery.

Characteristic of blood vessels

- Numerous blood vessels are present.
- Wall of the vessel is thin
- Wall is lined by flattened endothelium
- Wall is devoid of contractile muscular and elastic layers
- The vessels therefore do not contract on cutting and bleed profusely.

BLOOD SUPPLY

- Enlarged maxillary artery
- Ascending pharyngeal artery
- Vidian artery
- Branch of Internal carotid artery
- Vertebral artery
- Bleeding is caused by disruption of parenchyma of swelling or feeding vessels or it can be spontaneous

CLINICAL FEATURES

- Spontaneous, recurrent, intractable bleeding from the nose. The bleeding may be dangerous to life.
- Nasal obstruction
- Nasal discharge
- Headache (chronic sinusitis, dural compression, invasion of sphenoid sinus).
- Rhinolalia clausa
- Anosmia, hyposmia
- Deafness due to eustachian tube obstruction.
- Otalgia
- Interference with deglutition, respiration
- Anaemia
- Anterior rhinoscopy
  - Nodular, lobulated mass
  - Reddish in colour
  - Mostly unilateral, at times bilateral nasal extension
  - Mucopurulent secretions
  - Bowing of septum
- Posterior rhinoscopy
  - Pinkish red mass filling the nasopharynx

Extensive disease

- Splaying of nasal bones
- Swelling of temple and cheek
- Fullness between ascending ramus of mandible and side of maxilla
- Trismus
- Bulging of parotid gland
- Proptosis, falling vision
- Classical frog face

SPREAD OF NASOPHARYNGEAL ANGIOFIBROMA

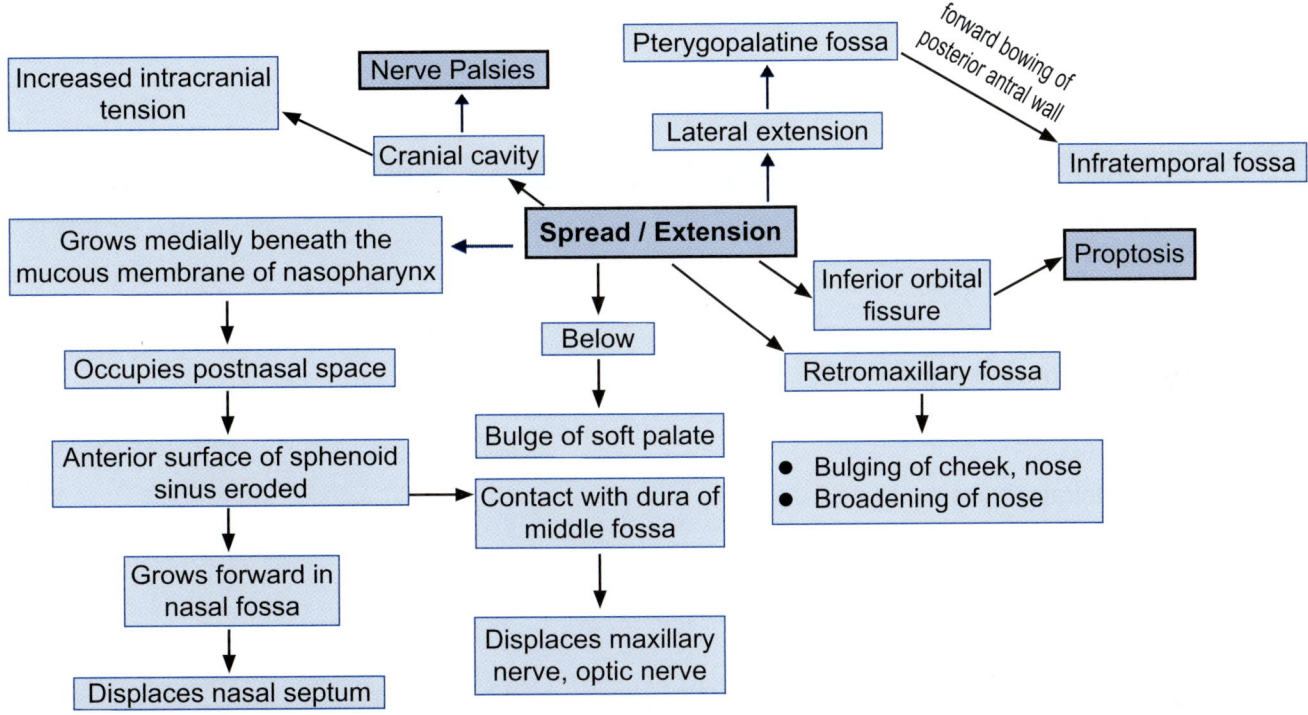

DIAGNOSIS

1. History-recurrent epistaxis
2. Seen in males
3. Appearance of the mass
4. X'ray lateral view nasopharynx
   - Soft tissue mass in nasopharynx without any air shadow between it and the cervical vertebrae
5. C.T. scan
   - Extent of growth
   - Erosion of bones
   - Intracranial extension
   - Invasion of sphenoid sinus, pterygopalatine fossa
   - Forward bowing of posterior antral wall (angiofibroma filling pterygopalatine fossa)
6. Carotid angiography
   - To find vascular supply: vascular blush in postnasal space
   - Collaterals

- Feeding vessel embolization
- No BIOPSY is taken because of risk of severe haemorrhage

COMPLICATIONS

- Haemorrhage
- Shock
- Sepsis
- Intracranial complications

DIFFERENTIAL DIAGNOSIS

- Antrochoanal polyp
- Chordoma
- Tumours of postnasal space
- Large adenoids

TREATMENT

1. Hormone therapy
   - Testosterone
   - Oestrogen

   Action
   - Maturation of collagen in the tumour
   - Reduction in vascularity
2. Radiotherapy is for
   - Inoperable intracranial extensions
   - Recurrent tumours
3. Action
   - Hardening of tumours due to reduction in vascularity
4. Surgical excision

Approaches

SURGICAL APPROACH	COMMENT
Transpalatal	• This approach is for tumours just in nasopharynx
Lateral rhinotomy	• Tumour in nasopharynx and in infratemporal fossa
Combined Transnasal Transantral achieved by Weber Ferguson incision	• For extensive tumours

PRINCIPLES OF SURGERY IN COMBINED APPROACH

- To sufficiently expose the maxillary antrum
- Removal of all walls of the maxillary antrum especially the medial wall including the perpendicular plate of palatine bone
- The orbital floor and upper alveolar arch can be left intact
- The nasal cavity, antrum, infratemporal fossa, pterygopalatine fossa and nasopharynx are converted into a single large cavity
- The maxillary artery is ligated first followed by tackling the tumour in the infratemporal fossa, antrum and then the nasopharynx. Removal of perpendicular plate of palatine bone uncaps the part of the tumour occupying the sphenopalatine foramen

COMPLICATIONS

- Palatal fistula
- Crusting in nose
- Anaesthesia of cheek
- Ectropion of eyelid
- Recurrence

NASOPHARYNGEAL CARCINOMA

It forms 80% of all head and neck cancers and 18% of all malignancies. It is commonly seen in China

It is seen more in males than females. M:F=2-3:1

It has a bimodal age group presentation, seen in 10-20 yrs and 55-65 yrs. of age.

Nasopharyngeal carcinoma
• China
• Far East Asia
• South East Asia
• Europe
• India
- Manipur
- Assam

ETIOLOGY

1. Genetically determined susceptibility
2. Epstein-Barr virus infection. (It is said that Epstein-Barr virus genomes get integrated into nasopharyngeal mucosal cells and form a tumour)
3. Nasopharyngeal carcinogenic agents
   - Ingestion of salted fish
   - Smoke of incense burning
   - Soot from lamps
   - Unburnt kerosene
   - Preserved vegetables
   - Nitrosamines and nitro-precursors
   - Chinese herbal medicine
   - Cigarette (tobacco) smoking
   - Industrial chemicals
   - Metal smelting
   - Furnaces
   - Formaldehyde
   - Wood dust

PATHOLOGY

It arises from the crypts and squamous/respiratory epithelium lining the nasopharynx.

Types of nasopharyngeal tumours

Epithelial	Nasopharyngeal carcinoma Adenocarcinoma Adenoid cystic carcinoma Mucoepidermoid carcinoma
Lymphoid	Malignant lymphoma Burkitt's lymphoma Hodgkin's lymphoma Plasmacytoma
Soft tissue	Fibrosarcoma, angiosarcoma Rhabdomyosarcoma
Bone / cartilage	Chondrosarcoma, Osteosarcoma
Miscellaneous	Melanoma, Chordoma, Craniopharyngioma

Gross

- Polypoidal mass
- Ulcerative mass
- Infiltrative mass

Histopathology:

- Squamous cell carcinoma
- Undifferentiated carcinoma
- Non-keratinizing carcinoma

CLINICAL FEATURES

- Bilateral nasal obstruction
- Cervical metastasis
- Epistaxis
- Headache
- Deafness, tinnitus, otalgia
- Nerve palsies, Horner's syndrome
- Metastasis

> **Trotter's Triad:**
> - Pain on ipsilateral side of face
> - Ipsilateral palatal palsy
> - Ipsilateral conductive deafness

  - Loco regional: paranasal sinuses, orbit, parotid gland, infratemporal fossa, parapharyngeal space
  - Distant: bone, lung, liver (thoraco lumbar spine is the most common site)

Nasopharyngeal cancer is known to give rise to secondaries with the primary area hidden **(occult cancer)**. The lymph node group affected rapidly increases in size and spreads to other groups.

The first nodal station is the retropharyngeal node which is not palpable clinically. The nodes thus first palpable are the jugulodigastric or the apical node under the sternocleidomastoid. Epistaxis and ozaena due to tumour necrosis is seen in advanced stages. Pain is seen when the tumour erodes skull base or in sphenoid sinus sepsis. Trismus is seen when the pterygoid muscles get involved. Cranial nerves IX and X get most commonly involved. Cranial nerves III, IV and VI are next to be affected within the cavernous sinus. Otitis media with effusion causing tinnitus occurs gradually.

Spread of nasopharyngeal carcinoma

CHART I

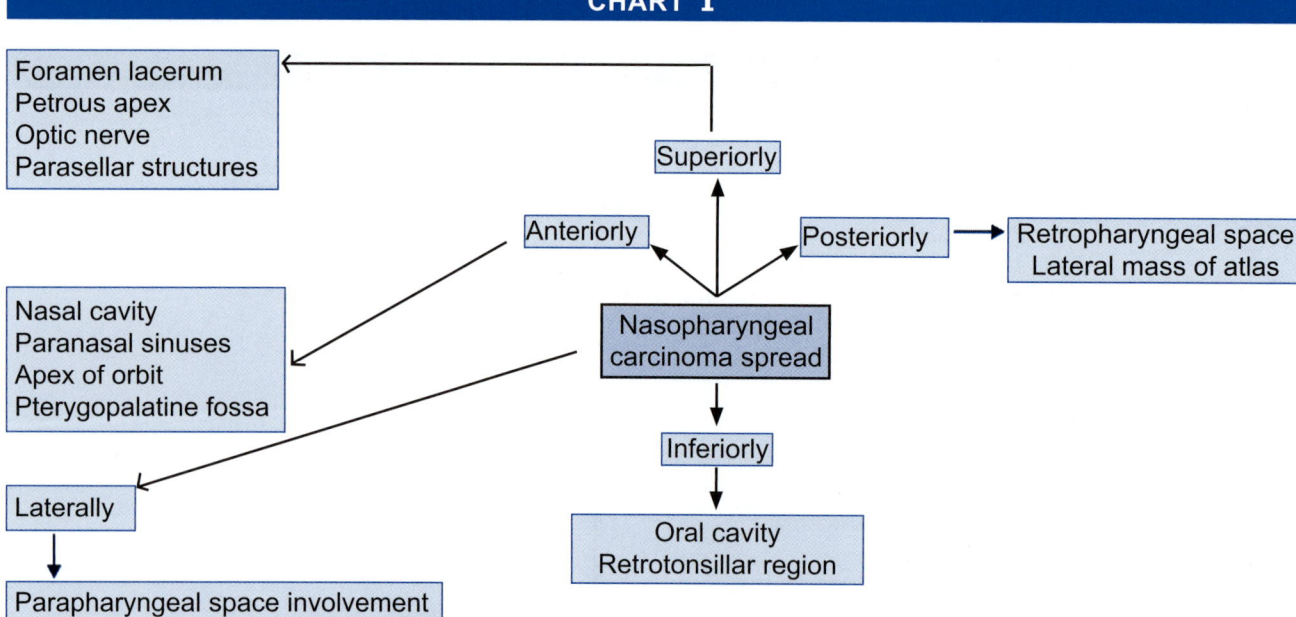

Parapharyngeal space involvement can be:

1. PRESTYLOID

Involvement of

- Mandibular nerve
- Pterygoid muscles
- Deep lobe of parotid gland

2. POST STYLOID COMPARTMENT

- Vascular compression of carotid sheath
- Invasion of cranial nerves IX, X, XI, XII and Cervical chain

CHART II

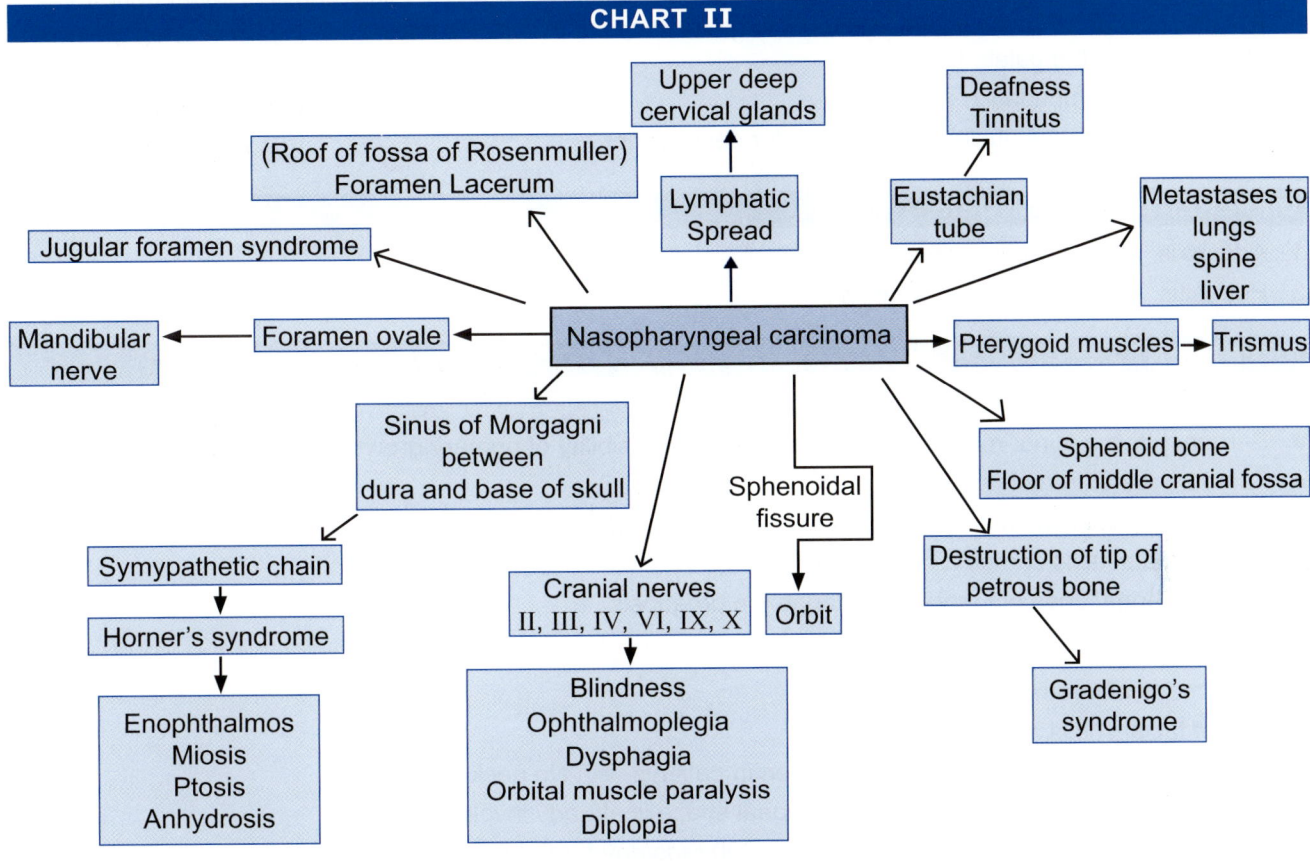

DIAGNOSIS

1. Delay in diagnosis can occur because of:

   a) Occult nature of the carcinoma

   b) Bizarre symptoms

   c) Nasopharynx is a relatively inaccessible space

   d) First metastasis is to clinically non palpable retropharyngeal node.

2. Posterior rhinoscopy
3. Digital palpation of nasopharynx
4. Nasopharyngoscopy
5. X-ray lateral view / Submentovertical view of nasopharynx
6. C.T. scan / MRI
   - Obliteration of paranasopharyngeal soft tissue planes
   - Obliteration of fat in the paranasopharyngeal space.
   - Erosion of base-skull
   - Extension of tumour through carotid artery or foramen lacerum
   - Upward extension through floor of middle cranial fossa into cavernous sinus and parasellar region

- Asymmetry of muscle layers is seen in:
  - Neuromuscular infiltration by the carcinoma
  - Post radiotherapy cases.
- Ring enhancement seen in affected nodes due to central necrosis/peripheral vascularity.

7. EBV serology: High IgA titre to the viral capsid antigen (VCA), 1:10 is suggestive of nasopharyngeal carcinoma.

8. Biopsy under general anaesthesia is taken through a visible growth or a blind biopsy is taken from fossa of Rosenmuller and roof of nasopharynx with angled forceps or a biopsy is taken (with postnasal biopsy forceps) after retracting the palate forwards.

9. Pure tone and Impedance audiometry

10. X'ray chest and radionucleide bone scan for secondaries.

DIFFERENTIAL DIAGNOSIS

1. Adenoids   2. Plasmacytoma
3. Petrositis   4. Trigeminal neuralgia

TREATMENT

Principles

- Surgery plays a minor role because of relative inaccessibility of primary growth and early bilateral spread
- Tumours are extremely radiosensitive
- Presence of cervical metastasis does not alter the cure rate
- Distant metastasis carries a bad prognosis
- Chemotherapy does not markedly change the prognosis

Radiotherapy

- Main mode of treatment
- Use of facial shells is advocated
- Prophylactic neck radiation should be given in patients with No neck
- Treatment failure can occur if parapharyngeal space is already involved.
- Dosage is 5000-6000 rads over 5-6 weeks (200 rads/day for 5 days in a week)

Brachytherapy

- High dose is given to the tumour
- Intracavity Iridium-192 is used for residual/recurrent disease.

Complications of radiotherapy:

- Ablation of parotid gland
- Xerostomia
- Mucositis
- Radiation otitis media with effusion
- Dental caries
- Osteoradionecrosis (mandible, skull base)
- Radiation myelitis, encephalomyelitis
- Optic atrophy, retinitis
- Temporal lobe necrosis
- Hypopituitarism

SURGERY

The nasopharynx is a relatively inaccessible area making surgical intervention difficult

Reasons

- Situation is deep in the skull
- Internal carotid artery and carotid canal are in close proximity to lateral nasopharynx where most tumours recur

- Adequate removal of tumour requires drilling of clivus
- Lack of adequate surgical margins
- Post operative trismus is a problem

Surgical approaches to the nasopharynx

- Transnasal
- Transmaxillary
- Transpalatal
- Sublabial midfacial degloving
- Transfacial-maxillary swing
- Transmandibular-mandibular swing
- Infratemporal approach
- Transtemporal - sphenoidal
- Transpharyngeal
- Transcervical

APPROACH	PROCEDURE
Transnasal	• For removing tumours in maxillo-ethmoid region • Denker's extension of Caldwell-Luc can be tried • Lateral rhinotomy / Weber Ferguson improves exposure but is complicated by midfacial scarring • Lefort I osteotomy approach can be used by down fracturing entire hard palate and inferior maxilla • It may affect facial growth and damage non-erupted teeth
Trans palatal	• Shortest and most direct approach • Allows extension to sphenoid and choana • A 'U' incision on the palate extended to a 'S' type around the tuberosity of maxilla is taken. The greater palatine bundle is preserved and after elevating palatal mucoperiosteal flap, tumour is exposed
Sublabial midfacial degloving approach	• Allows enough exposure of nasal complex, nasopharynx and mid-third of face. • Gingivolabial incision is carried across from one maxillary tuberosity to the other • Soft tissues are elevated • Infraorbital nerves are preserved • Routine rhinoplastic incisions are taken • Septal-vestibular incision is connected to sublabial incision for degloving upto root of nose • The necessary bones are removed and the tumour tackled
Transfacial	Combines Weber-Ferguson-Long-mire incision with splitting of hard palate and multiple osteotomies detaching the maxilla

Prognostic factors

The prognosis depends on the following factors:

- Nodal disease
- Degree of differentiation

5 year survival rates are:

- 75% in early cases
- 15% in late cases

Women have high survival rate than men.

NASOPHARYNGEAL CARCINOMA

- Chinese race
- Occult cancer
- Early bilateral lymphatic spread
- Cervical metastasis occurs
- Neurological palsies common
- Very invasive tumour
- Metastasis very common
- Paradoxical tumour and nodal stage relationship
- Radiotherapy is treatment of choice.

CARCINOMA (MAXILLA) PARANASAL SINUSES

Sex

Men are more affected than women

M:F = 10:1

Age

50 yrs of age (lesser age group)

<20% of head and neck cancers

TYPE

- Squamous-cell – commonest
- Adenocarcinoma – rare
- Sarcoma – in children
- Burkitt's lymphoma – in children of South Africa

Carcinoma maxilla:

Bantu tribe of South Africa is more prone due to use of home-made snuff.

ETIOLOGY

Predisposing factors

1. Chronic inflammation (not a major factor)
2. Leukoplakia of palate
3. Irradiation to nose, sinuses in
   - Telangiectasia
   - Fibrous dysplasia
4. Inhalation of snuff
5. Exposure to wood dust in timber industries
6. Cutting and polishing of beach wood
7. Working in chrome, nickel and shoe industry

Premalignant conditions

- Ringertz tumour
- Squamous cell papilloma

SITES

- Maxillary sinus ⎤ 99%
- Ethmoid sinus ⎦
- Frontal sinus ⎤ 1%
- Sphenoid sinus ⎦

CLASSIFICATION

I. Ohngren's classification

An imaginary line drawn from medial canthus to angle of mandible and a perpendicular line through the pupil creates four zones for carcinoma maxilla bearing different prognosis.

FOUR ZONES ARE THUS FORMED	PROGNOSIS
• Antero inferior medial	Good, causes early symptoms
• Anfero inferior lateral	Poor
• Postero superior lateral	Poor
• Postero superior medial	Worst, spreads rapidly

II. Moffet (1952) classification

Upper group

- Arising from middle and superior meati

Lower group

- Alveolus
- Teeth
- Gums, extending into antrum

III. Ledermann's (1970) classification

- Two parallel lines are drawn across a frontal section of the skull. Upper line – passing through the orbital floor
- Lower line – through the floor of the antrum.
- Two vertical lines are drawn extending down from medial orbital wall on each side of nasal floor. These vertical lines separate ethmoids and nasal fossa
- The nasal septum separates the region into right and left sides.
- Three regions are thus formed
  - Supra structure
  - Mesostructure
  - Infrastructure

IV. TNM classification

T : Primary tumour

N : Regional nodes

M : Distant metastasis

1. Primary tumour (T)

Tx : Minimum requirements to assess the primary tumour cannot be met

T_0 : No evidence of primary tumour

Tis : Carcinoma in situ

T_1 : Tumour confined to the antral mucosa of the infrastructure with no bone erosion or destruction

T_2 : Tumour confined to the suprastructure without bone destruction, or to the infrastructure with destruction of medial or inferior bony walls.

T_3 : More extensive tumour invading skin of cheek, orbit, anterior ethmoid sinuses, or pterygoid muscles

T_4 :   Massive tumour with invasion of cribriform plate, posterior ethmoids, sphenoid, nasopharynx, pterygoid plates or base of skull.

2. Nodal involvement (N)

Nx   :   Minimum requirements to assess the regional nodes cannot be met.

N_0 :   No clinically positive nodes

N_1 :   Single clinically positive homolateral node 3 cm or less in diameter.

N_2 :   Single clinically positive homolateral node 3 cm to 6 cm in diameter or multiple clinically positive homolateral nodes none more than 6 cm in diameter.

N_{2a} :   Single clinically positive homolateral node (3 cm to 6 cm) in diameter

N_{2b} :   Multiple clinically positive homolateral nodes, none more than 6 cm in diameter.

N_3 :   Massive homolateral node(s), bilateral nodes or contralateral node(s) (> 6cm)

N_{3a} :   Clinically positive homolateral node (s), one more than 6 cm in diameter

N_{3b} :   Bilateral clinically positive nodes (in this situation, each side of the neck should be staged separately)

N_{3c} :   Contralateral clinically positive node(s) only.

3. Distant metastasis (M)

Mx   :   Minimum requirements to assess the presence of distant metastasis cannot be met

M_0 :   No (known) distant metastasis

M_1 :   Distant metastasis present

V. Clinical classification

Antro – alveolar

Antro – ethmoidal

VI. Classification according to site of origin

Primary   :   Arising from maxilla

Secondary   :   Involving maxilla from surrounding structures like the nose, alveolus, palate.

CLINICAL FEATURES

Symptoms

- Absent in early stages (growth when confined to antrum)
- Discomfort over face
- Dull pain over cheek
- Anaesthesia or paraesthesia of cheek
- Swelling of nose and maxillary region.

Characteristic of Mass / Anterior rhinoscopy

- Visible mass in nostril
- Nodular, irregular mass
- Friable mass
- Ulceration is common
- Bleeds on touch
- Fast growing

SPREAD

- Lymphatics from the nose pass backwards to a plexus in the lateral wall of the posterior choana
- The lymphatics then drain to retropharyngeal and deep jugular nodes. Retropharyngeal nodes are difficult to detect clinically and require C.T. scan for assessment.

- If the skin is involved, the glands get affected soon. The submaxillary and internal jugular glands are affected first followed by the mediastinal glands.
- Glandular enlargement occurs late in the disease
- Distant metastases are rare

DIAGNOSIS

- High degree of suspicion in early cases
- Visible mass on anterior rhinoscopy
- Mass over cheek
- Exophthalmos
- Palatal ulceration
- Loose teeth
- Glands in neck
- Radiological evidence
- Biopsy

DIFFERENTIAL DIAGNOSIS

1. Gumma
   - Destructive lesion involving cartilage and bone
   - VDRL positive
2. Lupus
   - Apple jelly nodules on septum
   - X'ray chest for tuberculosis

INVESTIGATIONS

Apart from routine investigations, the following specific investigations may be required:

- Biopsy: The various methods are:
  - Directly with Luc's forceps if nasal mass is seen
  - Through intranasal antrostomy if growth is not visible
  - Caldwel-Luc operation is not preferred for biopsy for fear of implanting malignant cells
  - Intranasal antrostomy is preferred since it acts as a drainage channel. The anterolateral wall is removed at surgery or even for irradiation.
  - Endoscopic biopsy is preferred nowadays
- X'ray paranasal sinuses may show:
  - Soft-tissue mass
  - Bony erosion
- C.T. Scan / MRI to show
  - Extent of growth
  - Spread
  - Erosion / destruction of walls of antrum
- Cytology from antral lavage washings

TREATMENT

- Surgery
- Radiotherapy
- Chemotherapy

SURGERY

Removal of tumour by:

- Palatal fenestration
- Denker's operation
- Moure's lateral rhinotomy
- Maxillectomy
  - Partial
  - Total
  - Radical
  - Extended radical

Contraindications

- Involvement of base-skull
- Involvement of pterygoid plates
- Involvement of cranial nerves
- Inoperable glands
- Trismus
- Presence of Horner's syndrome
- Distant metastasis
- Poor general condition
- Poor cardiac and pulmonary reserve.

RADIOTHERAPY

Indications

- Anaplastic carcinoma
- Sarcomas

Contraindication

- Involvement of malar bone

Advantages of radiotherapy

- Reduction in size of tumour
- Reduction in vascularity of tumour
- Prevents tumour dissemination

Mode of administration

1. Preoperative radiotherapy
2. Postoperative radiotherapy
3. Sandwich treatment (pre and post operative)

CHEMOTHERAPY

It is mainly palliative in nature and the following agents are used:

- 5-fluorouracil
- Methotrexate
- Antimetabolites

Immunotherapy is also palliative in nature.

LARYNX

1. HISTORY AND EXAMINATION

1. Change in voice

Hoarseness of voice is one of the commonest disorders seen. Other alterations in voice are those of strength, pitch, tone and quality. Hoarseness implies a rough, husky voice. It is due to lesions affecting the vocal cords. It is seen in patients with vocal abuse eg:- hawkers, teachers. Hoarseness is mainly due to laryngeal inflammation, tumours, trauma or vocal cord mobility disorders. Hoarseness in elderly can be due to malignancy. Hysterical female patients may have functional aphonia.

2. Dyspnoea

Obstructive pathology in the larynx produces dyspnoea. Stridor is noisy breathing due to obstruction to airflow. Stertor is low-pitched sound produced by obstruction above the level of the larynx. It is due to vibration of the tissues of pharynx, nasopharynx and soft palate. Stridor is a harsh sound produced due to laryngeal, tracheal or bronchial obstruction.

Expiratory obstruction usually produces a wheezing sound during respiration. Respiratory obstruction is characterized clinically by an increased respiratory rate, indrawing of larynx and trachea into mediastinum, intercostal, suprasternal and subcostal retraction.

Differential diagnosis of Stridor

Congenital (Laryngeal / tracheal / bronchial)

- Laryngomalacia
- Webs
- Stenosis
- Tracheomalacia
- Cysts
- Vocal cord paralysis
- Haemangiomas

Inflammatory

- Laryngitis
- Laryngo tracheobronchitis
- Epiglottitis
- Tuberculosis
- Diphtheria

Traumatic

- Corrosive burns
- Iatrogenic
- Blunt injury
- Penetrating injury

Neoplastic

- Papillomas
- Carcinomas

Foreign body

- Laryngotracheobronchial
- Oesophageal

Miscellaneous

- Allergy
- Mediastinal tumours.

3. **Cough**

Dry cough is due to laryngeal irritation. Productive cough is seen in lower respiratory tract infections. Blood-stained, foul smelling sputum is seen in malignancies. Laryngeal foreign bodies, laryngitis, tracheitis are common causes of cough production.

4. **Dysphagia and odynophagia**

Dysphagia is seen more in pharyngeal disorders. In laryngeal pathology, supraglottic tumours especially involving the aryepiglottic folds produce dysphagia. Odynophagia is seen in neoplasms with secondary infection and in laryngeal tuberculosis.

5. **Foreign body sensation and clearing of throat (hawking)**

It is seen in laryngitis, vocal cord polyps and early malignancy.

6. **Swelling in the neck**

It is seen in secondaries in the neck, neoplasm spreading outside of larynx and in perichondritis.

7. **History suggestive of etiology:**
   - Tobacco intake by chewing or smoking
   - Alcoholism
   - Vocal abuse seen in singers, hawkers and teachers.
   - Tuberculosis, syphilis

EXAMINATION OF LARYNX

Inspection

The larynx is inspected for any mass, fullness, fistula and movements during deglutition and respiration. It gets indrawn during inspiration in laryngeal obstruction. Tracheal obstruction does not produce such changes. Laryngeal framework may get distorted in certain tumours, malignancies and inflammatory conditions.

Palpation

It is done with both hands standing behind the patient. The patients head should be slightly flexed to relax the neck muscles. The hyoid bone and the thyroid and cricoid cartilages are identified. The cartilages are palpated for thickening, tenderness and any broadening.

The thyroid gland lies over the thyroid cartilage from the second to fourth tracheal rings. It is examined for its consistency, swellings within, tumour or any pulsations. Its movement is examined at deglutition and protrusion of tongue.

The larynx is examined for **laryngeal crepitus**. It is the grating sensation which is produced when the larynx is moved laterally (side to side) on the vertebral column. It is present normally and is absent in postcricoid malignancy and retropharyngeal lesions, because the larynx gets pushed forwards and its movements over the vertebral column do not occur.

A systematic examination of the neck nodes is carried out.

Internal examination of the larynx is done by indirect laryngoscopy. It is an out-patient procedure.

INDIRECT LARYNGOSCOPY

The patient is explained the procedure. The patient and the examiner are both seated facing eachother. A head mirror with a light source, indirect laryngoscopy mirror, gauze pieces to hold the tongue, spirit lamp to warm the mirror are the instruments needed for the procedure. The light is focussed on the patient's mouth. An indirect laryngoscopy mirror of adequate size is warmed on a spirit lamp or in hot water to prevent fogging on its surface. Its warmth is tested on the examiner's hand. The patient opens his mouth and protrudes the tongue which is held by a gauze piece between the left thumb and middle finger. The left index finger retracts the upper lip.

Patient is asked to breathe quietly (through his mouth). The warmed mirror with the mirror facing downwards is held in the right hand like a pen and gently introduced from the angle of mouth, above the tongue surface. It is slowly taken behind and finally rested against the base of the uvula.

By tilting the mirror and gently lifting the uvula, the following structures are seen:

1. Base of tongue
2. Valeculla
3. Epiglottis (lingual surface)
4. Posterior aspect of arytenoids
5. Aryepiglottic folds
6. True and false vocal cords
7. Anterior and posterior commissures
8. Upper tracheal rings and subglottis may be seen
9. Pyriform fossa and part of posterior pharyngeal wall

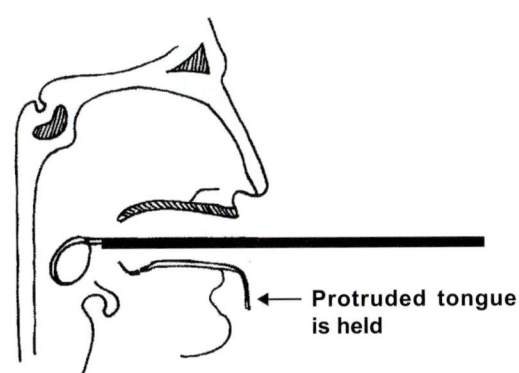

← **Protruded tongue is held**

METHOD OF PERFORMING INDIRECT LARYNGOSCOPY

The mobility of the vocal cords is examined during phonation by asking the patient to say "ee". The true vocal cords appear as ivory white ribbon-like bands and the false cords appear as dull-red bands. The tension, position and adduction of vocal cords is seen on phonation and deep inspiration. The vocal cords are examined for any redness, nodules, polyps, ulceration, carcinoma etc. In cases with overhanging epiglottis, the anterior commissure may not be seen.

The epiglottis is pinkish white and the arytenoids are pink in colour.

The pyriform fossa, lying on either side of the epiglottis between the aryepiglottic fold and the lateral pharyngeal wall are common sites for foreign bodies. They lodge in the pyriform fossa because of contraction of the cricopharyngeus muscle. Pooling of saliva in the pyriform fossa occurs due to obstruction to swallowing below the pyriform fossa **(Jackson's sign)**.

Difficulties encountered in indirect laryngoscopy are:

1. Patient co-operation is essential
2. Gag reflex gets elicited if the mirror touches the posterior part of tongue or posterior pharyngeal wall
3. In cases with overhanging epiglottis, anterior commissure is difficult to visualise.
4. It is difficult to perform in children, unco-operative adults and obese patients with a short neck.
5. The tongue may obstruct the view of the vocal cords during phonation.
6. In cases with overhanging epiglottis, direct laryngoscopy is indicated to see the anterior commissure.
7. Anterior commissure, ventricle and subglottic areas are not adequately visualised.

Uses:

1. For diagnosis of laryngeal pathology
2. Removal of foreign body from posterior $\frac{1}{3}$rd of tongue, valeculla and pyriform fossa.
3. To take biopsy from suspected lesions in larynx and hypopharynx.
4. To perform direct laryngoscopy and bronchoscopy, local anaesthesia can be given via indirect laryngoscopy.
5. Removal of small lesions or cauterisation of small ulcers.

Other methods of examination of larynx:

1. Direct laryngoscopy
2. Stroboscopy
3. Microlaryngoscopy
4. Fibreoptic laryngoscopy
5. Laryngogram
6. Tomography
7. X'ray neck
8. C.T. scan / M.R.I.

VOCAL NODULE

SYNONYMS

1. Singer's nodule
2. Screamer's nodule
3. Chronic nodular laryngitis

It is seen in people who overuse and abuse their voice, like teachers, singers and hawkers

PATHOLOGY

There is hyperplastic thickening of the epithelium because of vocal trauma (vocal abuse). Subepithelial haemorrhages occur beneath the hyperplastic epithelium. At this stage, the nodules are soft. The subepithelial collection gets slowly organized and leads to formation of firm nodules. This occurs at the junction of anterior $\frac{1}{3}$ rd with posterior $\frac{2}{3}$ rds of the vocal cords. It is at this junction that the vocal cords are put to maximum stress or work-load.

FEATURES OF THE NODULE

1. Greyish white in colour
2. Bilateral
3. Symmetrical

TREATMENT

1. Absolute voice rest for 2-3 weeks, soft nodules may regress.
2. Removal of the nodule by micro laryngoscopy
3. Speech therapy

VOCAL CORD POLYP

Vocal cord polyps are commonly seen in adults and affects males more than females. They are thought to be due to trauma caused by overuse of voice. They are seen in hawkers, factory workers, teachers and people who shout against background noise.

PATHOLOGY

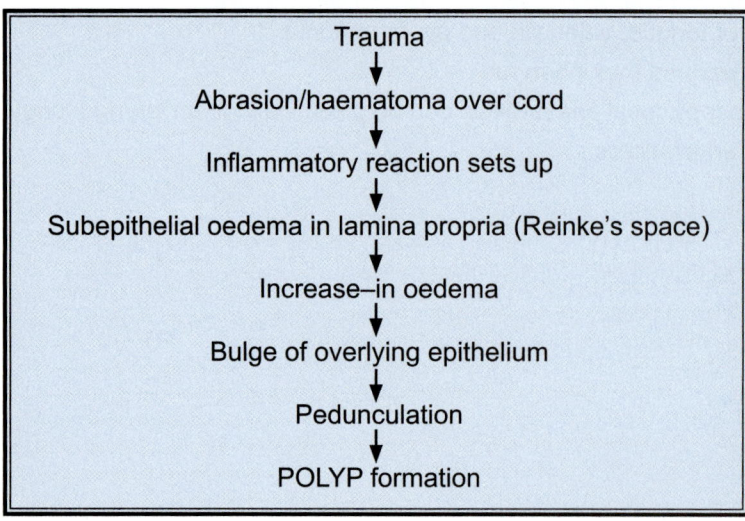

Trauma
↓
Abrasion/haematoma over cord
↓
Inflammatory reaction sets up
↓
Subepithelial oedema in lamina propria (Reinke's space)
↓
Increase–in oedema
↓
Bulge of overlying epithelium
↓
Pedunculation
↓
POLYP formation

HISTOLOGICAL TYPES:

- Gelatinous
- Transitional
- Telangiectatic

FEATURES

- Pink in colour
- Pedunculated or sessile lesion
- Usually near the anterior commissure
- Moves with respiration and coughing
- Causes hoarseness of voice of gradual onset and of long duration
- A large polyp can cause choking spells

TREATMENT

- Removal of the polyp by microlaryngoscopy with microsurgical instruments
- The polyp has to be properly grasped, pulled medially and trimmed off by scissors without damaging the underlying cord.
- Post operative speech therapy

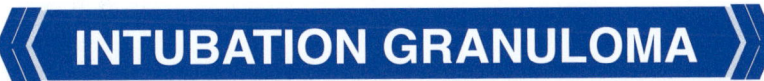

INTUBATION GRANULOMA

ETIOLOGY

- Prolonged intubation in general anaesthesia
- Blind intubation causing trauma.
- Prolonged surgery on a lightly anaesthetised patient in whom vocal cords keep brushing against the tube.

PATHOLOGY

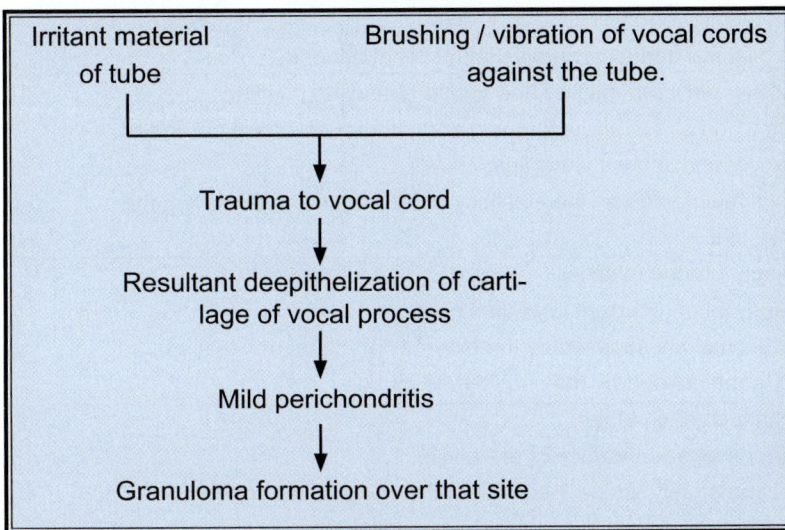

SITES

- Vocal process
- Anterior commissure

FEATURES

- Past history of surgery
- Typical site
- Hoarseness of voice

TREATMENT

Removal of granuloma under micro laryngoscopy. If the underlying cartilage is infected, it needs to be removed to help new mucosa to grow over it.

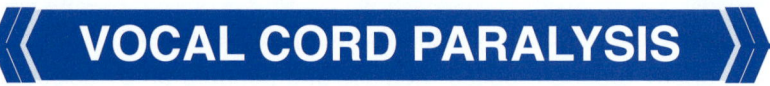

VOCAL CORD PARALYSIS

The lesion could be central or peripheral. Central causes could be supranuclear or nuclear in origin.

VOCAL CORD POSITIONS

1. Median
2. Para median
3. Cadaveric
4. Gentle abduction
5. Full abduction

POSITION	COMMENT
Full abduction	• Normal position • Seen in forced / deep inspiration.
Gentle abduction	• Normal position • Seen in quiet respiration • Also seen in bilateral adductor paralysis-functional aphonia.
Intermediate / cadaveric	• Cord lies halfway between midline and gentle-abduction position. • Position seen when all the abductors and adductor muscles are paralysed. • Cords are flaccid and show a wavy line. • This position is maintained by the elasticity of the capsule surrounding the cricoarytenoid joint.
Para median	• Cord lies adjacent to the midline • Complete paralysis of recurrent laryngeal nerve • The cricothyroid muscle supplied by the external laryngeal nerve is spared. • This position is maintained by the cricothyroid muscle.
Abductor chink	• Cords almost touch each other • Abductors are paralysed. Adductors are active. • Cords do not completely adduct because of the tilting of the arytenoid cartilages forward due to relaxation of the cricoarytenoid posticus muscle.
Median / phonatory position	• Vocal cords close the glottis • Abductors are paralysed. Adductors are active. Cords fall forward.

PALSY	ETIOLOGY	FEATURES	TREATMENT
1. Superior laryngeal nerve palsy.	• Direct trauma in operations of the neck • Tumours in the neck • Complication of Diphtheria.	• Rough, feeble, toneless voice • Easily fatiguable voice • Unaffected respiration. • Wavy margin of cord because of cricothyroid paralysis • Unilateral cases: Cord shorter and higher than the opposite and disappears under the ventricular fold on respiration. • Bilateral cases: Rima glottidis has an irregular outline • Analgesia of larynx can lead to aspiration.	Electric stimulation
2. Unilateral superior and recurrent laryngeal nerve paralysis	Lesion in the vagus nerve above the level of superior laryngeal nerve.	• Feeble voice • Respiration unaffected • Cord in cadaveric position • Cord also atonic, flaccid **Incomplete paralysis** • Abductor fibres succumb • Adductor action intact • Cord in midline because of unopposed action of adductors • Tensor muscle keeps the cord taut • Voice is normal because of the other cord **Complete paralysis** • Hoarse voice • Cadaveric position of cord • Affected side cord appears shorter because of tilting of the arytenoid cartilage. **Compensation** • Normal cord moves to the opposite side. Complete compensation does not occur in the posterior part. • Harsh voice	Aim: To bring the paralysed cord to midline **Teflon injection in affected cord** **Cricoarytenoid arthrodesis:** The joint is opened, roughened and arthrodesis is carried out with a Montgomery screw.
3. Bilateral combined paralysis of superior and recurrent laryngeal nerves.	• Lesion of cerebral cortex • Lesion of medulla affecting bulbar centre - Haemorrhage - Thrombosis - Embolism - Syphilis	• Uncommon • Voice is completely lost • Glottis is wide • Aspiration is common • Respiration is unaffected • Bad prognosis	• Tracheostomy • Cricopharyngeal myotomy. • Total laryngectomy

PALSY	ETIOLOGY	FEATURES	TREATMENT
	- Tumours of base of skull - Nasopharyngeal carcinoma - Glomus tumours ● Lesion affecting vagus nerve in the neck.		

4. Unilateral recurrent laryngeal nerve paralysis.	**Left side paralysis**
	● Carcinoma oesophagus
	● Carcinoma bronchus
	● Carcinoma thyroid
	● Operations
	  - Thyroidectomy
	  - Radical neck dissection
	  - Cardio-pulmonary surgeries.
	● Enlarged left atrium
	● Malignant tumours in thorax.
	● Aortic aneurysm
	● Peripheral neuritis
	● Diphtheria
	Right side paralysis
	● Carcinoma thyroid
	● Carcinoma apex of lung
	● Thyroidectomy
	● Tuberculosis
	● Subclavian aneurysm
	● Peripheral neuritis.
		● Minimal hoarseness of voice
		● Paramedian position of cord.
			● No treatment in minimal voice disturbance
			● Compensation occurs by 6 months
			● Teflon paste injection can be given in non-recovered cases.

5. Bilateral paralysis of recurrent laryngeal nerve (Bilateral abductor paralysis).	Total thyroidectomy	● Sudden palsy: stridor ● Gradual onset: adaptation ● Cords are almost in the midline by the unopposed action of adductors. ● Sooner or later, respiratory embarassment occurs.	● Immediate relief with **tracheostomy.** ● Permanent tracheostomy with a speaking valve can be used to retain voice. ● Spontaneous recovery can occur by 6 months. ● Surgical procedures providing adequate airway but not an adequate voice can be tried on patients after 6 months, not willing to carry on with the tracheostomy. Operations: ● External arytenoidectomy ● Arytenoidectomy and cordopexy.

PALSY	ETIOLOGY	FEATURES	TREATMENT
			• Arytenoidoplasty and cordopexy. A gap of 4 mm. is created at the posterior end in the above. **Brien's king's operation:** Attaching the omohyoid muscle to the arytenoid cartilage through a window in the thyroid cartilage. The function of the vocal cord may get restored. **Kelly's operation:** The arytenoid is displaced laterally and fixed. **Woodman's operation:** The arytenoid is rotated laterally and anchored to the thyroid cartilage and sternomastoid. **Endolaryngeal arytenoidectomy** **Nerve muscle implants:** Implanting descendens hypoglossi nerve into posterior cricoarytenoid muscle. **Laterofixation of vocal cords.**
6. Bilateral adductor paralysis (Functional / hysterical aphonia)	Occurs in young anxious, nervous emotionally unstable females. (20-25 yrs) Paresis of adductor muscles is due to derangement of cortical centres.	• H/o sudden loss of voice which was normal till then. • Normal movements of vocal cords on respiration. • Gap is present in between the vocal cords on phonation due to lack of patient's efforts to produce voice.	• Psychotherapy

⟪ CARCINOMA LARYNX ⟫

- Common in old age (50-60 yrs.)
- Males are more affected than females
- Third most common cancer among males.

ETIOLOGY

1. Smoking
2. Alcohol
3. Abuse of voice
4. Irradiation for laryngeal papilloma
5. Occupational exposure to asbestos, dust
6. Heredity

PREMALIGNANT CONDITIONS

1. Erythroplakia
2. Laryngeal papillomatosis
3. Vocal cord polyp
4. Chronic laryngitis
5. Keratosis of larynx
6. Leukoplakia of larynx

CLASSIFICATION

I. **UICC classification**

Supraglottis	Laryngeal surface of epiglottis
	Aryepiglottic folds
	Arytenoids
	False cords
	Ventricle
Glottis	Vocal cords
	Anterior commissure
	Posterior commissure
Subglottis	Starts 10 mm below the free margin of vocal cord
	Extends to inferior edge of cricoid cartilage.

Cancer affecting any of these regions does not affect the other until late due to natural barriers to cancer spread. These embryologically separate units can thus be treated separately.

II. **Ledermann's classification**

In this classification, marginal zone is included to supraglottis, glottis and sub glottis.

Marginal zone: -   Tip of epiglottis

-   Aryepiglottic fold

III. **Isambert (1876) and Krishabuer's (1879) classification**

Intrinsic	Involves Larynx proper
	False cords
	True cords
	Sub glottic region
Extrinsic	Posterior pharyngeal wall
	Laryngopharynx
	Postcricoid region

IV. **TNM classification**

Tis : Carcinoma in situ

SUPRAGLOTTIS

Tx : Tumour cannot be assessed by rules.

T0 : No evidence of primary.

T1 : Confined to one subsite with normal vocal cord mobility.

T2 : Involving more than one subsite of supraglottis or glottis with normal vocal cord mobility.

T3 or : Limited to larynx with vocal cord fixity and/or extension to postcricoid area, medial wall of pyriform sinus, pre-epiglottic space.

T4 : Massive tumour extending beyond the larynx to involve oropharynx, soft tissues of neck, or causing destruction of thyroid cartilage.

GLOTTIS

Tx : Tumour cannot be assessed by rules.

T0 : No evidence of primary.

T1 : Confined to vocal cord(s) with normal mobility (includes involvement of anterior or posterior commissures).

T1a : Limited to one vocal cord.

T1b : Involving both vocal cords.

T2 : Supraglottic and/or subglottic extension of tumour with normal or impaired cord mobility.

T3 : Confined to larynx with fixation of vocal cord.

T4 : Massive tumour with thyroid cartilage destruction and/or extension beyond the confines of the larynx into oropharynx or soft tissues of the neck.

SUBGLOTTIS

Tx : Tumour cannot be assessed by rules.

T0 : No evidence of primary.

T1 : Confined to subglottic region.

T2 : Extending to vocal cords with normal or impaired cord mobility.

T3 : Tumour confined to larynx with cord fixation.

T4 : Massive tumour with cricoid or thyroid cartilage destruction and/or extension beyond the confines of the larynx.

REGIONAL LYMPH NODES (N)

No : No evidence of regional lymph node involvement

N1 : Single ipsilateral mobile lymph node (< 3cm)

N2 : Ipsilateral involvement of multiple nodes (< 6cm)

N2a : Multiple ipsilateral mobile lymph nodes (< 6m)

N2b : Bilateral mobile lymph nodes (< 6m)

N2c : Contralateral mobile lymph nodes (< 6m)

N3 : Lymph nodes >6cm in size

DISTANT METASTASES (M)

M0:   No evidence of distant metastases

M1:   Distant metastases present

N STAGE	SINGE / MULTIPLE	FIXED /MOBILE	IPSILATERAL / CONTRALATERAL	SIZE (CM)
N0	-	-	-	-
N1	Single	Mobile	Ipsilateral	<3 cm
N2	Single / Multiple	Mobile	Ipsilateral	3-6 cm
N2a		Mobile	Ipsilateral	3-6 cm
N2b		Mobile	Bilateral	3-6 cm
N2c		Mobile	Contralateral	3-6 cm
N3	Single / Multiple	Fixed / mobile		>6 cm

STAGING

I	T^1	N^0	M^0
II	T^2	N^0	M^0
III	T^3	N^0	M^0
	T^1		
	T^2 $-N_1$		M^0
	T^3		
IV	T^4	N^0	M^0
	any T $-N^2$		M^0
	$-N^3$		M^0
	any T	any N	M_1

DIAGNOSIS

1. **Endoscopy and biopsy:**
   a) To visualise extent of disease, including subglottic extension.
   b) Biopsy taken at margins is important to study criteria for conservation procedure.

2. **CT Scan:**
   It is the best radiographic technique
   1. to assess invasion of the ventricle, pre-epiglottic and paraglottic spaces, the post cricoid region, subglottic and extralaryngeal extension.
   2. to assess fixation of the vocal cord.
   3. for evaluation of cartilage invasion (it is difficult to assess due to uneven pattern of ossification of the laryngeal cartilage).
   4. may help to assess metastatic disease in the neck.

CLINICAL FEATURES

FEATURE	COMMENT
Change of voice	Glottic cancers
Hot potato voice	Supraglottic cancers
Dyspnoea-inspiratory	Sub glottic cancers (narrowest part)
Dysphagia	Growth involves cricopharyngeal sphincter
Odynophagia	Cancer involving epiglottis
Cough with expectoration	
Blood-stained sputum	
Referred ipsilateral otalgia	(via X^{th} Cranial nerve)
Choking on swallowing food	Aspiration Cancer epiglottis causing mechanical fault in closure of laryngeal inlet Cancer pyriform fossa involving superior laryngeal nerve causing sensory loss.

Signs: - Halitosis
   - Growth on IDL
   - Cervical lymphnodes enlarged
   - Loss of laryngeal crackle.
	Laryngeal crackle: Larynx is moved in a transverse direction over the cervical vertebrae and no crackling sound indicates extralaryngeal spread of carcinoma.

FEATURES OF GROWTH

CANCER SITE	GROWTH CHARACTERISTICS	CLINICAL SIGNS	TREATMENT

Supraglottis	• Exophytic growth
	• Arises from epiglottis
	• Small nodule over ary-epiglottic folds
	• Red swelling over false cords
	• Growth invades the pre-epiglottic space
	• Regional lymph nodes get involved
	• Rich network of lymphatics is present Spreads to the glottis in late stages
	• In epiglottic cancer, both sides of neck gets involved with metastasis.
	• Poor prognosis as early lymph node spread
	• Fixation of cord indicates invasion of cricoarytenoid joint or thyroarytenoid muscle.
		• Husky and muffled voice
		• Lymph nodes in neck
			• Cancer epiglottis
			   - Supraglottic laryngectomy
			   - Radical cervical lymphadenectomy if glands are palpable
			   - Radiotherapy is not used as primary mode of treatment
			• Cancer aryepiglottic fold
			   - Supraglottic laryngectomy with neck dissection
			• Cancer false cords
			   - Radiotherapy
			   - Total laryngectomy for recurrences

Glottis	• Localized congestion, ulcer or a small mass over the vocal cord
	• Occurs over anterior third of vocal cord
	• Spreads along the edge anteriorly more than posteriorly
		• Change of voice
		• Hoarse and aphonic voice
		• Progressive hoarseness
			• T1 tumours
			   - Radiotherapy
			   - 95% success rate
			• Tumours of small size (2.5 cm)
			   - Laser surgery
			   - Laryngofissure and cordectomy

CANCER SITE	GROWTH CHARACTERISTICS	CLINICALSIGNS	TREATMENT

	• Spreads to anterior, posterior commissures and opposite cord in late stages
	• Least spread occurs upwards
	• Cords becoming fixed due to involvement is rare because of dearth of glottic lymphatics
	• Rarely Delphian node (cricothyroid node) may get involved.
	• Excellent prognosis
	  - As it is localized for a long time
	  - Length of vocal cord is 2 cm
	  - Presents early
			- Vertical hemilaryngectomy

Subglottis	• These rare tumours occur from under surface of vocal cord to lower border of cricoid
	It occurs:
	• Primarily in subglottic region
	• Direct spread from glottic region
	• Metastasis from distant organs.
	It spreads to:
	• Thyroid gland
	• Trachea
	• Strap muscles
	• Paratracheal glands
	• Vocal cords may become fixed by direct invasion
		Emergency presentation with dyspnoea and stridor	• Poor results
			• Increase chances of recurrence
			• Combined treatment
			  - Radiation
			  - Total laryngectomy
			  - Surgery for fixed vocal cord and nodal metastasis cases
			  - Neck dissection
			  - Paratracheal glands are also removed
			  - High tracheostomy in emergency cases.

Transglottis	Metastasis occur to paratracheal and mediastinal lymph nodes rather than in the neck • Cancer involving all three regions of larynx • Aggressive tumours • Metastasizes to thyroid gland, cervical lymph nodes and strap muscles. • Fixed vocal cord occurs in invasion of cricoarytenoid joint. • Poor prognosis		Total laryngectomy with/without neck dissection

DIAGNOSIS

1. Endoscopy / Biopsy
   - Extent of disease-subglottic extension
   - Biopsy from margins
   - Deeper biopsy in submucosal spread ie; small lesions with decrease cord mobility
   - Debulking can be carried out at endoscopy.

2. C.T. Scan: It is indicated for the following:
   a. To study extension to: Ventricle, pre epiglottic, paraglottic, post cricoid, subglottic and extra laryngeal regions
   b. Fixation of vocal cord
   c. Invasion of cartilage: Thyroid cartilage invasion excludes radiotherapy or conservative surgery as treatment of choice
   d. Metastasis in neck

DIFFERENTIAL DIAGNOSIS

- Tuberculous laryngitis
- Syphilitic laryngitis
- Vocal nodules
- Vocal cord polyps
- Vocal cord palsy
- Leukoplakia
- Vocal cord granuloma

INVESTIGATIONS

- Complete blood count
- Biopsy
- Direct laryngoscopy
- X'ray chest, neck
- C.T. scan
- VDRL test

TREATMENT

PRINCIPLES

Supraglottic carcinoma

T1 and T2

- Radiation for T1 carcinomas
- Supraglottic horizontal partial laryngectomy for deeply infiltrating lesions of false cords and infrahyoid epiglottis
- Radiation followed by salvage surgery.

T3 and T4

- Wide field laryngectomy with cervical lymph node removal (level 2, 3 and 4 on either side)
- Post operative radiotherapy: for all lesions extending to pharyngeal wall, valeculla, base tongue and pyriform sinus

Glottic cancer

- Radiation therapy is preferred in early glottic cancers (T1, T2)
- Surgery (Total laryngectomy) is preferred for advanced carcinomas (T3, T4)
- Total laryngectomy is the treatment for post radiation residual/recurrent cancers
- Premalignant lesions of glottis are treated by complete stripping of mucosa of vocal cord by microsurgery or laser. Repeated stripping may be required for recurrences.
- Radiotherapy is not very effective in carcinoma-in-situ cases.
- Endoscopic CO_2 Laser for early glottic carcinoma equals radiotherapy cure rates.

  Advantages of CO_2 laser treatment
  - Precision
  - Bloodless surgery
  - Decrease oedema

- Recurrence in radiated patients does not follow usual patterns of spread
- Stomal recurrence occurs from residual tumour in soft tissues surrounding trachea and paratracheal nodes

T2 and early T3 lesions

Vertical hemilaryngectomy

Radiotherapy: quality of voice is better

T3 Lesions

Cordal fixation: Laryngectomy

Indications of post operative radiotherapy

- Cartilage invasion
- Subglottic extension
- Gross / microscopic tumour at surgical margin
- Positive nodes in neck
- Tumour in soft tissues of neck

T4 Lesions

- Wide field laryngectomy with / without radical neck dissection
- Ipsilateral thyroid lobe may also be removed

Subglottic carcinoma

- Radiation for early lesions
- Surgery for fixed vocal cord and nodal metastases
- Stomal recurrence results from residual tumour in soft tissues surrounding trachea and para tracheal nodes.

SURGERIES FOR LARYNGEAL CARCINOMA

Vertical Partial Resection

- Cordectomy
- Lateral, partial laryngectomy (laryngofissure)
- Frontolateral partial laryngectomy
- Extended fronto lateral partial laryngectomy
- Frontal partial laryngectomy

Horizontal Partial Resection

- Epiglottectomy
- Supraglottic partial laryngectomy
- Extended supraglottic partial laryngectomy

Total Resection

- Total laryngectomy
- Total laryngectomy with partial pharyngectomy or glossectomy
- Total laryngo-pharyngo-oesophagectomy with reconstruction

RADIOTHERAPY

- External beam radiotherapy
- Cobalt 60 is the source
- Dose 6000-7000 rads, (200 rads/day for 5 days in a week) over 6-7 weeks
- Protection of cervical spine with shields is needed.

CHEMOTHERAPY

Palliative treatment for dysphagia and pain relief

TREATMENT PROFILE

Stage I – Radiotherapy
Preservation of function of larynx

Stage II – Surgery / Radiotherapy
Equal results

Stage III – Surgery with pre / post operative radiotherapy

Stage IV – Palliative treatment

PALLIATIVE TREATMENT

- Nasogastric feeding
- Palliative chemotherapy
- Palliative radiotherapy
- Tracheostomy
- Antibiotics, analgesics

REHABILITATION OF POST-LARYNGECTOMY PATIENT

- Voice rehabilitation
- Socio-economic rehabilitation
- Care of permanent tracheostomy

ORAL CAVITY AND OROPHARYNX

1. HISTORY AND EXAMINATION

1. Dysphagia

It means difficulty in swallowing. It can result from diseases of the oral cavity, oropharynx and oesophagus. Difficulty in mastication is due to inflammatory or infective lesions of the oral cavity.

- Onset, duration, progress
- To solids / liquids
- Associated with odynophagia / not

Differential diagnosis of dysphagia

DYSPHAGIA

I. Organic

1. **Extraoesophageal**

   a. Oral
   - Stomatitis
   - Ulcero membranous conditions
   - Dyspeptic ulcers
   - Cleft palate
   - Ludwig's angina
   - Carcinoma
   - Palatal palsy

   b. Oropharyngeal
   - Tonsillitis
   - Quinsy
   - Foreign bodies
   - Carcinoma
   - Bulbar palsy
   - Retropharyngeal abscess
   - Parapharyngeal abscess
   - Plummer-Vinson syndrome

   c. Others
   - Trismus
   - Nasal tumours
   - Nasal packing
   - Maxillofacial trauma

2. **Oesophageal**

   a. In the lumen (Luminal) and in the wall (Intrinsic)

   i) **Congenital**
   - Web
   - Stricture
   - Tracheo-oesophageal fistula
   - Foreign body

   ii) **Neoplastic**
   - Benign tumours like leiomyoma
   - Malignant neoplasms
   - Malignant strictures

   iii) **Infective / Inflammatory**
   - Oesophagitis
   - Benign strictures

   iv) **Traumatic**
   - Corrosive poisoning leading to oesophagitis and stricture formation
   - Iatrogenic trauma at neck surgeries

   v) **Neurological**
   - Myasthenia gravis

- Paralysis of oesophagus
- Spasm of cricopharyngeal sphincter
- Tetanus
- Achalasia cardia
- Diffuse spasm of oesophagus

b. **Outside the wall (Extrinsic / Extraluminal)**

External compression by:
- Tumours of thyroid gland-benign / malignant
- Pharyngeal pouch / diverticulum
- Cervical lymph node metastasis
- Cervical spondylosis (Cervical dysphagia)
- Retrosternal goitre
- Dysphagia lusoria (pressure on the oesophagus by an aberrant blood vessel)
- Mediastinal tumours and lymph nodes (Hodgkin's disease, malignancy)
- Cardiomegaly
- Pericardial effusion

II. Non-organic
- Functional / Globus hystericus

2. Odynophagia
Odynophagia means painful deglutition. It is mainly due to inflammatory lesions of oropharynx and supraglottis
- Unilateral / bilateral
- Intermittent / continuous
- Referred to ear

Differential Diagnosis of odynophagia:
- Stomatitis
- Glossitis
- Tonsillitis
- Pharyngitis
- Quinsy
- Retropharyngeal abscess
- Parapharyngeal abscess

3. Foreign body sensation in throat
This happens due to presence of an actual foreign body, secretions or tumour causing irritation in the throat

Causes:
1. Post nasal drip
2. Granular pharyngitis
3. Viral/bacterial pharyngitis
4. Foreign body throat
5. Styalgia-Eagle's Syndrome
6. Malignant tumours
7. Idiopathic
8. Functional

4. Lump in throat
It is seen in
- Malignancy
- Spasm of cricopharyngeal sphincter
- Cervical spondylosis
- Pharyngeal pouch

5. Nasal regurgitation and nasal twang
Nasal regurgitation is regurgitation of ingested material to the nose.

It occurs due to inadequacy of velopharyngeal sphincter leading to incomplete closure of nasopharynx from the oropharynx. It occurs in palatal paralysis and in abnormal communication between oral and nasal cavities.

Nasal twang in voice is known as Rhinolalia aperta. It is due to excessive escape of air into the nose during speech due to velopharyngeal insufficiency. It is usually associated with nasal regurgitation

6. Rhinolalia aperta

It is seen in the following conditions:

1. Cleft palate
2. Short palate
3. Palatal paralysis
4. Palatal perforation
5. Following adenoidectomy (in submucous cleft patients)

Pharyngeal paralysis leads to dysphagia along with aspiration into trachea.

Rhinolalia clausa is decrease in nasal component of voice.

It is seen in the following conditions:

1. Nasopharyngeal tumours
2. Enlarged adenoids

7. Muffled voice

Muffled voice results due to mechanical obstruction to speech and articulation by tumours within. It is seen in base tongue, epiglottic and hypopharyngeal tumours. The speech is characteristically known as "hot-potato speech", (a person trying to speak with a hot potato in his mouth).

8. Increased salivation

It is inability to swallow the saliva completely due to pain (odynophagia) or difficulty in swallowing (dysphagia).

The saliva may be blood-stained in cases of malignant tumours with ulceration or erosion.

9. Halitosis

Halitosis is foul smell emanating from the mouth. It is due to poor oral hygiene.

It is seen in:

● Dental caries
● Aphthous ulcers
● Malignancy

10. Trismus

Inability to open the mouth is seen in cases with submucous fibrosis and cases of carcinoma with invasion to retromolar trigone.

11. Paraesthesia / anaesthesia of area of chin lateral to midline. It indicates invasion of inferior alveolar nerve by a tumour

After noting down chief complaints, ask the following history:

H/o '6 S'

- Smoking
- Spices
- Spirit
- Syphilis
- Sharp tooth
- Speckled candidiasis

These "6 S' predispose to pathological lesions and carcinoma in the oral cavity and oropharynx.

EXAMINATION OF ORAL CAVITY AND OROPHARYNX

Inspection

The clinical examination is done using a light source (Bull's lamp) and a head mirror.

The lips are first examined to see any colour changes, ulceration or tumours. The patient is asked to open the mouth and the oral vestibule is inspected. Halitosis may be present. Oral hygiene is noted. The corner of the mouth is inspected for any fissures. Small painful ulcers on the lips and cheek are usually associated with dyspepsia. A tongue depressor is used to retract the cheek. The opening of the parotid duct (as a papillae at the root of the upper second molar tooth) has to be looked, for evidence of pus. The teeth, gums and the cheeks are inspected for signs of caries, infection, pus, ulcer or any growth. The patient is asked to lift the tip of the tongue and the orifices of the submandibular duct and floor of mouth are seen. The duct orifices are inspected for redness, oedema and pus by pressing on the gland.

The tongue is inspected for any superficial glossitis and any ulcer with its size, shape, surface and relation to the surrounding part is noted. Movements of the tongue are inspected for paralysis or neoplastic infiltration. The palate is examined for its colour, clefts, ulceration or any swellings. Pallor of palate is seen in anaemia or tuberculosis.

The oropharynx is now examined by depressing the anterior $\frac{2}{3}^{rd}$ of the tongue with a tongue depressor. The tongue depressor should not be put on the posterior $\frac{1}{3}^{rd}$ of the tongue to avoid gagging.

The faucial pillars are inspected for redness. Pressure by the tongue depressor squeezes the debris from the tonsillar crypts in chronic tonsillitis. Lingual tonsil, if hypertrophied appears as a second tonsil on each side of the base of tongue.

The whole oropharyngeal mucosa is examined for its colour, ulceration or membrane formation. Any swelling or neoplasm is noted for its size, shape, colour, surface, and surrounding area. Movements of the soft palate are observed by asking the patient to say "Ah". Post-nasal discharge may be seen trickling behind the soft palate on the posterior pharyngeal wall. It is seen in inflammatory conditions of the nose, paranasal sinuses and the nasopharynx. The posterior pharyngeal wall is examined for granulations or a bulge as seen in retropharyngeal abscess.

PALPATION

Finger palpation is required to examine inside the oral cavity.

First bidigital palpation of the submandibular salivary gland and its duct is done for any calculus and gland hypertrophy. A submandibular salivary gland is bimanually palpable, a submandibular lymph node is not.

Palpation of the tongue kept within the oral cavity and floor of mouth is done for any tumour infiltration. Any ulcer, swelling and surrounding induration is palpated for. Palpation of base tongue and tonsils is done to rule out infiltrative growths. Digital examination of the tonsil is done to detect any calculus in the supratonsillar crypt. An elongated styloid process may be felt on palpation through the tonsillar fossa.

An important area of palpation is the **Tonsillo-lingual sulcus**. This is the junction between the anterior pillar and the tongue where malignancy is commonly hidden. It is known as the **Graveyard of oropharynx** as it frequently hides malignancy which can be missed if cautious examination of oropharynx by way of palpation is not carried out.

There are certain other sites also where malignancy can be easily missed if not adequately examined. These sites are referred to as the Surgeon's Graveyard.

Another area of importance is the retromolar trigone. It is an area of mucosa covering the ascending ramus of the mandible, roughly triangular in shape. Its base is the posterior surface of the last molar tooth and the apex is the tuberosity of the maxilla. Laterally and above is the ascending ramus of the mandible joining the gingivobuccal sulcus. Medially is the mucosa of the gingivolingual sulcus and the mucosa of the inner surface of the lower alveolus.

Surgeon's Graveyard:
1. Tonsillo-lingual sulcus
2. Valeculla
3. Pyriform fossa
4. Floor of mouth
5. Nasopharynx

This area is examined by using two tongue depressors, one to retract the cheek laterally and the other to retract the tongue medially. This area is important as it is difficult to see this site clinically and an early cancer may be missed.

Palpation of the neck for lymph nodes completes the examination.

2. OROANTRAL FISTULA

Definition

It is an abnormal communication between the oral cavity and the maxillary antrum

Etiology

- Dental: Extraction of upper molars or premolars.
- Traumatic: Injury to palate, gums, teeth
- Maxillofacial injuries.
- Inflammatory : - Osteomyelitis of antral floor
  - Osteoradionecrosis of maxilla.
  - Sinusitis
- Neoplastic: Carcinoma maxilla
- Iatrogenic: Caldwell-Luc surgery
- Palatal fenestration surgery in the past

Sites of oroantral fistula

- Sublabial
- Palatal
- Alveolar

Clinical Features

- History tooth extraction, surgery etc.
- Foul smell and taste in mouth due to drainage of pus in oral cavity.
- Change of taste
- Nasal regurgitation of fluid / food particles (oro nasal fistula)
- Fistulous opening seen in oral cavity. Granulation tissue may be present within the opening or surrounding inflammation may be seen
- Probe may pass in the fistulous tract

Diagnosis

- Clinical features
- Fistulogram: Instillation of radioopaque dye into the tract outlines the tract and its openings on radiography.

Treatment

- Local hygiene
  - Antibiotic / Antiseptic gargles
  - Systemic antibiotics
- Primary closure with sutures
- Inferior meatal antrostomy can provide
  - Adequate drainage of sinus
  - Antibiotic washes can be given

  A small fistula can heal by the above measures by secondary intention and granulation tissue formation.

- Use of local flaps for closure
    - Palatal flap
    - Buccal mucosal flap

3. SUBMUCOUS FIBROSIS

DEFINITION

It is an insidious chronic disease of unknown etiology, characterized by gradually increasing fibrosis of submucosa of oral cavity, pharynx and occasionally the oesophagus

Geographical distribution:

It is seen in Indians, Indians living abroad and also reported from Ceylon, Malaysia, Nepal, South Vietnam.

Common sites of affection:

- Buccal mucosa
- Retromolar trigone
- Soft palate
- Tonsils
- Faucial pillars
- Lips, uvula, floor of mouth

Larynx is always free from the disease. Respiratory distress never occurs.

ETIOLOGY

Exact etiology is unknown but following factors have been mentioned

I. Hereditary predisposition

II. Prolonged local Irritation
    1. Betel nut
    2. Betel nut lime
    3. Paan
    4. Tobacco (Desa 1957)
    5. Chillies (Desa 1957)

III. Deficiency diseases
    1. Vit B complex (Roy 1952)
    2. Vit A (Krishnamoorthy 1970)

IV. Defective Iron metabolism

V. Localised collagen disease (Rao 1962)

VI. Reaction to bacterial infections
    - Klebsiella Rhinoscleromatis (Sengupta 1952)
    - Streptococcal toxin (Mukherjee and Biswas)

1. **Hereditary predisposition**

   Found in Indians and Indians living abroad. Thus a genetic factor is suspected

2. Prolonged local irritation

1. Betelnut
   - Acts by mechanical and chemical irritation
     a. Mechanical - Nut is hard and its sharp jagged edges cut into mucosa. It causes superficial ulceration which heals by fibrosis
     b. Chemical - Arecolins - alkaloid present in areca catechu nut. It is a local irritant and also acts on nerve endings in oral mucosa - Neurotrophic changes

2. Betelnut with Lime

   It contains arecolins, lime and tannic acid. It causes local irritation, damage to mucosa, vesiculation and ulceration. Commonly chewed is paan.

3. Kapuri Tobacco

   Incidence of SMF is high in Manipuri district associated with habitual consumption of camphor containing tobacco.

4. Chillies

   Allergic reaction to chillies is an important factor. Capsicin - an active ingredient from capsicum has been shown to be an irritant

3. Deficiency disease

It is characterised by repeated vesiculation and ulceration of oral cavity.

The deficiency could be the effect of defective nutrition due to impaired food intake in advanced cases.

4. Localised collagen disorder

This localised collagen disease of the oral cavity is similar to retroperitoneal and mediastinal fibrosis.

5. Defective iron metabolism

- Hiranandani (1970) reported achlorhydria in cases of SMF
- Microcytic hypochromic anaemia with increase serum Fe has been reported by Millard (1966) in SMF

6. Reaction to bacterial infection

Rise in mucopolysaccharides and mucoprotein - represent reactants in active stage of disease

Desa - cultured fluid from vesicles, found it to be sterile

Sengupta - reported growth of Klebsiella rhinoscleromatis in cases of SMF and suspected that this may be a factor in its causation

PATHOLOGY

Histopathologically, there are connective tissue and epithelial changes. In the connective tissue, there is progressive accumulation of fluid, constriction of blood vessels, hyalinization of collagen and fibrosis. The epithelium shows progressive atrophy, hyper and parakeratosis. Pathologically it is divided into very early, early, moderately advanced and advanced cases.

CLINICAL FEATURES

Insidious in onset

Clinical stages

1. Stage of stomatitis and vesiculation
2. Stage of fibrosis
3. Stage of sequelae and complications

STAGES	SYMPTOMS	SIGNS
1. Stage of stomatitis and vesiculation	• Burning sensation of oral mucosa • Inability to eat spicy foods • Increase / Decrease salivation	• Vesicles, ulcerations • Granulating spots on cheek, palate, pillars
2. Stage of fibrosis	• Difficulty in opening mouth • Difficulty in protruding tongue • Difficulty in blowing out cheeks, whistling • Nasal twang of speech - Rhinolalia aperta (decrease palatal movements)	• Vesicles on soft palate, anterior pillars, buccal mucosa, mucosa of lips • Vesicles - are painful, and when rupture, leave superficial ulcers • Culture of fluid from vesicles is sterile
3. Stage of sequelae and complications	This stage is similar to stage of fibrosis. Oral mucosa loses its natural suppleness.	• Oral mucosa - Whitish, blanched or mottled. • Soft palate - Whitish. Decrease mobility. Fibrous bands originate from pterygomandibular raphe to anterior faucial pillar • Trismus is seen due to contraction of fibrous tissue underneath the mucosa. • Faucial pillars - Thick, short and hard. Tonsils pressed between fibrosed pillars • Progressive narrowing and inability to open mouth fully.

INVESTIGATIONS

- Complete haemogram   -   Decrease Hb
  -   Increase Eosinophils
- ESR is raised in 50% of individuals
- Routine urine and stool examination
- Blood biochemistry
- Serum protein: decrease Albumin, increase Y-Globulins
- X-ray chest
- Electromyography
  - Gives an exact state of contractility of muscles. EMG of Temporalis, Buccinator, etc is done.
    Use - To differentiate in SMF whether pathology is contraction due to fibrosis or is sustained contraction of muscles.
- Exfoliative cytology
  - Morphological characteristics are examined

TOLUIDINE BLUE STAINING

It is metachromatic drug of thiazine group. Malignant cells which contain more DNA than RNA have got affinity to this dye. Dye reacts metachromatically with malignant cells delineating the abnormal cells which can be biopsied.

PAS staining shows increase PAS +ve granules in connective tissue.

SMF as a Pre Cancerous Condition: -

1. Frequency of leukoplakia is 6-8 times more common in SMF
2. In South India about ½ of cancer patients show SMF
3. Expectancy of life is not reduced unless SMF is associated with malignancy.
4. There is a chance of recurrence after relief of early symptoms, hence close follow-up is essential.
5. Long term follow-up shows it to be turning malignant by 6-10%.

MANAGEMENT

PREVENTIVE MEASURES

a. Abstaining from ingestion of irritants Eg. Betelnut, Pan parag, Tobacco, Chillies etc.
b. Maintenance of proper oral hygiene
c. Vitamin supplements
d. Well - balanced diet

MEDICAL TREATMENT

Submucosal injections of

- Fibrinolysins
- Gold
- Vit A and D and
- Corticosteroids

1. **Steroids: -**
   a. Cortisone given in doses of 20 mg or 100 mg daily for a total of 1500 - 2500 mg. can be given orally / parenterally
   b. Hydrocortisone with lignocaine can be - injected in oral cavity and soft palate
   It is most effective in early / moderately advanced cases

   Mode of action:
   1. Immuno suppressive action
   2. Decreases inflammation
   3. Decrease fibroblastic proliferation - Prevents fibrosis

2. **Hyalase: - (Hyaluronidase)**
   - Acts on Hyaluronic acid and decreases its formation which plays an important role in formation of collagen
     Regime (Kacher and Venkatachalam)
     1500 u of Hyalase + 1 ml of 2% lignox - Twice weekly for first 3 weeks
     followed by 1500 u of Hyalase + 4 ml of dexamethasone - Twice weekly for 7 weeks

3. **Placental extract and dexamethasone can be given for 6 weeks.**
   Improvement by these injections is temporary.

4. **POTABA: -** (Potassium Amino Benzoic Acid)
   It decreases collagen formation and inturn decreases fibrosis.

SURGICAL TREATMENT

Indications:

1. Severe trismus
2. Dysplastic / neoplastic changes

a. Excision of fibrotic bands

Always done under general anaesthesia

It is difficult or impossible to intubate if patient has severe trismus

Means of giving anaesthesia:

1. Blind awake intubation is done through nose
2. Retrograde rail roading technique
3. Tracheostomy

Procedure

Forceful opening of mouth with the help of jaw stretchers is done. Incision is taken on the mucosa from the angle of mouth to anterior pillar, taking care not to damage the parotid duct. Incision is deepened down to the muscle and associated fibrous tissue with muscle is incised.

Postoperatively physiotherapy is given in the form of active and passive wide opening of mouth. Wound at site of division heals in 4-6 weeks.

b. Excision of fibrotic bands with split thickness skin grafting

Excision of fibrotic bands is done in a similar fashion followed by split thickness skin grafting of raw surface to cover the defect. Graft is immobilised over a sponge bolus. Mouth is kept open with a pair of small smooth rubber anaesthesia props to produce an inter incisor distance of 35-40 mm.

Postoperatively, patient is fed via a Ryles tube for 7 days

- Daily mouth opening exercises are done
- Nocturnal props are used for 4 weeks.

c. Excision of fibrotic bands with split thickness skin grafting with bilateral temporalis myotomy or coronoidectomy

Rationale of temporalis myotomy: Secondary contracture formation occurs in temporalis tendon, muscle and in the pterygomandibular raphe which is the principal cause of trismus

d. Excision of fibrotic bands with reconstruction

Indication: - Severe trismus with interincisor distance < 1 cm

An ideal tissue for reconstruction is

i. Adequate in amount
ii. Has less tendency to fibrosis and contraction
iii. Maintains its vascularity until healing is achieved.

Reconstruction is done with:

1. Bilateral full thickness nasolabial flaps
2. Tongue flaps.

Advantages of a tongue flap:

i. It is available near the site
ii. It is vascular
iii. Less tendency to contraction
iv. It is the only mucosa left in the oral cavity without fibrosis

4. ULCERS OF THE TONGUE

- Dr. Rajiv Joshi

D / D

1. Dyspeptic or aphthous ulcer
2. Traumatic or dental ulcer
3. Malignant ulcer
4. Tuberculous ulcer
5. Syphilitic ulcer
6. Simple ulcer due to glossitis
7. Post-pertussis ulcer
8. Herpetic and pseudo herpetic ulcers
9. Chronic non-specific ulcer

1. Dyspeptic ulcer:
- Occurs at any age
- Seen usually at the tip but may occur at any site with or without abscess in the lip or cheek
- Single or multiple
- Small and circular
- Edge of the ulcer has an oedematous hyperaemic zone
- Floor is white
- Thin and watery discharge
- Pain and tenderness present
- Generalised features of dyspepsia

Investigation - To R/O malabsorption syndromes

Rx: Ulcers respond to high doses of Vit A, C, B complex
Correction of dyspepsia.

2. Traumatic or dental ulcer:
- Can occur at any age
- Usually at the margin of the tongue, commonly towards the back
- Single
- Any shape according to shape of traumatic agent
- Depth and size is moderate
- Edge of the ulcer is oedematous
- Floor is covered with slough
- Discharge is often purulent
- Induration is present
- Pain and tenderness is marked
- Presence of a sharp tooth or ill-fitting denture
- Neck lymph nodes are firm and tender if, secondarily infected

Investigations: for presence of sharp tooth or ill-fitting denture-X-ray / OPG

Rx: Usually heals after removal of source of irritation

3. **Malignant ulcer**
   - Seen in elderly
   - Usually seen at the margin and common in ant. $\frac{2}{3}^{rd}$
   - Single or multiple
   - Raised, rolled out and everted edge
   - Floor covered with necrotic debris and looks dirty grey
   - Discharge is offensive
   - Painless initially, painful later with pain referred to the ear
   - LN enlarged, stony hard and fixed in late stage
   - Excessive salivation, difficulty in articulation and speech

   Rx - Surgery or Radiotherapy.

4. **Tuberculous ulcer:**
   - Young adults
   - Multiple sites - tip, margin, dorsum
   - Shallow ulcer of moderate size
   - Oval or circular
   - Discharge-apple jelly nodules
   - Undermined edges
   - Floor covered with pale granulation tissue
   - Painful
   - Lymph nodes are enlarged and matted with or without cold abscess
   - Associated tuberculosis of the lungs or larynx with features of TB toxaemia

   Rx: AKT

5. **Syphilitic ulcer:**
   - Seen in tertiary stage of syphilis
   - Dorsum of the tongue
   - Single
   - Oval or circular
   - Punched out edges
   - Floor deep with washed leather slough
   - Slightly indurated
   - Discharge greyish-white
   - Painless
   - Lymph nodes are enlarged, shotty and discrete-usually epitrochlear, occipital lymph nodes are involved

   Investigations: Sr - VDRL

   Rx: Antisyphilitic doses of Penicillin

6. **Simple ulcer due to glossitis:**
   - Occurs in chronic superficial glossitis
   - Usually single known as 'Smoker's patch'
   - Burning pain during food intake present

7. **Post-pertussis ulcer:**
   - Occurs in children following whooping cough
   - Confined mostly to the phrenum linguae

8. **Herpetic ulcers:**
   - Common in children and young adults
   - Occurs due to herpetic-affection of lingual nerve.
   - Acute, unilateral neuralgic pain on affected side - vesicle - ulcer

9. **Chronic non-specific ulcer:**
   - Seen in individuals with poor oral hygiene
   Rx: Correction of poor oral hygiene and high dose of vitamins

Note on lymphatic drainage of tongue:

Tip	-	Submental nodes
		Bilateral drainage
Post ⅓	-	Upper deep cervical lymph nodes (Jugulodigastric), Bilateral drainage
Ant ⅔	-	Unilateral drainage to submandibular nodes and then to deep cervical chain

Ultimately all the lymph drainage from the tongue reaches the jugulo-omohyoid lymph node in the deep cervical chain

Important Characteristics:

a. Lymphatics draining the ant ⅔rd of the tongue and floor of the mouth traverse the periosteum of the mandible on their way to submental and submandibular lymph nodes. Hence part of the mandible is removed during radical dissection

b. Lymphatics decussate in the midline, hence contralateral lymph nodes may be involved. It is necessary that glands on both sides be dealt with in Rx of Ca tongue.

c. Lenthal Cheatle showed that the lymphatics draining the tongue which pierce the mylohyoid and tongue muscles are of exceptionally large calibre. Hence in Ca tongue embolic spread is more common due to squeezing of the malignant cells (by activity of the tongue musculature) through these large lymphatic vessels without being held up in them.

d. Because of the secluded position and consequent late diagnosis, growths of the posterior ⅓rd of tongue show the highest incidence of cervical metastasis.

e. Septic infection which invariably occurs in the malignant ulcer may cause a non-malignant enlargement of the lymph nodes under the jaw.

5. CARCINOMA OF TONGUE

Common lesion and accounts for more than 15% of HFN malignancies and more than 50% of all intraoral malignancies.

Aetiology: M: F 3:1

5th-6th decade usually

Predisposing factors

1. Chronic irritation caused by
   - **S**harp tooth or ill fitting dentures
   - **S**moking - particularly pipe smoking
   - **S**pirits - excessive alcohol intake
   - **S**pices
   - **S**epsis - poor oral hygiene / oral health
2. **S**yphilis
3. **S**uperficial glossitis - Chronic
4. **S**essile papilloma
5. **S**yndrome Plummer - Vinson

Precancerous lesions

1. Leukoplakia
2. Erythroplakia
3. Chronic superficial glossitis
4. **S**yphilitic ulcer
5. **S**essile papilloma
6. Melanoplakia (rarely)

Macroscopic features

1. Ulcerative type - raised, irregular, rolled or everted margins, a sloughing yellow grey base and induration of surrounding tissues.
2. Papilliferous or warty types
3. Fissured or cracked type with induration - usually follows chronic superficial glossitis or syphilis
4. Nodular type - a submucous nodule or plaque - oral, raised plaque with keratin flakes on the surface
5. Frozen tongue - indurated tongue or wooden tongue

Microscopic features

Ant ⅔rd   - Squamous cell carcinoma

Post ⅓rd   - Lymphoepithelioma or basal cell Ca or transitional cell Ca

Ant ⅔rd	**Post ⅓rd**
1. Epidermoid Ca	- Lymphoepithelioma
2. Lymphatic spread is ipsilateral except tip	- Lymphatic spread is bilateral
3. Ulcerative growth (primary presentation)	- Primary (silent)
	- Malignant secondaries (active lesion)
4. Different Rx portal	- Always subjected to radiotherapy

Metastases

1. Local spread: Through substance of tongue
   - To floor of mouth (Ant ⅔rd)
   - To mandible (Junction of ant ⅔rd and post ⅓rd)
   - To tonsil, epiglottis, soft palate, larynx, cervical spine (Post ⅓rd)
2. Lymphatic spread: Occurs early by embolisation than by permeation and follows lymphatic drainage of tongue.
3. Haematogenous spread (rare): More from post ⅓rd, occurs only in 2% of cases to lungs.

Symptoms

Early cases are virtually symptomless or there is a painless lump / irregularity or ulcer on the surface of the tongue.

More advanced cases present with:

1. Enlarging ulcer, pain in the tongue

   Pain - infection and ulceration
   - Lingual nerve involvement
   - Pain referred to the ear (auriculotemporal nerve which is also a branch of mandibular division of trigeminal nerve).
   - Post ⅓rd Ca-Odynophagia

     Pain in the back of the tongue
2. Excessive salivation-Pain promotes salivation. Saliva may be blood stained
3. Dysphagia and difficulty in mastication
   - Still, lumpy, partially fixed tongue makes swallowing difficult. More pronounced in Ca Post ⅓rd
4. Foetor oris: - Due to poor oral hygeine and secondary bacterial stomatitis

   Necrosis-infection (offensive odour)
5. Ankyloglossia: - Frozen tongue leading to inability to protrude the tongue.
   - Deviation to one side is due to fixation by extensive infiltration of floor of mouth
6. Difficulty in speech
   - Inability to articulate properly is due to extensive carcinomatous infiltration of the tongue and / or floor of the mouth.
7. Alteration in voice especially in post ⅓rd Ca
8. Lump in the neck (due to secondary deposits in draining lymph nodes)

   Signs - Site and character of the lesion (macroscopic features)
   - Palpate for induration, mobility of the lesion and of the tongue
   - Cervical lymph node enlargement

   D / D - Other types of ulcers on tongue
   - Rare tumours of tongue
   - Papilloma, lymphangioma, haemangioma, neurofibroma, lingual thyroid

Terminal event or death occurs due to

1. Aspiration bronchopneumonia from superadded oral sepsis
2. Haemorrhage from the growth
   - Erosion of lingual artery
   - Erosion of carotid artery or internal jugular vein in post ⅓rd Ca or by metastatic lymph nodes.
3. Malignant cachexia
4. Starvation and exhaustion from a combination of
   - Pain, dysphagia, odynophagia

- Compression of pharynx, oesophagus by metastatic lymph nodes
- Anorexia resulting from infected fungating ulcer in mouth

5. Asphyxia due to airway obstruction from enlarged and fixed carcinomatous lymph nodes or due to oedema of glottis which is due to an extension of the lymphatic oedema around a growth at the back of the tongue

Management

Investigation :
- Routine
- Sr. VDRL
- Laryngoscopy to see post $\frac{1}{3}^{rd}$ of tongue especially the region of the valeculla
- Pus swab for SCAST from ulcer
- X-ray of the mandible to rule out bone involvement
- Biology - Documentary evidence of growth
  - Type of growth
- L. N. FNAC
- X-ray chest for pneumonia / secondaries in lung
- OPG

Rx-Preliminary measures :
- Oral hygiene is established
- Dental Rx of carious teeth
- Teeth-scaling and polishing
- Extraction of teeth if they block radiation
- Frequent antiseptic mouth washes
- Antibiotics to prevent and control secondary infection, correction of nutritional and metabolic disorders
- Correction of anaemia, respiratory status
- Improvement of general condition

Prophylactic Rx:
- Remove source of chronic irritation
- Excision of unresolving or suspsicious areas of leukoplakia
- Biopsy of suspicious lesion

Treatment in Ca tongue

1. Surgery : Indications
   - Surgically resectable growths
   - LN involvement (mets - freely mobile LN)
   - Ca supervening in cases of leukoplakic patch
   - Growth involving the jaw or in close proximity of bone

Modalities of Sx Rx are:

1. Partial Glossectomy
2. Hemiglossectomy
3. Subtotal glossectomy (removal of ant $\frac{2}{3}^{rd}$ of tongue)
4. For N1 neck - Hemiglossectomy + hemimandibulectomy + RND (radical neck dissection) Commando operation followed by reconstruction with a pectoralis major myocutaneous flap (PMMF) or pectoralis major osteocutaneous flap (PMOM)

   For No neck one may do a glossectomy with a suprahyoid block as a staging procedure

2. Radiotherapy:

It is treatment of choice in post $\frac{1}{3}^{rd}$ Ca (by teletherapy only because this part is anatomically difficult, both for surgery and interstitial therapy).

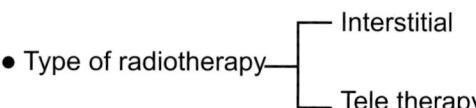

- Type of radiotherapy — ⌐ Interstitial
  └ Tele therapy

- Dosage 6000 rads

Indications for RT:

- Post $\frac{1}{3}^{rd}$ Ca
- Inoperable growth with fixed lymph nodes
- Recurrence of growth after surgery

Contra indications

- Involvement of bone
- Growth in close proximity of bone
- Mobile lymph nodes

3. Chemotherapy
   a. Regional arterial Amphotericin
   b. Prince - Hill regime
      Bleomycin, Adriamycin, Vincristin.
      Other drugs used are
      - Cisplatin
      - Methotrexate
      - Endoxan

Management of LNs:

1. For No neck - Suprahyoid block as a staging procedure
2. For N1 neck - Commando operation
3. For N3 neck - RT with SOS salvage block dissection of cervical nodes.

For N_2 neck
Full block on side followed by modified neck dissection on the other side along with adjuvant RT or CT

Palliation : Indicated in large unresectable primary fixed lymph nodes.
- Irradiation
- Mouth washes to reduce local infection and foul small of necrotic lingual carcinoma
- Antibiotics
- Control of pain and apprehension with adequate analgesia and sedation with morphine
- Tracheostomy in respiratory obstruction
- Feeding with a nasogastric tube in patients with dysphagia

Prognosis : Depends on site, stage and lymph node involvement
1. Site   : a. Growth in ant $\frac{2}{3}^{rd}$ - 50% 5 yr. survival rate
              b. Growth in post $\frac{1}{3}^{rd}$ - 10% 5 yr. survival rate.
2. Stages   : a. Early stage - 60% 5 yr. survival rate
              b. Late stage - 15% 5 yr. survival rate
3. Nodes   : a. If involved - 15% 5 yr. survival rate
              b. If not involved - 60% 5 yr. survival rate

Radical Neck Dissection [RND] is En Bloc removal of all the cervival L.N. + Fibrofatty tissue in neck + the structures which are:

1. Sternomastoid
2. Omohyoid / digastric
3. Accessory nerve
4. Internal jugular vein
5. Sub mandibular gland
6. Tail of parotid gland

6. CLEFT LIP AND PALATE

- Dr. Uday Bhatt

HISTORY

Name, Age, Sex, Religion, Occupation, Address.

Cleft lip is more common in males and cleft palate in females.

Chief Complaints

CLEFT LIP + ALVEOLUS (Cleft of primary palate):

H/o deformity of lip and palate.

H/o cosmetic problems.

H/o additional complaints.

H/o occlusal problems (cleft alveolus).

H/o difficulty in speech / articulation (bilateral cleft lip).

H/o sucking problems (usually no problem in cleft of primary palate).

CLEFT PALATE

H/o deformity of palate.

H/o cosmetic problems (maxillary hypoplasia).

H/o difficulty in suckling because of failure to generate negative intraoral pressure.

H/o occlusal problems.

H/o nasal regurgitation of fluids.

H/o speech problems - hypernasality, nasal escape, unintelligibility (in associated velopharyngeal insufficiency).

H/o articulation problems.

H/o recurrent middle ear infections.

H/o upper respiratory tract infections (occasional).

Submucous cleft

H/o Speech and articulation problems.

H/o Symptoms of velopharyngeal insufficiency.

H/o Nasal regurgitation.

H/o Hypernasality / nasal twang in voice.

H/o Risk factors: (Cleft lip and palate)
Maternal:

H/o increased maternal age during pregnancy.

H/o smoking, alcoholism, phenytoin therapy in mother.

H/o deficiency of vitamin A, riboflavin, folic acid etc. in mother.

Foetal:

H/o hypoxia during embryogenesis.

Genetic:

H/o family history.

H/o consanguinous marriages.

H/o syndromes : - Treacher Collins syndrome.
- Trisomy of group D, G, E chromosomes.

Past / Personal / Family History

To lay special emphasis on:

- Past H/o of middle ear infections / secretory otitis media.
- Past H/o of any medical / surgical management with their result / benefits.
- Family H/o of similar siblings / syndromes.

Clinical Examination

General Examination

As per routine format with emphasis on:

- Pallor (because of feeding problems).
- Signs of upper respiratory tract infection (because of possible regurgitation).

Local Examination

Description of Anatomy of cleft:

- Unilateral / bilateral
- Complete / incomplete
- Primary / secondary / both

Cleft lip: Describe:

- Obliquity of cupid's bow.
- Hypoplasia of vermilion.
- Ill-defined white roll.

Cleft alveous: Describe:

- Through which teeth the cleft is passing.
- Collapse if any of alveolar arch.
- Occlusion defect.

Cleft palate: Describe:

- Cleft anatomy in detail.
- Whether vomer touching any of the shelves.
- Movement of soft palate, posterior pharyngeal wall on phonation.
- Passavant's ridge.
- Shortness of palate.
- Hypoplasia of maxilla.
  Also describe the tongue, tonsil and oral hygiene in each.

Submucous cleft describe:

- Intact oral and nasal mucosal layer.
- Description of middle muscle layer.
- Bifid uvula present.
- A zone of transillumination - zona pellucida seen in the midline from the oral side if light is thrown in the nostrils.
- Palpate for midline bony defect.

Examination of nose
- Flaring of nostrils.
- Hypoplastic alar cartilages.
- Oblique columella.
- Round and asymmetric tip
- Deviated septum.
- Signs of rhinitis.

Examination of ear

Bilateral affection

Signs of secretory otitis media.
- Dull bluish ear drum.
- Retracted tympanic membrane.
- Air-fluid level may be seen.

Signs of chronic suppurative otitis media:
- Bilateral safe, central perforation.
- Active mucosal disease may be present.

MANAGEMENT OF CLEFT PALATE

At birth, parental counselling and presurgical orthopaedics are carried out. Presurgical orthopaedics includes means to realign the alveolar segments and to retract the protrusion of the premaxilla.

Lip repair is ideally carried out at 3 months of age and palate repair between 6 and 12 months of age. The first phonemes, that require closure of the velopharynx are used between 6 and 9 months of age of the child, therefore repair should ideally precede this age. The palatal repair can be carried out by Veau's technique or Von Langenbeck's method.

Veau's method

In this method bone deep oral mucosal incisions are made on the sides of the cleft and on the palatal surface to raise flaps based on the greater palatine artery.

After raising mucoperiosteal flaps, the nasal mucosa, soft palate musculature and the nasopharyngeal mucosa is mobilized. The mobilization should be adequate to let the flaps reach the midline with ease. The three layers are sutured separately.

By mobilization of flaps, defects are created laterally which heal by secondary intention.

Cleft palate repair may be complicated by haemorrhage, affection of growth of mid-face and postoperative fistula formation.

SUBMUCOUS CLEFT PALATE

It is a condition characterized by a triad of:
1. Bifid uvula
2. Palatal muscle diastisis
3. Bony notch in the hard palate

   They can be overt or occult. Usually the oral and nasal mucous membranes are intact and the muscle layer is deficient giving rise to a white translucent zone in the palate.

7. CHRONIC TONSILLITIS

SYNONYMS

- Chronic follicular tonsillitis
- Parenchymatous tonsillitis
- Hypertrophic tonsillitis
- Lacunar tonsillitis

It is chronic inflammation and infection of faucial tonsils

It is commonly seen in children between 3-8 yrs. of age.

ORGANISMS

- Bacteria
  - Streptococcus
  - Staphylococcus
  - Diphtheroids
  - Pneumococcus
- Virus

ETIOLOGY

1. Recurrent acute tonsillitis
2. Subclinical tonsillar infections aggravated by diseases like measles, scarlet fever etc.
3. Excessive ingestion of carbohydrates.

PREDISPOSING FACTORS

- Overcrowding
- Contact with person with tonsillitis
- Immunodeficiency
- Ingestion of cold eatables (causes localized vasoconstriction and lowered immunity)
- Pollution
- Foreign body embedded in the tonsil

CLINICAL FEATURES

- Dysphagia / odynophagia: repeated attacks associated with fever and symptom free interval in between.
- Fever
- Cough
- Difficulty in breathing
- Affects speech
- Poor appetite
- Halitosis

TONSILLAR SIGNS

- Enlarged tonsils project beyond the anterior pillar, meeting in the midline-kissing tonsils. These hypertrophied tonsils (**parenchymatous type**) can give rise to choking attacks on feeding, in children
- Congestion of bilateral anterior pillars.
- Tonsils may be atrophic, small, hidden within the pillars-**Fibrosed Tonsils**. This is seen in elderly people
- Pus may extrude out from the crypts on pressure over the tonsils-**Lacunar Tonsillitis** (**Irwin Moore's Sign**).
- Non-tender and palpable jugulodigastric lymph nodes. (palpable just below and behind the angle of mandible).

CHRONIC TONSILLITIS

Cardinal signs

- More than 4-5 attacks of acute tonsillitis in a year
- Hypertrophied tonsils
- Congestion of anterior pillars
- Pus exuding from crypts on pressure over the tonsils
- Enlarged, non-tender jugulo-digastric lymphadenopathy

TREATMENT

Medical treatment

- Antibiotics
- Anti-inflammatory analgesics
- Antiseptic gargles
- Antiseptic throat paints
  - Mandl's paints
- General measures
  - Good nutrition
  - Exercise
  - Fresh air

Surgical treatment

- Tonsillectomy is the treatment of choice.

8. LINGUAL TONSILLITIS

The lingual tonsil is an aggregate of lymphoid tissue situated posteriorly at the base of the tongue. It is bounded by circumvallate papillae anteriorly and epiglottis posteriorly.

Hypertrophy of lingual tonsil occurs more in women. Acute and chronic forms occur. It is affected in the same manner as the faucial tonsil. It can occur due to early removal of faucial tonsils in children.

CLINICAL FEATURES

- Severe dysphagia
- Foreign body sensation in throat
- Indirect laryngoscopy will show enlarged, hypertrophied tonsils at the base of the tongue.

TREATMENT

- Antibiotics
- Local application of throat paint
- Removal of the tonsils by Lingual tonsillotome
- Cryosurgery
- Diathermy reduction of size
- Laser application

9. ADENOIDS

Synonym: Nasopharyngeal tonsil

Adenoids is the hypertrophied mass of lymphoid tissue situated at the junction of the roof and posterior wall of nasopharynx.

The mass of lymphoid tissue is termed as 'Adenoids" only when it is hypertrophied. It is difficult to differentiate between physiological hypertrophy and pathological enlargement.

It usually undergoes atrophy by puberty (13-14 yrs.)

ETIOLOGY

- Hereditary
- Cold climate
- Specific infection like tuberculosis.
- Physiological hypertrophy may be seen between 3-10 yrs.

FEATURES

- Pink, globular mass
- Vertical ridges on its surface
- No crypts
- Lined by columnar ciliated epithelium
- No capsule

SYMPTOMS

Local (Due to adenoid hypertrophy and infection):

- Bilateral nasal obstruction
- Snoring
- Mouth breathing
- Rhinolalia clausa
- Frequent rhinorrhoea
- Epistaxis
- Feeding problems in children
- Adenoid facies (seen if nasal obstruction persists for a long time)
- Conductive deafness due to eustachian tuble block
- Enlarged cervical glands
- Bronchitis
- Otitis media
- Gastrointestinal disturbances

General

- Anorexia
- Lethargy

Features of adenoid facies

- Sunken eyes
- Narrow pinched nostrils
- Open mouth
- Gothic (high-arched) palate
- Crowded teeth
- Loss of nasolabial fold
- Dull mask-like face
- Rhinorrhoea
- Everted upper lip
- Protruding teeth
- Drooling of saliva

Aural manifestations in Adenoids:

Otalgia

Secretory otitis media

Acute otitis media

Atelectasis

ET block

Chronic otitis media

- Poor physical and mental development
- Bed-wetting
- Pigeon chest
- Protruberant abdomen

DIAGNOSIS

- H/o nasal obstruction, rhinorrhoea
- Pink globular mass with vertical ridges on posterior rhinoscopy
- Bilateral retracted eardrums
- X'ray postnasal space shows soft tissue mass.

DIFFERENTIAL DIAGNOSIS

- Thornwaldt's cyst
- High arched palate

Detection of Adenoids
Posterior rhinoscopy
Digital palpation
Examination under GA
X'ray soft tissue nasopharynx

COMPLICATIONS

1. Adenoid facies
2. Otitis media with effusion
3. Recurrent acute otitis media
4. Rhinolalla clausa
5. Chronic sinusitis
6. Sleep apnoea syndrome
7. Decrease mental/physical development

TREATMENT

Medical
- Adequate nutrition
- Antibiotics
- Anti inflammatory analgesics
- Decongestant nasal drops

Surgical
- Adenoidectomy
- Myringotomy with grommet insertion.

Neck

1. SWELLINGS IN THE NECK

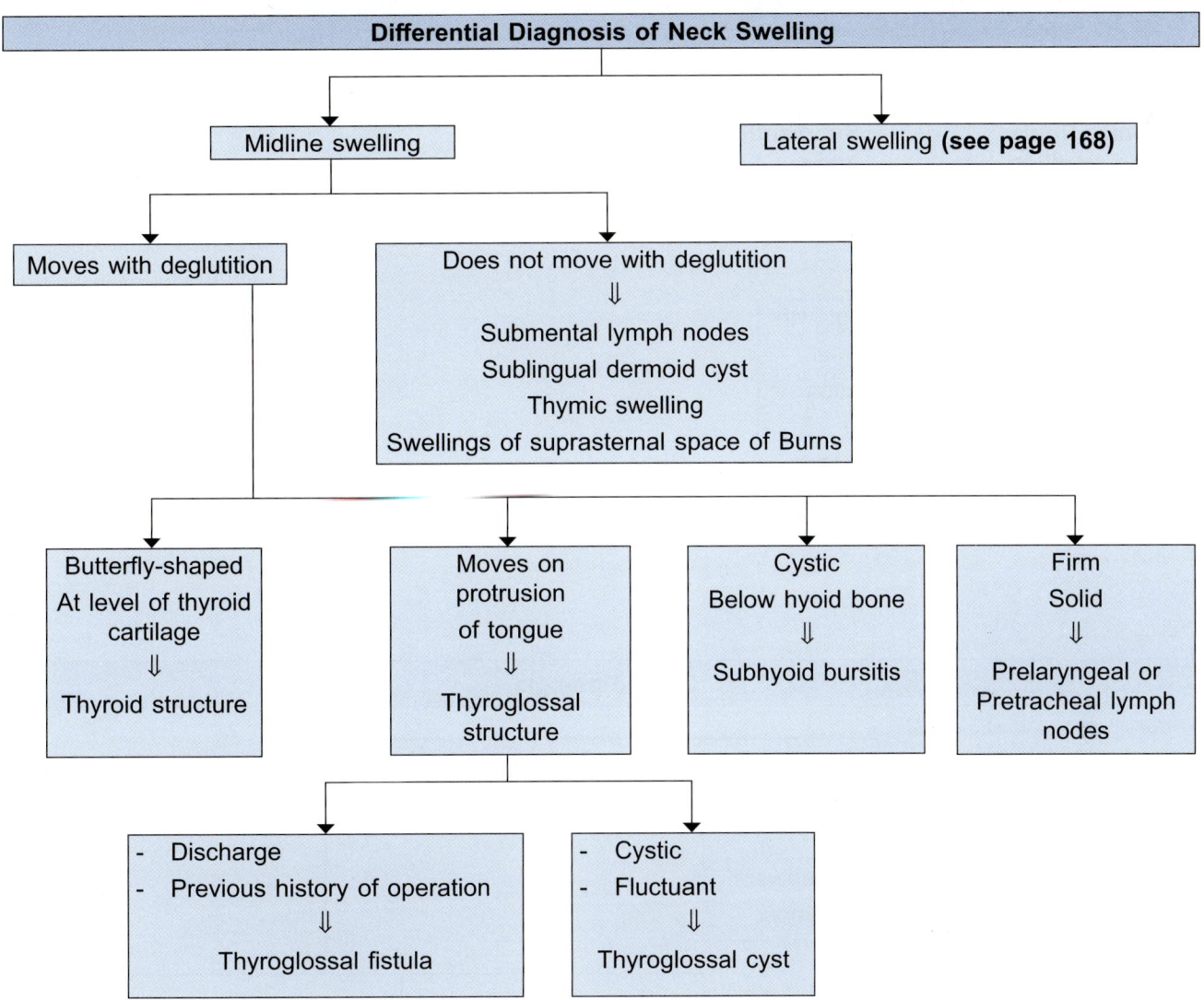

Differential Diagnosis of Neck Swelling

- Midline swelling
- Lateral swelling **(see page 168)**

Midline swelling:
- Moves with deglutition
- Does not move with deglutition
  ⇓
  Submental lymph nodes
  Sublingual dermoid cyst
  Thymic swelling
  Swellings of suprasternal space of Burns

Moves with deglutition:

- Butterfly-shaped
  At level of thyroid cartilage
  ⇓
  Thyroid structure

- Moves on protrusion of tongue
  ⇓
  Thyroglossal structure

- Cystic
  Below hyoid bone
  ⇓
  Subhyoid bursitis

- Firm
  Solid
  ⇓
  Prelaryngeal or Pretracheal lymph nodes

Thyroglossal structure:

- Discharge
- Previous history of operation
  ⇓
  Thyroglossal fistula

- Cystic
- Fluctuant
  ⇓
  Thyroglossal cyst

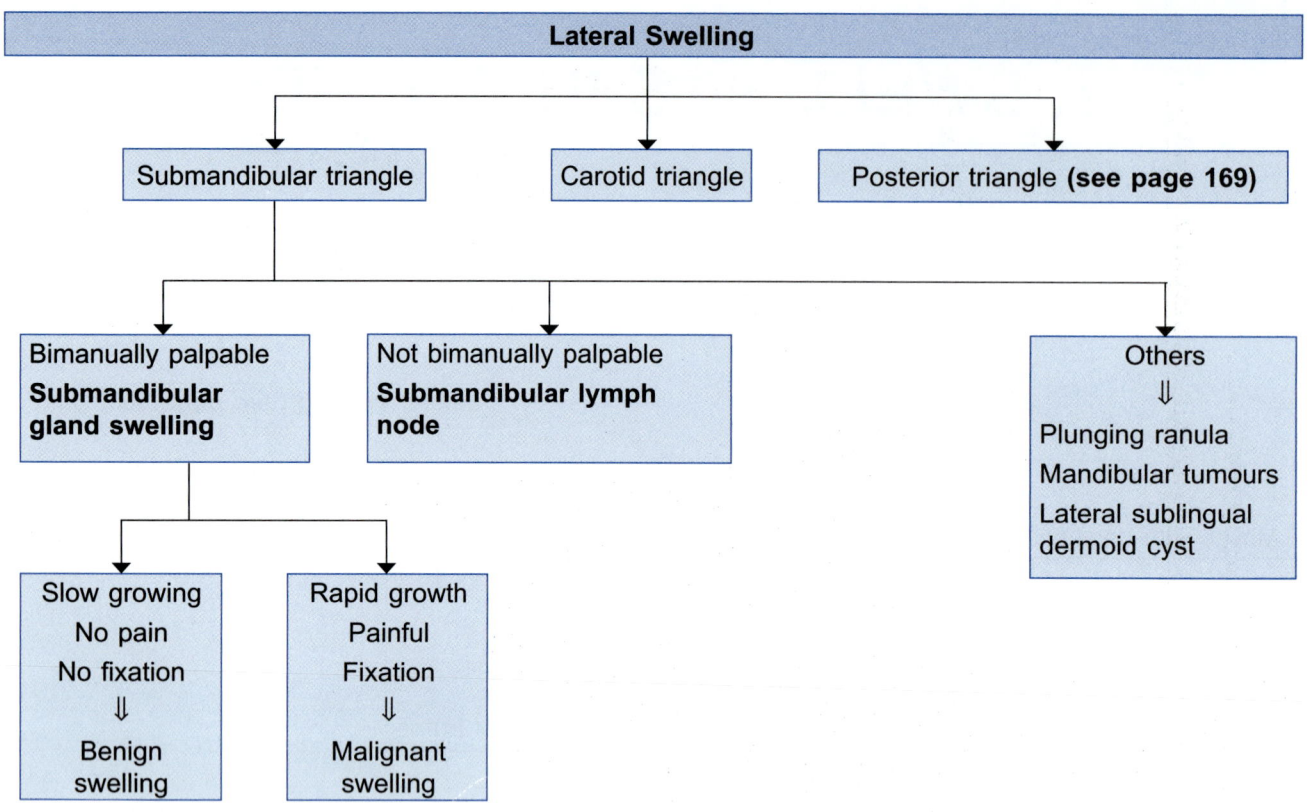

Lateral Swelling

- Submandibular triangle
- Carotid triangle
- Posterior triangle **(see page 169)**

Submandibular triangle:

- Bimanually palpable **Submandibular gland swelling**
  - Slow growing
  - No pain
  - No fixation
  ⇓
  Benign swelling

  - Rapid growth
  - Painful
  - Fixation
  ⇓
  Malignant swelling

- Not bimanually palpable **Submandibular lymph node**

- Others
  ⇓
  Plunging ranula
  Mandibular tumours
  Lateral sublingual dermoid cyst

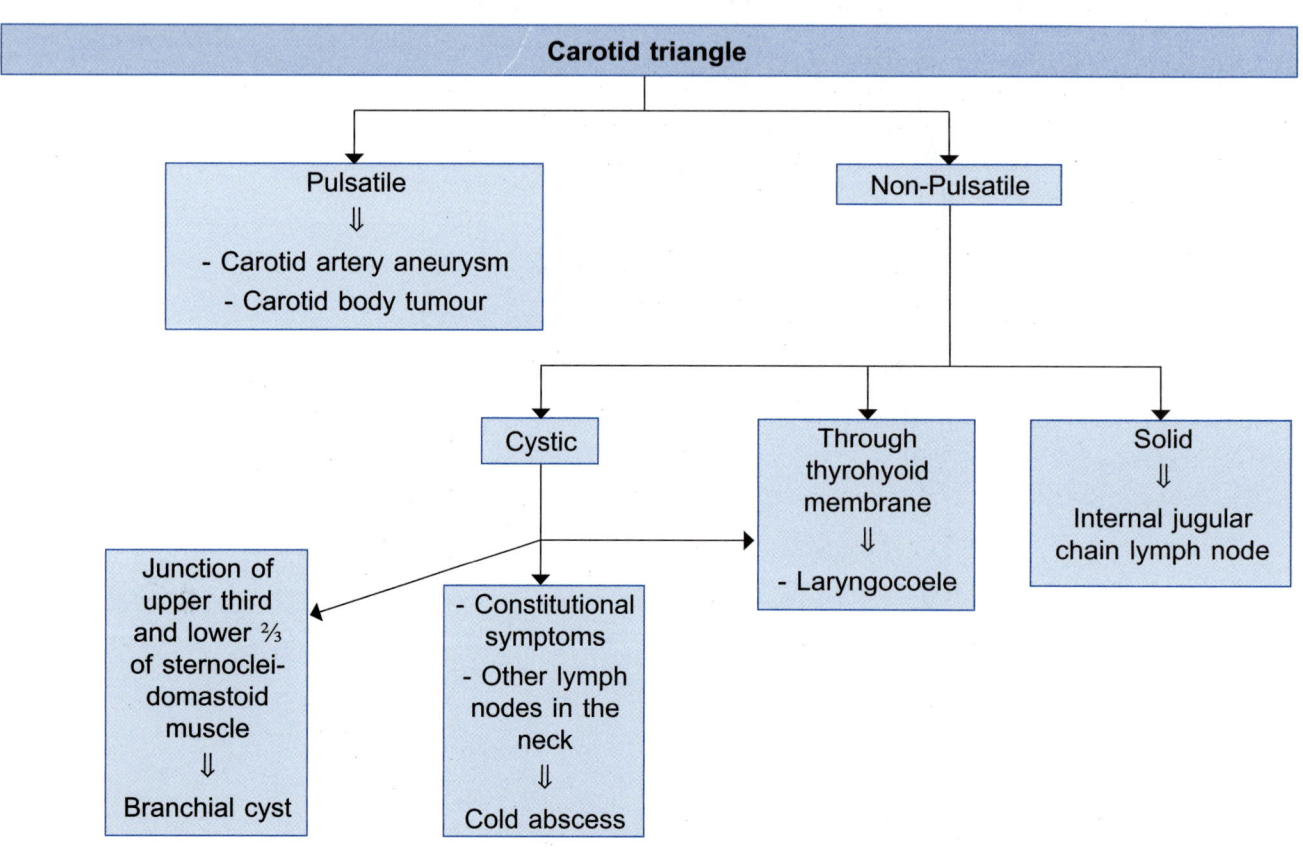

Carotid triangle

- Pulsatile
  ⇓
  - Carotid artery aneurysm
  - Carotid body tumour

- Non-Pulsatile
  - Cystic
    - Junction of upper third and lower ⅔ of sternocleidomastoid muscle
      ⇓
      Branchial cyst
    - Constitutional symptoms
    - Other lymph nodes in the neck
      ⇓
      Cold abscess
  - Through thyrohyoid membrane
    ⇓
    - Laryngocoele
  - Solid
    ⇓
    Internal jugular chain lymph node

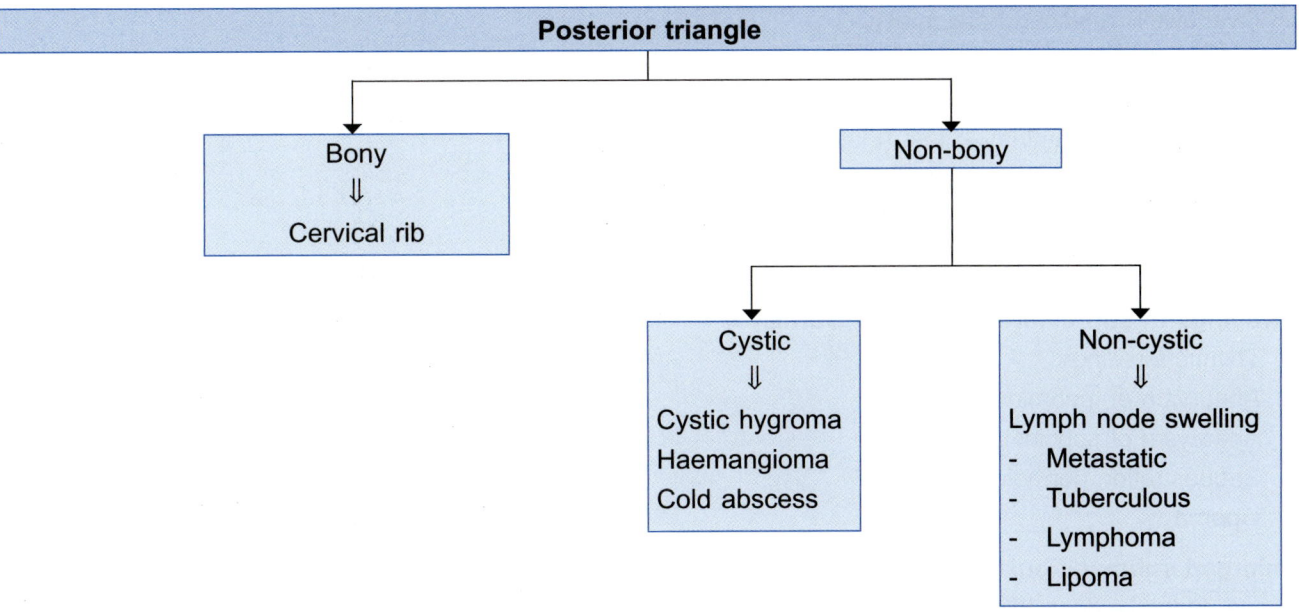

Sublingual dermoid cyst

It is a sequestration dermoid cyst occurring in the midline due to sequestration of ectodermal cells at the site of fusion of two mandibular arches. It is lined by squamous epithelium and contains sebaceous and sweat glands, but no hair.

A lateral variety also exists, arising from the 2nd branchial cleft.

Features:

- Swelling in submental region (midline variety is more common)
- Soft, cystic swelling
- Painless
- Seen in young age group
- Positive fluctuation test
- Negative transillumination test as it contains thick cheesy material

Treatment:

Excision by intraoral approach

Pretracheal and prelaryngeal lymph nodes

These lymph nodes get enlarged in the following conditions:

1. Laryngitis: In acute laryngitis, the nodes are tender and soft
2. Tuberculosis
3. Carcinoma of larynx: Metastatic nodes are hard in consistency
4. Papillary carcinoma of thyroid: It spreads via lymphatics to these nodes. The nodes would be firm to hard.

Subhyoid bursitis

The subhyoid bursa as the name suggests is located just below the hyoid bone in front of the thyrohyoid membrane. Inflammation of this bursa results in a tender swelling with collection of inflammatory fluid within. It can develop into an abscess.

Features:

- Midline subhyoid swelling
- Tender

- Oval swelling placed horizontally
- Soft, cystic
- Positive fluctuation test
- Negative transillumination test (Fluid inside is not clear)
- Swelling moves up with deglutition

Treatment:

Complete excision

Swellings in suprasternal space of Burns

1. Thymic swellings
2. Aneurysm of innominate artery
3. Aneurysm of subclavian artery
4. Sequestration dermoid cyst
5. Lipoma

Enlarged submandibular lymph nodes

These nodes lie deep to the deep fascia. They are not bimanually palpable unlike the submandibular salivary gland.

They get enlarged due to the following conditions:

1. Acute lymphadenitis: Due to dental caries causing soft, and tender enlargement of the nodes.
2. Tuberculous lymphadenitis: The nodes are firm and matted with central caseous necrosis
3. Metastasis from carcinoma of oral cavity mainly from the cheek and tongue. The nodes are hard and may be fixed.
4. Non-Hodgkin's lymphoma: The nodes are firm and rubbery in consistency

2. THYROID GLAND

- Dr. Rajiv Joshi

HISTORY

Name, age, sex, occupation, residence, religion.

Residence - Endemic areas: Foot hills of Satpuda, Ratnagiri, Subhimalayan region, Dhule, Nashik

Endemicity >10% general population

Age:
- Young - primary / physiological
- Middle aged - secondary

Endemic Areas
● Satpuda foothills
● Ratnagiri
● Dhule
● Nasik
● SubHimalayan region

Sex - Goitre commoner, in females

H/O - Swelling and onset of symptoms:

- Onset - (simultaneous or otherwise, to differentiate between primary and secondary thyrotoxicosis.)
- Sudden increase in size:
  - Malignancy
  - Haemorrhage.
  - Long duration of swelling: Multinodular goitre, Colloid goitre.

Symptoms:

- Pain in the gland : Inflammation

    Malignant change. eg: Follicular carcinoma in MNG

H/o:

1. Pressure symptoms:

- Trachea   - Inspiratory stridor
                                       - Dyspnoea
- Oesophagus   - Dysphagia
- Recurrent laryngeal nerve   - Hoarseness of voice / dysphonia
- Carotids   - Transient Ischemic attacks (TIA) / syncope
- Carotid sheath and cervical sympathetic trunk - Horner's syndrome: in Ca thyroid
- Pressure symptoms due to retrosternal goitre - Superior mediastinal compression syndrome

2. Endocrine status of the gland:

SYSTEM	HYPERTHYROIDISM	HYPOTHYROIDISM
1. **Central nervous system**	Irritability, anxiety, insomnia / altered sleep habits, restlessness Later - hyperreflexia, fine tremors	Lethargy, somnolence Normal contraction with sustained relaxation. Quadriceps Sign: feeling of give away of knees while climbing down stairs.
2. **Cardio vascular system**	Palpitations, high output cardiac failure (LVF) causing pericardial effusion, oedema feet and dyspnoea.	Congestive Cardiac failure / (RVF) causing effusions and dyspnoea.
3. **Gastrointestinal system**	Increased appetite with loss of weight, diarrhoea (Increased Basal Metabolic rate)	(N) appetite and gain in weight, constipation.

171

SYSTEM	HYPERTHYROIDISM	HYPOTHYROIDISM
4. **Skeletal system**	Weakness Wasting of muscle Osteoporosis	Weak and Flabby muscles.
5. **Skin**	Heat intolerance Warm and moist skin (increased perspiration)	Cold intolerance Skin-cold and dry, cool, pale, rough, doughy with periorbital oedema In anxiety - skin is cold and moist
6. **Genito - Urinary System**	Oligo menorrhoea Amenorrhoea	Polymenorrhagia, increased frequency of micturition
7. **Ophthalmic**	Exophthalmos, bulging of eyes with failure to close eyelids.	
8. **Respiratory system** There is dyspnoea due to pressure of the gland and CCF. There is cough (CCF/LVF) and recurrent URTI.		

Conditions where appetite increases with loss of weight:
- Hyperthyroidism
- Early Tuberculosis
- Diabetes mellitus
- Hypertrophic pyloric stenosis.

---

3. **Etiology:**
   - Drugs:
     - INH
     - Iodides
     - PAS
     - Thiouracil
   - Residence - to rule out endemic goitre
   - Irradiation:
     - H/o irradiation of neck-in adults for carcinoma
     - In children for thymoma / Hodgkin's lymphoma.
     - In young for Hodgkin's disease.
   - Stressful episodes in life:
     - Puberty
     - Pregnancy
     - Bad obstetric history
     - Mental stress.
   - Excessive ingestion of - Cabbage
     - Cauliflower   - Contaminated fish
     - Kale   - Turnip
     - Brassica family - Spinach

Etiology
- Drugs
- Endemic
- Stress
- Irradiation
- Goitrogens
- Familial

- Excessive flourine uptake
- Family h/o - enzyme linked disorders.

4. Investigations done and treatment taken:
Investigations:
- FNAC - may cause tenderness.
- X-ray neck
- USG neck
- Thyroid scan
- CT scan
- Indirect laryngoscopy (IDL)
- Blood investigations.

Treatment:
- Drugs - antithyroid drugs
- Surgery
- Irradiation

> **Positive Response to treatment:**
> - Increase in appetite
> - Weight gain
> - Decrease in sleeping pulse rate
> - Decrease T3, T4 levels.

5. Malignant changes and metastatic symptoms:
- Skeletal mets   -   Bone pains
  - Pathological fractures
  - Paraparesis
- Pulmonary mets   -   Dyspnoea
  - Haemoptysis, cough
- Cranial mets   -   Headache, convulsions, motor deficit
- Liver mets   -   Jaundice, ascites, lump in abdomen (hepatomegaly)
- Lymph node mets -   Painful lymphadenopathy with ulceration

6. Evidence of other hormonal deficits e.g. secondary sex characteristics

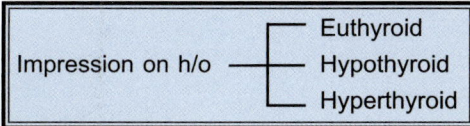

Impression on h/o
- Euthyroid
- Hypothyroid
- Hyperthyroid

Past History:
- Previous surgery
- Medical therapy for toxicity

Family History:
- Familial cause :   Deficiency of enzyme dehalogenase
  Medullary carcinoma thyroid
- Pendred syndrome   :   Goitre + congenital deafness
  Hypothyroidism
  Absence of enzyme peroxidase

GENERAL EXAMINATION

- Built and nourishment (usually poor) Look for :   Pallor
  Lymphadenopathy

- Temperature:
  - Increases in hyperthyroidism
  - Decreases in hypothyroidism
- Pulse rate: Tachycardia during active examination is meaningless. It is difficult to differentiate tachycardia due to thyrotoxicosis and anxiety

  To differentiate - sleeping pulse rate is taken. Sleeping pulse rate is taken either 4 hours after sleep (REM sleep) / by sedating the patient with diazepam - for a full 1-3 minutes for 3 consecutive days at around the same time and the average is calculated.

  (Patients with II° thyrotoxicosis have cardiac arrhythmias and hence taken for 3 minutes over 3 days)

  Importance of sleeping pulse rate
  - Helps to grade severity of thyrotoxicosis

    90-100   -   mild

    100-110 -   moderate

    > 110   -   severe
  - Helps judge response to treatment

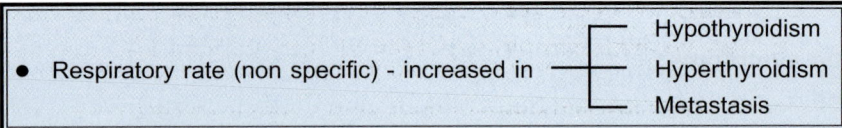

- Blood Pressure: Changes seen in secondary thyrotoxicosis.
- Tremors: Fine tremors of the hand are elicited by asking the patient to extend his upper extremities with palms facing downwards and fingers stretched apart. A piece of paper is kept over the stretched fingers. They are seen in Graves' disease
  - Tongue tremors
  - Uvula tremors

Tremors: Site:
● Hand / fingers
● Tongue
● Uvula

- Oedema feet: Congestive cardiac failure, pretibial myxoedema
- Lymphadenopathy - cervical in :   -   Thyroiditis

                                    -   Carcinoma
- Raised Jugular Venous Pressure in congestive cardiac failure.
- Examination of oral cavity for: Lingual thyroid

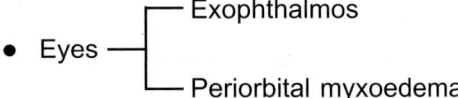

- Eyes ┬─ Exophthalmos

       └─ Periorbital myxoedema
- Skin changes, if any

LOCAL EXAMINATION

Inspection - Single, ovoid swelling, in the midline of the neck, which moves with deglutition, of size _____ cms x _____ cms, and extending from the hyoid bone above, to _____ cms above suprasternal notch (vertical extent) and from one sternomastoid to the other (lateral extent).

Swelling:
- Number
- Size
- Shape
- Movement with deglutition
- Extent

- Surface: Smooth / nodular

> **Surface: Goitre**
>
> - Smooth   :   • Adenoma
>   - Puberty goitre
>   - Graves' disease
> - Nodular: Multinodular goitre
> - Irregular: Carcinoma thyroid

- Skin over the swelling
  - Scars / sinuses
  - Pulsations
  - Dilated veins

> **D/D of midline neck swellings which move with deglutition.**
> - Thyroid gland swelling
> - Thyroglossal cyst
> - Laryngocoele
> - Subhyoid bursitis
> - Prelaryngeal lymph nodes (Delphian lymph nodes)
> - Pretracheal lymph nodes
> - External Ca of larynx

GOITRE	THYROGLOSSAL CYST
• Moves with deglutition • Does not move with protrusion of tongue	• Moves with deglutition • As well as with protrusion of tongue (tested after fixing the mandible)

> **Goitre is differentiated from rest by:**
> - History
> - FNAC
> - Thyroid scan

> ["Any midline swelling of neck which moves with deglutition is thyroid swelling unless proved otherwise.]

> **Situations when thyroid will not move with deglutition:**
> - Carcinoma thyroid
> - Subacute / Riedel's thyroiditis
> - Post operative thyroid.
> - Post irradiation.
> - Large goitre which retrosternal extension.

Platysma sign:

In carcinoma thyroid, nodules in skin occur with puckering / dimpling on tensing the platysma.

Pemberton's sign

1. Inspection
2. Percussion

Inspection:

- Ask patient to raise his arms and look for   :   Congestion of face
                                                                      Engorgement of neck veins
                                                                      Respiratory discomfort

Direct percussion:

Over manubrium sterni produces a dull note in retrosternal goitre

Types of retrosternal goitre		
• Substernal	:	Lower limit of gland can be seen on deglutition.
• Intra thoracic	:	Lower limit of gland can't be seen even on deglutition
• Plunging	:	Swelling appears on coughing and goes down again.

Clinical Importance of Retrosternal Goitre

- Superior mediastinal compression syndrome (SMCS)
- Anti-thyroid drugs are given with caution since gland may increase in size and precipitate or exacerbate SMCS.

    Diagnosis   -   Xray chest
                           -    CT scan.

Surgical approaches:

- Kocher's (skin crease) incision, as vascular control has to be achieved in the neck.
- Gland can then be removed piecemeal.
- A sternal split may be required for extremely large and vascular RSG.

PALPATION OF THYROID GLAND

Normally thyroid gland is not palpable.

4 methods of palpation:

- From back of the patient with cups of hand (standard)
- Lahey's method.
- Pizillo's method
- Crile's method.

- **Palpation from behind (Standard method)**
    Advantages:
    - Concavity of hand fits into convexity of neck.
    - Palpation is facilitated with pulp of fingers which are more sensitive.
    - Patient is less anxious than when palpated from front.
    - Gland palpation is better with neck flexed, since platysma and other muscles are relaxed

- **Lahey's method:**
    - Thyroid is palpated from front with neck flexed.
    - One lobe is made prominent by pushing the gland on other side and then palpated.
    - Similarly palpated on other side.

- **Pizillo's method:**
    - Employed in fat females with short neck.
    - Neck extended (no hyperextension)
    - Gland palpated from front.

- **Crile's method:**
  - For solitary thyroid nodule.
  - Palpation with flat of thumb.

On Palpation:

- Findings of inspection are confirmed.
- **Temperature over gland is increased in**:
  - Thyroiditis
  - Vascular tumours
  - Thyrotoxicosis
- **Tenderness is present in**:
  - Thyroiditis
  - Malignancy (due to to haemorrhage and necrosis)
- **Thrill** :
  - Felt at superior pole of gland.
  - Present in thyrotoxicosis because of hyperdynamic circulation and numerous A-V fistulae.
- **Consistency**:
  - Stony hard - Malignancy, Riedel's thyroiditis
  - Rubbery - Hashimoto's thyroiditis
  - Firm - Colloid goitre
  - Soft - Graves' disease
- **Mobility** : - Fixed in malignancy.

  Palpation of cervical lymphnodes is to be carried out to rule out hard, fixed lymph nodes seen in thyroid carcinoma.

Relation to Surrounding Structures:

- Trachea: Pressure effect on trachea is tested by:
  - Kocher's test - compression of the gland and hence of trachea leading to an inspiratory stridor is a positive test.

    Positive test is seen in long standing benign goitres.

    Negative test: malignancy.

> **Scabbard Trachea:**
> Pressure atrophy of posterior wall
> Benign enlargement of thyroid gland.

  Pressure on the lateral sides of the gland causes narrowing of tracheal lumen and therefore inspiratory stridor.

  In Malignancy - trachea flattens out and pressure on lateral sides of the swelling causes an increase in diameter of the tracheal lumen and therefore no stridor is seen.

- Shift of trachea - Traile's sign

  Traile's sign: Prominence of sternomastoid on the side of shift of trachea.

- Carotids -

  In a normal individual carotid pulsations are palpable against the tubercle of the transverse process of C6 vertebra (Chassagnaec tubercle). A positive Berry's sign is one in which carotid pulsations are not palpable.

  Berry's sign:

POSITIVE	NEGATIVE
Malignancy Reidel's thyroiditis	Benign goitre

- **Sternomastoids:**

  Extent of the gland and involvement of sternomastoid is tested by contracting the sternomastoid against resistance.

  With patient sitting in front of you, put right hand to check the patient's right sternomastoid.

- **Cervical sympathetic trunk:**

  Involved in malignancy - Horner's syndrome

PERCUSSION

Direct percussion over manubrium sterni

Dullness - Plumberton's sign positive in retrosternal goitre

Resonance - normal

> **Horner's Syndrome:**
> - Ptosis
> - Miosis
> - Anhydrosis
> - Loss of ciliospinal reflex

AUSCULTATION

Bruit heard over the superior pole of gland in toxic goitre

Bruit is heard over superior pole:

- Superior thyroid artery is a direct branch of external carotid artery
- Superior thyroid artery is more superficial than the inferior artery

Examination of other systems:

- For endocrine status
- Metastasis
- Complications

- **Per abdomen:**
  - Hepatosplenomegaly in Hashimoto's thyroiditis
  - Hepatomegaly due to metastasis in carcinoma thyroid (present usually if lung mets are also present)
- **Cardiovascular system:**
  - Ejection systolic murmur in thyrotoxicosis.
  - Loud S1, S2.
  - Pericardial rub in congestive cardiac failure
- **Central nervous system**

  Cranial metastasis.

  Hyperthyroidism - hyperreflexia / i.e. brisk contraction and relaxation

  Hypothyroidism - normal contraction and sustained relaxation.
- **Musculo skeletal system:** Wasting of muscles - hypothyroidism
- **Respiratory system:** Crepitations in congestive cardiac failure in thyrotoxicosis.
- **Eye signs:**
  1. **Exophthalmos:**

> **Causes of Exophthalmos in thyrotoxicosis:**
> - Increased intraorbital congestion.
> - Retroorbital fibrofatty and glycogen deposition.
> - Paresis of extraocular muscles which support the eyeball.
> - Exophthalmos producing substances.

Differential diagnosis of exophthalmos:
- Idiopathic
- Thyrotoxicosis.
- Cushing's syndrome
- Retroorbital tumours:
    - Retinoblastoma
    - Craniopharyngioma
    - Antral tumours
- Cavernous sinus thrombosis
- Haemangioma (pulsatile)
- Retinal artery aneurysm.

Eye signs in thyroid:
- Joffroy's sign
- Moebius sign
- Dalrymple's sign
- Nafzigger's sign
- Gifford's sign
- Ballet's sign
- Anroth's sign
- Jellinger's sign
- Stellwag's sign
- Von graeffe's sign
- Rosenbach's sign
- Becker's sign

Diagnosis of exophthalmos:
- With the patient. looking straight:
    - Normally: Either one limbus present at 6/12 O'clock position or none is seen
    - Exophthalmos: Both are seen simultaneously.
- Accurate diagnosis - Measurement by Kelly's exophthalmometer:
    - Distance between limbus and outer canthus of eye: is 16-23 mm
    - Exophthalmos: >23 mm. It does not hold good in squints.

Signs for exophthalmos:
- Joffroy's sign   : Absence of wrinkling of forehead on looking upwards with face inclined downwards
- Moebius sign   : Convergence of eye is difficult.
- Dalrymple's sign   : Increased width of palpebral fissure.
                                      Test: Finger brought suddenly from distance to nose.
- Nafzigger's sign   : Tangential view (from patient's back) over the forehead shows protruding eyeballs.
- Gifford's sign   : Difficulty in passively everting upper eyelid.
- Feeling of resistance : When pressure is applied to eyeballs (due to retroorbital congestion and fibrofatty deposition).

2. Ophthalmoplegia (Ballet's sign)

Inability to move the eyeball completely. The superior rectus and inferior oblique are particularly affected and range of movement is diminished. Patient cannot look up and out.

3. Chemosis (Anroth's sign):
- Oedema of the conjunctiva and lids.
- Caused by obstruction of normal venous and lymphatic drainage of the conjunctivae by increased retroorbital pressure.

4. Jellinger's sign: Pigmentation of skin of eyelids.

5. Eye signs due to increased sympathetic activity:
- Stellwag's sign: Retraction of the upper eyelid with infrequent blinking. This sign is caused by an overactivity of involuntary (smooth) muscle part of levator palpebrae superioris. If the upper eyelid is higher than normal and lower lid in its correct position, patient has no lid retraction.
- Von graeffe's sign:

  Lagging behind of upper eyelid on looking downwards

  If upper eyelid doesn't keep pace with eyeball as it follows a finger moving from above downwards (at accommodation distance), patient's eyelid has lid lag.
- Rosenbach's sign: Fine tremors of eyelid
- Becker's sign: Abnormal pulsations of retinal arteries on fundoscopy.

6. Epiphora
7. Diplopia
8. Photophobia.

DIAGNOSIS

- A - year old, male / female patient, a case of
- Toxic / non-toxic
- Multinodular goitre / diffuse, smooth / solitary thyroid nodule
- With / without pressure symptoms
- With / without retrosternal extension
- With / without eye signs.

INVESTIGATIONS IN A THYROID CASE

A. Haematological and biochemical:
- Haemoglobin: anaemia correction.
- Total / differential WBC count: If low counts, then anti-thyroid drugs are not given, since they may cause agranulocytosis.
- ESR: Increased in thyroiditis.
- BUN / Sr. creatinine: Increased levels in thyrotoxic myopathy.
- Serum cholesterol : - Increased in hypothyroidism.
  - Decreased in hyperthyroidism.
- Blood sugar ┬ Fasting
  └ Post-prandial (PP)
- Serum electrolytes.

- **Thyroid function tests:**
  - T3, T4 levels.
  - TSH estimation.
  - Estimation of thyroid antibodies / thyroid immunoglobulin (LATS)
    Increased in: - Hashimoto's thyroiditis
                   - Graves' disease
  - Antimitochondrial antibodies (AMA)
  - Thyrotropin releasing hormone (TRH) test

CLINICAL STATE	TSH	T_3, T_4
Hyperthyroidism	⇓	⇑
Hypothyroidism	Ⓝ/⇑	⇓
Euthyroid	Ⓝ	Ⓝ

In clinically euthyroid patient's, also estimation of T3, T4 is a must to detect subclinical hyperthyroidism, which may manifest as 'thyroid storm' during surgery. Also 6-10% of patients with a normal sleeping pulse rate may have latent Thyrotoxicosis.

B. Radiological:
  - X-ray neck
    - Anteroposterior
    - Lateral view
    - Position of trachea for intubation
    - Calcification in thyroid

D / D: Calcification in thyroid:
- Fine stippled calcification: Psammoma bodies in papillary carcinoma
- Sparse, coarse calcification: Long standing benign goitres.
- Calcification also seen in: - Medullary carcinoma
                               - Anaplastic carcinoma

  - X-ray chest (PA) : - Tuberculosis
                        - Retrosternal goitre
                        - Secondary metastasis in lung
  - USG of thyroid : - For morphology
                      - Solid / cystic lesions.
  - Thyroid scan (I^{125} and I^{131}) :
    - Activity (function) of gland.
    - Morphology of gland: especially in solitary nodule to rule out carcinoma
  - CT scan : - Neck - in carcinoma
              - Thorax - in retrosternal goitre

C. Miscellaneous:
  - **Electrocardiogram: Cardiac changes**

HYPOTHYROIDISM	HYPERTHYROIDISM
• Low voltage ECG	• Sinus tachycardia
• Bradycardia	• ST-T changes
• Inverted 'T' waves	• Arrhythmias

- **Sleeping pulse rate**
- **Indirect laryngoscopy:** In 2% of general population, there is intrinsic vocal cord palsy. These cases have to be detected, as well as those who have recurrent laryngeal nerve damage due to carcinoma for medicolegal purposes.
- **Ankle tendon reflex duration by**
  - Phototomyography
  - Electromyography

  Hyperthyroid - brisk contraction and relaxation

  Hypothyroid - normal contraction and sluggish relaxation

  ### Diagnosis of:
  - Physiological goitre
  - Colloid goitre
  - Carcinoma

- **FNAC -** limited role in:
  - MNG
  - Follicular ca - cannot differentiate between follicular adenoma and carcinoma
- - BMR - obsolete now
  - Presently, **Resting energy metabolism (REM)** is estimated.

    Both these are increased in case of hyperthyroidism.
- Kelly's exophthalmometer - exophthalmometry.

TREATMENT

Overall view

A. Diffuse, smooth, non-toxic goitre:

(ie. either physiological / endemic goitre)

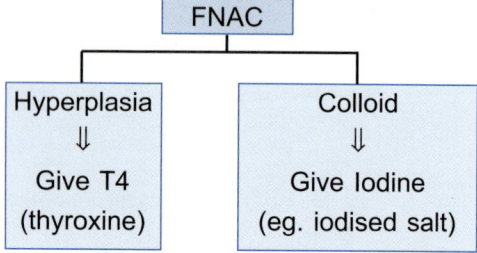

B. Solitary thyroid nodule: Refer pg 177

C. Primary toxic goitre:
- Medical treatment followed by medical treatment throughout.
- Medical treatment followed by surgical treatment.

D. Secondary toxic goitre:
- Medical treatment always.

1. MEDICAL RX

A. Supportive Rx:
- Admit patient (thyrotoxic) in a cool (A/c), quiet, cosy corner of the ward - to allay anxiety and irritability

- Tepid water sponging to decrease temperature
- Oral / I.V. fluids.

Correction of catabolic state:

- High protein diet.
- Vitamins
- Correction of anaemia - haematinics

B. Drugs:

- Diazepam - sedative and anxiolytic 10 mg Hs.
- Antithyroid drugs:
  - Carbimazole - 40 mg / day in divided doses and to suppress TSH - thyroxine in low doses (0.1 mg)

Disadvantages of carbimazole:

- Long duration of treatment
- Expensive
- Takes longer time to act
- Prolonged use causes   :   - Agranulocytosis,
  - Drug rash
  - Sore throat
  - Diarrhoea
- Makes gland more vascular and causes enlargement of gland, hence to be given with caution in retrosternal goitre / when pressure symptoms are present.
- Patient may slip under effect of drug and relapse again.
- Regular monitoring of CBC is required.
- Propylthiouracil 100-150 mg / day in divided doses and little doses of T4 to suppress TSH.

C. Propranolol: 20-40 mg TDS

Contraindication   :   - Bronchial asthma
  - Congestive cardiac failure
  - Myocardial ischaemia
  - Arrhythmias and heart block

D. Lugol's iodine: given 10 days prior to surgery. Dose 5-15 drops / day discontinued 2 days before the operation.

Response to therapy is judged by:

- Sleeping pulse rate
- Patient's sleep pattern
- Weight gain
- Confirmation by biochemical levels of T_3, T_4, TSH

Lugol's iodine (orally)

- It makes the gland firmer and hence easy to handle during surgery
- It decreases vascularity of gland.

  Precaution: since it causes an increase in size of gland, it is to be given with caution in patients with retrosternal goitre.

- It is also indicated during a thyroid storm.

2. SURGICAL MODALITY OF TREATMENT - SUBTOTAL THYROIDECTOMY (STT)

Indications for surgery (3F's)

- Medical Rx not fancied - for socioeconomic or other reasons like patient's incompliance.
- Medical Rx fails.
- Medical Rx not feasible.

  eg:-   Multi-nodular toxic goitre

- Diffuse goitre with pressure effects.
- Side effects of medical treatment
- Retrosternal goitre

Contraindications for surgery:

- High risk patients
- Thyrocardiac patients
- Recurrence of thyrotoxicosis after previous surgery

Advantages of surgery:

- Radical cure of disease is obtained
- Suitable for patients < 35 years

- Suitable when medical Rx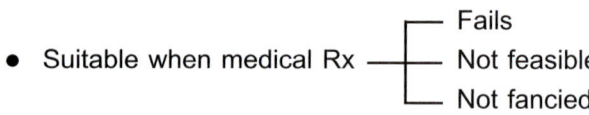
  - Fails
  - Not feasible
  - Not fancied

Disadvantages of surgery:

- Complications - haemorrhage, recurrent laryngeal nerve damage etc.
- Recurrence - due to inadequate removal of gland.

3. RADIOACTIVE IODINE THERAPY

The isotope used is I131 which emits β rays which destroys the thyroid cells. The isotope gets concentrated in the thyroid gland.

Dosage :   8-10 millicuries on empty stomach.

Indications :
- High risk patients
- Thyrocardiac patients
- Recurrence of thyrotoxicosis after previous surgery / drug treatment. (hot nodule)

Contraindications:
- Patients < 40 years of age
- Pregnancy

Advantages :
- Easy mode of administration
- Ideal for high risk and thyrocardiac patients

Disadvantages:
- Radiation thyroiditis
- May induce malignant changes
- Development of hypothyroidism
- Requires strict follow-up and patient should be intelligent enough to void urine in a safe place
- Infertility (therefore contraindicated before 40 years of age)
- Relatively small group of patients can be subjected to this mode of treatment

TREATMENT: (OF INDIVIDUAL CASES)

- **Hot nodule:**
  - Antithyroid drugs
  - After patient becomes euthyroid / toxicity controlled - hemithyroidectomy
  - If patient refuses surgery - radioactive I_2 treatment to ablate the nodule

- **Warm nodule:**
  - Usually patient left alone and kept under observation.
  - If patient worried about cosmesis : - Hemithyroidectomy (or)
    - Resection and enucleation

- **Cold nodule:**

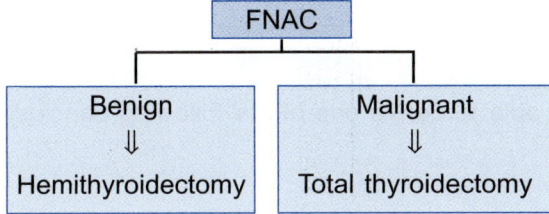

- **Diffuse smooth non-toxic goitre:**

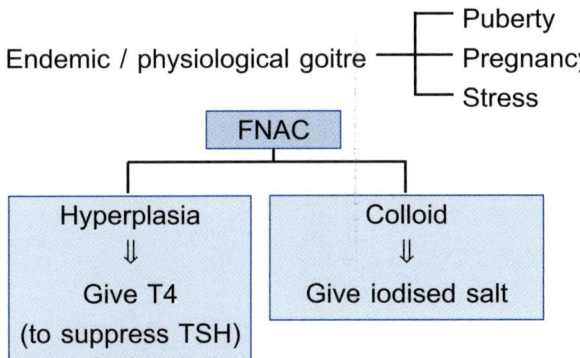

Indications for Sx:
- Cosmetic disfigurement
- Pressure symptoms
- Failure of conservative line of Rx

  Surgical treatment - subtotal thyroidectomy (STT)

  (formerly - partial thyroidectomy was done)

- **Multi nodular non-toxic goitre:**

  Rx always surgical because:
  - Doesn't respond to conservative treatment, this being an autonomous gland.
  - Compression symptoms common with multinodular goitre
  - Cosmetic disfigurement
  - Chances of secondary thyrotoxicosis are high.
  - Chances of developing malignancy are more (follicular ca)

    Surgical Rx - subtotal thyroidectomy (STT)

- **Diffuse smooth toxic goitre:**

  (Graves' disease / primary thyrotoxicosis)

3 modalities of Rx :   ● Medical

                        ● Surgical - subtotal thyroidectomy

                        ● Radioactive I_2 treatment

- **Multinodular toxic goitre (Secondary thyrotoxicosis)**
  - Medical treatment to control toxicity
  - Surgery - subtotal thyroidectomy after control of toxicity

- **Ca thyroid - Total thyroidectomy**

  In toxic goitre, patient is put on medical line of treatment to control toxicity to prevent development of thyrotoxic crisis on operation table.
  - Once toxicity is reasonably controlled, patient is subjected to surgery 6 weeks after control.
  - 7-10 days prior to surgery, patient is administered Lugol's iodine

SCHEME FOR THE DIAGNOSIS OF A THYROID SWELLING

After examination of the patient with goitre, one should be able to derive one of the following conclusions about the gland and its activity.

The Gland:
- Contains one palpable nodule (solitary thyroid nodule)
- Contains >1 palpable nodule (multinodular goitre)
- Diffusely enlarged (smooth / hyperplastic)

Activity of the gland:

Normal, hyper / hypo secretion

Normal - euthyroid (non-toxic)

Hyper -thyrotoxicosis (toxic)

Hypo - myxoedema

- **If only one swelling is palpable it may be:**
  - The only palpable nodule of multinodular goitre.
  - Whole of one lobe is usually involved by Hashimoto's Thyroiditis
  - Benign adenoma:
    - Papillary
    - Follicular
  - Carcinoma
  - Cyst caused by haemorrhage into a necrotic nodule

- **If more than 1 swelling palpable:**
  - Multinodular goitre
  - Anaplastic carcinoma

- **If there is diffuse homogenous enlargement of whole gland (hyperplasia)**
  - Graves' disease / primary thyrotoxicosis
    - Slight to moderate enlargement, diffuse, smooth, soft with a bruit
  - Hyperplastic colloid goitre
    - Moderate to gross enlargement, bosselated, no bruit
  - Thyroiditis

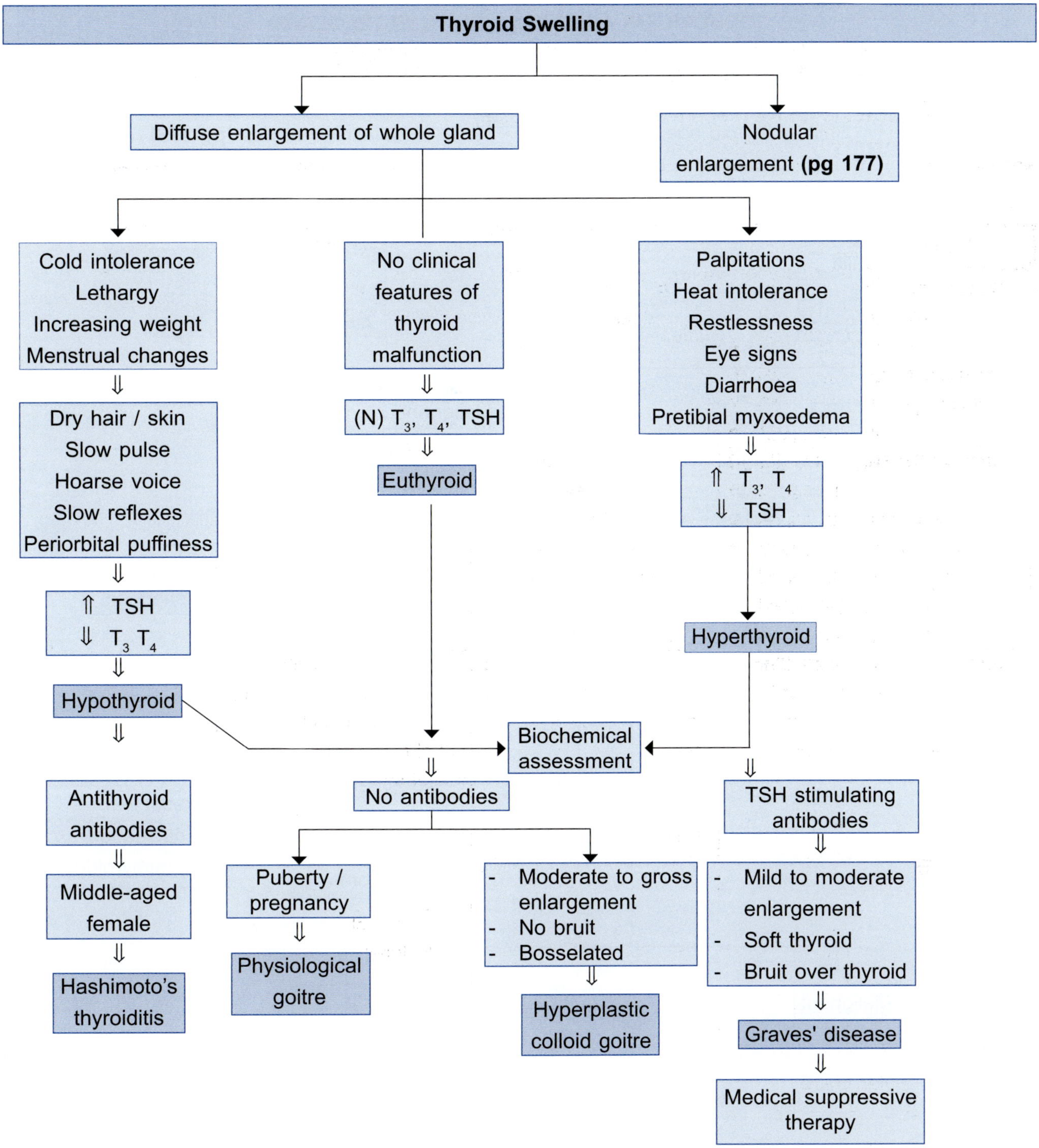

Thyroid Swelling

Diffuse enlargement of whole gland

Nodular enlargement (pg 177)

Cold intolerance
Lethargy
Increasing weight
Menstrual changes
⇓
Dry hair / skin
Slow pulse
Hoarse voice
Slow reflexes
Periorbital puffiness
⇓
⇑ TSH
⇓ T_3 T_4
⇓
Hypothyroid
⇓
Antithyroid antibodies
⇓
Middle-aged female
⇓
Hashimoto's thyroiditis

No clinical features of thyroid malfunction
⇓
(N) T_3, T_4, TSH
⇓
Euthyroid

No antibodies

Puberty / pregnancy
⇓
Physiological goitre

- Moderate to gross enlargement
- No bruit
- Bosselated

Hyperplastic colloid goitre

Palpitations
Heat intolerance
Restlessness
Eye signs
Diarrhoea
Pretibial myxoedema
⇓
⇑ T_3, T_4
⇓ TSH
⇓
Hyperthyroid

Biochemical assessment

TSH stimulating antibodies
⇓
- Mild to moderate enlargement
- Soft thyroid
- Bruit over thyroid
⇓
Graves' disease
⇓
Medical suppressive therapy

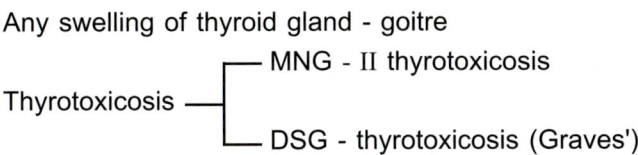

Any swelling of thyroid gland - goitre

Thyrotoxicosis ─┬─ MNG - II thyrotoxicosis
                     └─ DSG - thyrotoxicosis (Graves')

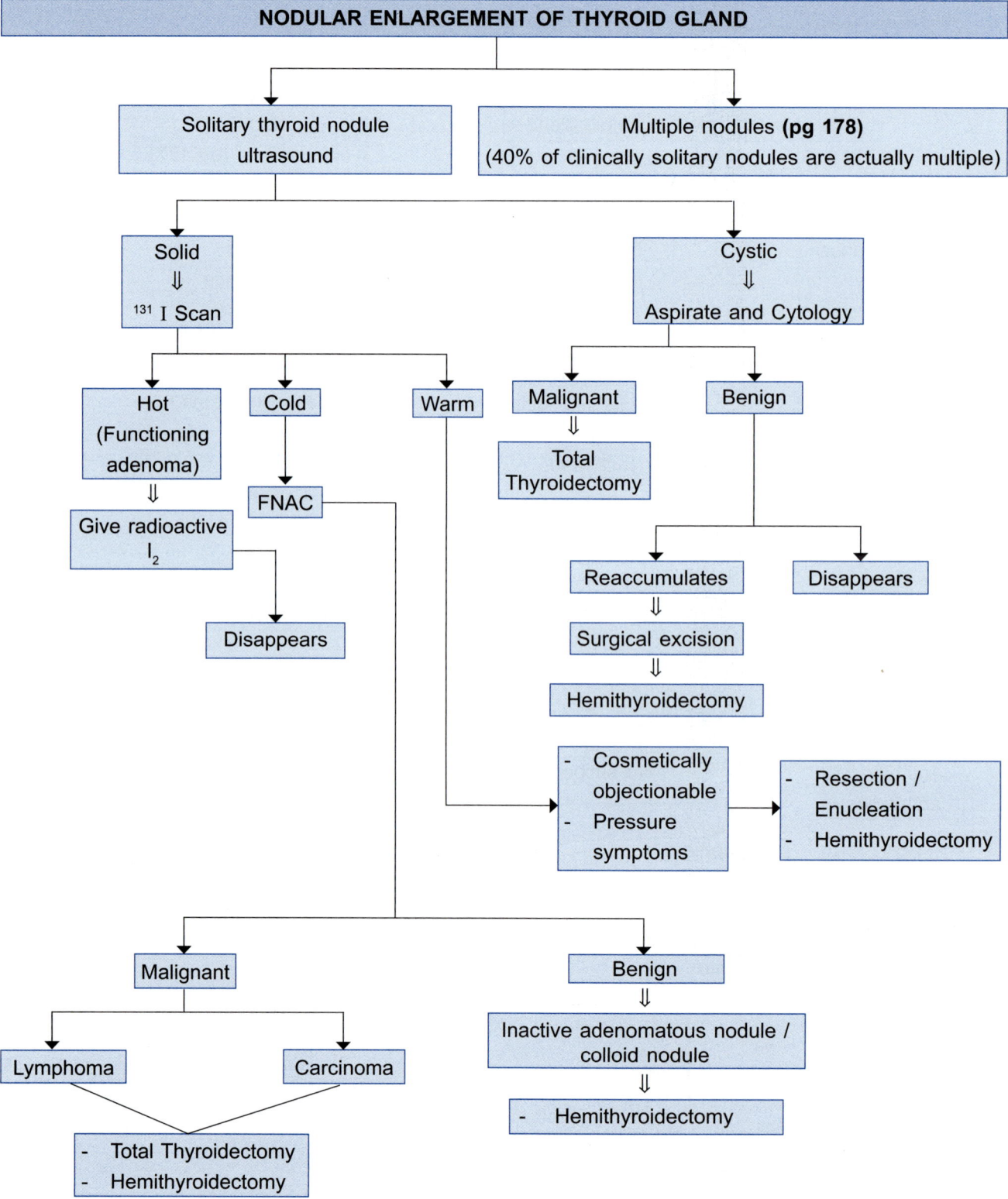

NODULAR ENLARGEMENT OF THYROID GLAND

Solitary thyroid nodule ultrasound

Multiple nodules **(pg 178)**
(40% of clinically solitary nodules are actually multiple)

Solid
⇓
^{131} I Scan

Cystic
⇓
Aspirate and Cytology

Hot
(Functioning adenoma)
⇓

Cold

Warm

Malignant
⇓

Benign

Give radioactive
I$_2$

FNAC

Total
Thyroidectomy

Disappears

Reaccumulates
⇓
Surgical excision
⇓
Hemithyroidectomy

Disappears

- Cosmetically objectionable
- Pressure symptoms

- Resection /
  Enucleation
- Hemithyroidectomy

Malignant

Benign
⇓
Inactive adenomatous nodule /
colloid nodule
⇓
- Hemithyroidectomy

Lymphoma

Carcinoma

- Total Thyroidectomy
- Hemithyroidectomy

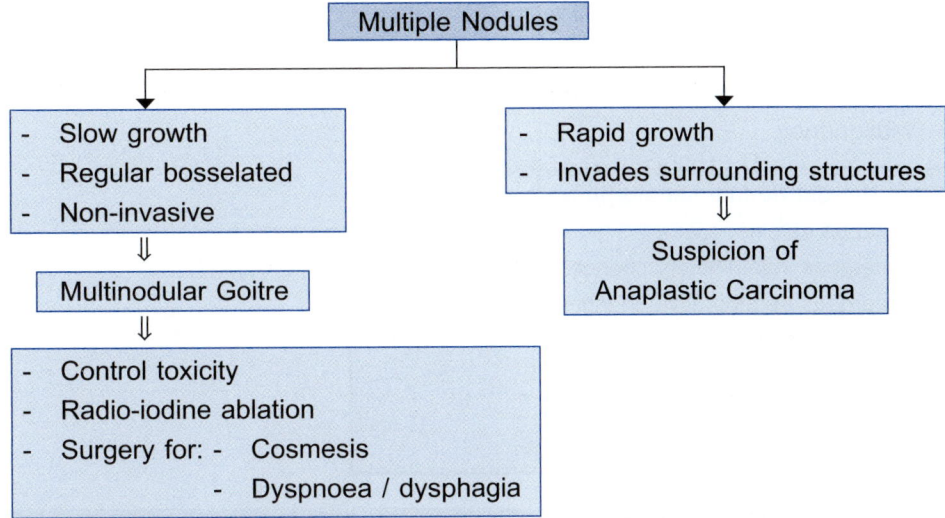

Synonym: Isolated thyroid swelling

Definitions

- It is a discrete, clearly defined swelling in the thyroid gland diagnosed by palpation. The surrounding tissue may be normal or a diffuse goitre may be present.
- A nodule is defined as an area of hyperplasia and involution following physiological / pathological changes in the thyroid gland.

Incidence: 3-4% of adult population.

Classification:

On basis of its appearance on the thyroid scintigram (i.e. thyroid scan)

1. Hot nodule : - 5% of all nodules
   - Causes hyperthyroidism
   - Predominantly observed in endemic regions in elderly.
   - Almost never malignant.
2. Cold nodule : - Commonest
   - Always considered malignant unless proved otherwise.
3. Warm nodule (neutral nodule)

Etiology:

- 3-4% of adult population
- F:M ratio 4:1
- 30-50 years age group
- External irradiation increases risk
- Positive family history increases risk

Clinical features:

- Isolated thyroid swelling
- Pain occurs due to:
   - Subacute thyroiditis
   - Haemorrhage / necrosis within nodule
   - Malignancy

- Hoarseness of voice occurs in:
  - Advanced carcinoma
  - Large benign nodule impinging on recurrent laryngeal nerve
  - Malignancy

Solitary thyroid nodule should be treated because:
- It could be carcinogenous
- It undergoes inflammatory changes
- It undergoes degenerative changes
- It bleeds in itself
- It produces pressure effects
- For cosmetic reasons
- It may be a part of a multinodular goitre

GOITRE

Causes of goitre

WITH HYPERTHYROIDISM	WITHOUT HYPERTHYROIDISM

• Graves' disease (primary thyrotoxicosis / hyperplastic toxic goitre)
• Toxic multinodular goitre (secondary thyrotoxicosis)
• Thyroiditis:
  - Chronic lymphocytic thyroiditis:
    - Autoimmune thyroiditis
    - Hashimoto's thyroiditis
  - Subacute thyroiditis
    - De quervains thyroiditis
  - Silent thyroiditis
	• Diffuse goitre of adolescence / pregnancy (hyperplastic non-toxic goitre / physiological goitre)
	• Endemic goitre (hyperplastic non-toxic goitre)
	• Drug induced goitre (hyperplastic non-toxic goitre)
	• Simple non-toxic goitre
	  - Multinodular
	  - Colloid
	  - Adenomatous
	• Thyroiditis
	  - Chronic lymphocytic thyroiditis:
	    - Autoimmune thyroiditis
	    - Hashimoto's thyroiditis
	  - Subacute
	    - De quervain's thyroiditis
	  - Riedel's thyroiditis
	  - Suppurative thyroiditis
	• Neoplasia:
	  - Anaplastic carcinoma
	  - Lymphoma
	• Dyshormonogenesis

A. WITH HYPERTHYROIDISM
- **Graves' disease / primary thyrotoxicosis:**
  - Diffuse, smooth toxic goitre
  - C/F : • Slight to moderate enlargement
    - Diffuse, smooth, soft with a bruit
    - Swelling and toxic symptoms appear simultaneously.
    - Sudden anxiety.
    - Increased appetite with loss of weight

- Eye signs marked
- Manifestations essentially of central nervous system
- Diagnosis is confirmed biochemically by:
  - Measurement of serum T3 and T4 levels. Ideally free T3 and T4 levels should be measured but facilities for such measurements aren't easily available
  - In patients with possible mild thyrotoxicosis in whom T3 and T4 measurements are equivocal, simplest way of establishing / excluding diagnosis is a thyrotropin releasing hormone (TRH) test. It is done by giving I.V. TRH. It stimulates release of pituitary TSH (peak response at about 20 minutes). Little / no TSH response occurs in thyrotoxicosis. This simple test has largely replaced radioiodine uptake studies in possible thyrotoxicosis.

- **Toxic nodular goitre:**
  - Less common cause of toxicity than Graves' disease.
  - Less severe, occurs mainly in older women.
    - **C/F** : • Swelling appears first followed by toxic symptoms over a period of time.
      - Manifestations are essentially cardiovascular.
      - It is rarely associated with extra thyroidal manifestations as exophthalmos.

  Diagnosis:
  - Multinodular gland
  - Biochemically confirmed toxicity

PRIMARY THYROTOXICOSIS (GRAVES' DISEASE)	SECONDARY THYROTOXICOSIS (TOXIC MULTI NODULAR GOITRE)
• Swelling and symptoms appear simultaneously	• Swelling first
• CNS manifestations	• CVS manifestations
• Eye signs prominent	• Eye signs less severe or absent
• Manifestations are of severe intensity	• Manifestations are of less severe intensity
• Younger women	• Older women
• Gland: diffuse, smooth	• Gland: multinodular

THYROIDITIS

1. **Chronic lymphocytic thyroiditis:**

   It is of two types:

   1. Autoimmune thyroiditis
   2. Hashimoto's thyroiditis

   It is most often seen in middle aged women.

   C/F : • Gland is enlarged, firm and bosselated.
   - Patients are usually clinically euthyroid, though hypothyroidism may occur at any time and the marginal thyroid function is commonly revealed by elevated TSH levels in the presence of normal T_4 levels.
   - Transient mild thyrotoxicosis / raised T4 levels occur infrequently

   Etiopathology:
   - Autoimmune thyroid disease, characterised by
     1. Presence of circulating thyroid antibodies.
     2. Lymphocytic infiltration on histology.
   - Elevated thyroid antibody levels are present in 75% of patients with Graves' disease and lymphocytic infiltration is also common. The spectrum of autoimmune thyroid disease includes Graves' disease together with the condition / conditions best termed - Chronic lymphocytic thyroiditis as well as myxoedema.

- Surgery, only if changes to lymphoma.
- May present as a solitary thyroid nodule when one whole lobe is involved.

2. **Chronic lymphocytic thyroiditis in subacute form (De quervain's)**

C/F : - Enlarged gland, painful and tender
- Fever
- Systemic upset with variable severity and duration

Ix : 1. Investigation of choice: FNAC
2. Cause of mild hypothyroidism, though thyroid function is more often normal.
3. Transient hyperthyroidism when present in De Quervains thyroiditis is the result of abnormal release of thyroid hormone.

CHRONIC LYMPHOCYTIC THYROIDITIS	SUBACUTE THYROIDITIS
1. Increased titres of thyroid autoantibodies	1. Absent / decrease antibody titre
2. Normal / increased radioactive I_2 uptake	2. Suppressed radio active I_2 uptake

3. **Riedel's thyroiditis:**

C/F   : • Gland stony hard.

Diagnosis : • Impossible to differentiate from anaplastic carcinoma
- Adjacent tissue infiltrated by pale, hard tumour like tissue.
- Histologically there is intense fibrous tissue deposition.

D/D   : • Ca thyroid.

Rx   : Surgery only if pressure symptoms cause:
- Respiratory distress
- Difficulty in swallowing
- Hoarseness of voice

4. **Suppurative thyroiditis**

C/F : • Gland enlarged, painful, extremely tender.
- Attributable to bacterial infection usually either staph / streptococcal.
- In most cases, source of infection is from a fistulous remnant of the 4th pharyngeal pouch.

5. **Silent thyroditis:**

- Atypical forms are without pain
- Systemic upsets are being increasingly recognised

Diagnosis of thyroiditis:

C/F : • Pain
- Fever
- Systemic upsets
- Firm, tender enlargement of thyroid

Ix : • Increased ESR
- Increased plasma globulin levels
- Decrease radio I_2 uptake in De quervain's and silent thyroiditis.
- Normal / increase radio I_2 uptake in autoimmune thyroiditis
- Normal response to TRH.

Rx : Essentially medical. The importance of thyroiditis as a cause of hyperthyroidism is that, destructive treatment, in particular surgery, should not be embarked upon, these conditions being self limiting.

B. WITHOUT HYPERTHYROIDISM

1. Adolescent diffuse goitre:

- Mild diffuse thyroid enlargement in the absence of abnormal thyroid function occurs in adolescent females and less often during pregnancy.
- Treatment - Physiologic goitre requires only reassurance.

2. Endemic goitre: (Mc Harrison theory of Iodine depletion in the soil because of running H_2O).

Etiology : Attributable to I_2 deficiency.

Incidence :
- Found in mountainous areas
- Increase incidence at foothills of Alps., sub Himalayan belt and foothills of Vindhyas (Ratnagiri's)

C/F :
- In young, the goitre is diffuse, but it progresses to nodule formation often with degenerative features.

> An endemic area is characterised by a prevalence of goitre of >10%.

3. Drug induced goitre:

- Goitrogens which interfere with thyroid hormone synthesis, resulting in over secretion of TSH which mediates the thyroid enlargement, are an uncommon cause of goitre.

> **Drugs causing goitre:**
> - Antithyroid drugs
> - Aminoglutethamide
> - Lithium carbonate
> - Sulfonylureas, sulfonamides / biguanides
> - Iodides
> - PAS (red rice grain like granules)
> - Fluorides
> - INH

4. Simple non-toxic goitre / colloid goitre

- Females : males ratio = 14:1
- Normal TSH levels
- There's an initial hyperplastic phase and excessive colloid accumulation with patchy involutation and subsequent development of nodules.

  Multinodular goitre may change to follicular carcinoma or anaplastic ca

  Nodules are:
  a. Cystic / contain colloid
  b. Solid and cellular: resembling true adenoma. Such nodules may develop autonomous function and may be responsible for hyperthyroidism

- Common features are:
  - Cyst formation
  - Haemorrhage
  - Necrosis
  - Fibrosis
  - Calcification
- Investigations: serum T_3, T_4 levels
- Ultrasound / thyroid scan are not required.

5. Dyshormonogenesis

It comprises rare inherited defects in thyroid hormone production, probably attributable to various enzyme deficiencies, that are an uncommon cause of goitre, often associated with hypothyroidism and usually present in childhood.

CLASSIFICATION

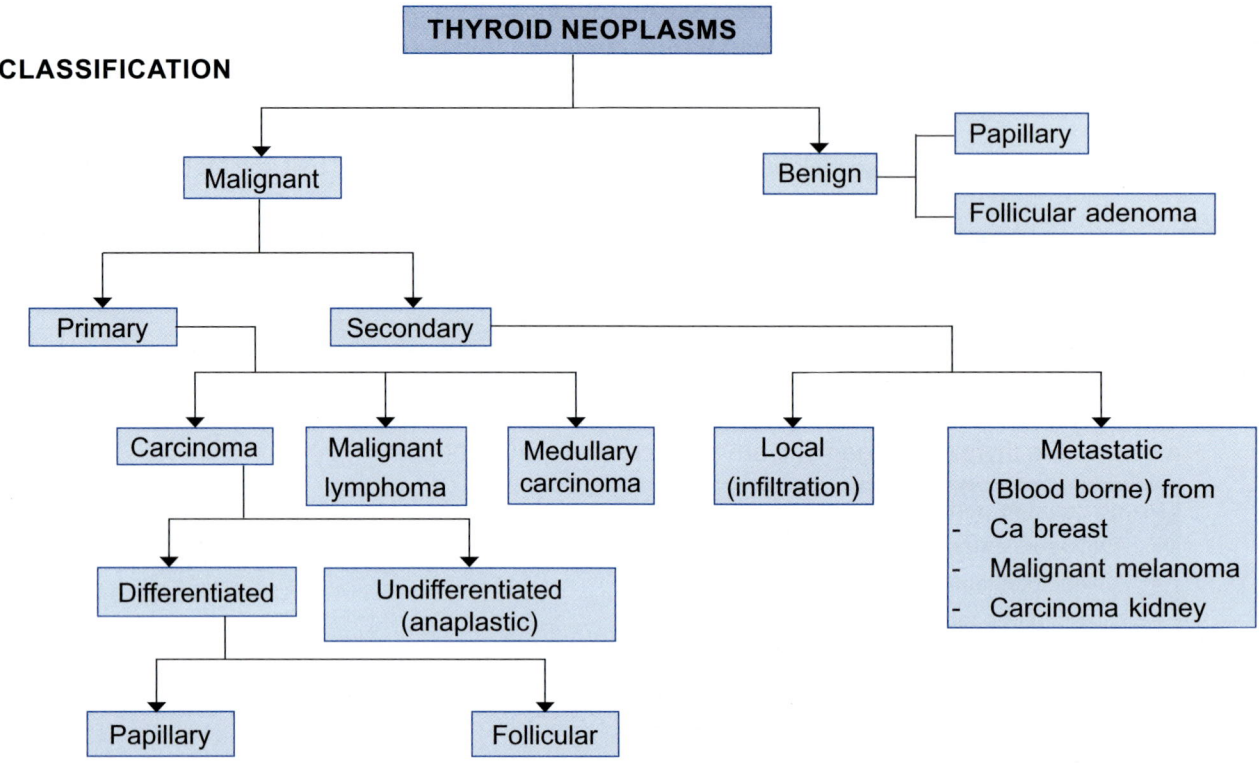

CARCINOMA THYROID

Etiology

- **Goitre** : There is a positive correlation between sporadic or endemic goitre of the multinodular type and follicular and anaplastic carcinoma. It is believed that increase TSH secretion may have a role to play.

- **Radiation** : Exposure of growing / fetal thyroid to radiation can lead to carcinoma thyroid especially, papillary carcinoma.

- **Genetic** : Heredo-familial incidence, especially seen in medullary carcinoma.

- **Autommune thyroiditis** : Leads to malignant lymphoma.

  C/F : Annual incidence - 20/1 million of population

  Sex ratio F:M = 3:1

Causes of carcinoma thyroid:
- Goitre
- Radiation
- Genetic
- Autoimmune

Presentation

- Solitary thyroid nodule.
- Clinically malignant gland (hard, fixed, irregular gland with evidence of direct spread).
- Goitre with a long history.
- Involved lymph node on the lateral side of the neck. Pain referred to the ear especially in infiltrating growths.
- Recurrent laryngeal nerve palsy
- Distant metastasis :
  - Jaundice, hepatomegaly
  - Pathological fractures, bone pains
  - Cough, haemoptysis, breathlessness

Diagnosis

- Every solitary thyroid nodule (cold) has to be taken as malignant unless proved otherwise.
- Many times diagnosis is obvious on clinical observation.
  - Thyroid scan: failure to take up radioactive iodine is characteristic of all thyroid carcinomas but also occurs in degenerating nodules and thyroiditis.
  - Thyroid antibody titre: often raised in malignancy.
  - FNAC
  - If no diagnostic test is confirmatory, exploration with frozen section is essential.

> **Thyroid scan cold nodule:**
> - Carcinoma
> - Degenerating nodules
> - Thyroiditis

SURGICAL PATHOLOGY

1. Papillary carcinoma

- Commonest
- It usually occurs in young adults
- Gross features: complex mass of papilliferous material lying in cystic spaces.
- Microscopic: glomerulus like papillary processes often arranged like a christmas tree.
- Many show some areas of follicular pattern.
- No signs of encapsulation.
- Spread: tumour is slow growing, but has a special tendency to spread via the lymphatics through the thyroid gland and outside to the nodes around superior and inferior thyroid arteries, the pretracheal lymph nodes and deep cervical nodes
- The tumour is TSH dependent and the primary tumour in thyroid may be minute and easily overlooked even when lymph nodes are involved.

> PL - papillary - lymphatic spread

- Fine calcific areas - psammoma bodies - are diagnostic features of papillary carcinoma.

> **Psammoma bodies are seen in:**
> - Papillary carcinoma of thyroid
> - Meningioma
> - Pheochromocytoma

2. Follicular carcinoma

- Less common
- It is usually seen in middle-aged females
- Gross: initially well capsulated, but local invasion and breach of capsule is always likely, cut section shows fleshy haemorrhagic and cystic areas.
- Microscopic: invasive and non-invasive tumour, colloid follicles filled with masses of epithelial cells or solid masses or trabeculae of cells.
- Spread: is essentially by blood stream (haematogenous), 50% of patients present with metastases to lungs and bones.

> FSH - follicular spreads through haematogenous

3. Anaplastic carcinoma

- Uncommon
- Occurs particularly in females > 60 years of age. Sometimes there is a goitre present for years
- Tumour grows rapidly and survival for longer than 6 months is unusual.

- Macroscopic: thyroid is hard and tender.
- Microscopic: there is considerable cell variation of giant cells, small round cells or spindle cells.
- Spread: rapid and predominantly by direct infiltration to local structures with the production of recurrent lymph nodes, sympathetic nerve lesions, dysphagia and respiratory obstruction.

> A. D. - anaplastic - direct spread

4. Medullary carcinoma

- Tumours of parafollicular / 'C' cells
- Usually occurs in 50-70 years age group and is very slow growing
- Gross: solid and circumscribed, cut surface is grey / yellow.
- Microscopic: variable amount of amyloid surrounding undifferentiated cells.
- Spread: is characteristically by lymphatic and blood stream.
- Patients with widespread medullary carcinoma have been shown to have enormously high levels of serum calcitonin.
- In some cases, tumour is familial and association with parathyroid adenomas, pheochromocytomas and multiple neuromas of the mucous membrane is present (MEN syndrome)
- Diarrhoea is a fearure in 30% of cases and this may be due to 5HT / Prostaglandins produced by tumour cells.

TREATMENT

- **Papillary carcinoma**
  - Because of multifocal nature of the disease - total thyroidectomy is usually advised.
  - Because of the high incidence of lymph node metastases; even in the occult tumours, the pretracheal and paratracheal nodes should be resected (Anterior compartment clearance). Other involved nodes (Berry picking) should be removed individually. Rarely is block dissection required. [RND on more involved side and MND on less involved side]. After operation, TSH production must be suppressed by full doses of thyroxine: 0.3-0.4 mg / day.
  - Recurrences are treated by radioactive I_2 for which tumour cells usually have a greater affinity once the gland has been removed.
  - Local deposits are managed by radiotherapy. If properly treated - the prognosis is extremely good.

  > **Advantages of total thyroidectomy:**
  > - Tumour markers will be helpful to detect metastasis or recurrences.
  > - Radioactive I_2 will be selectively taken especially by metastasis

- **Follicular carcinoma**
  - Because multiple foci are rare, wide excision by hemithyroidectomy is a good treatment.
  - Lymph nodes rarely require excision and although not particularly hormone dependent, full doses of thyroxine should be given in the post-operative period.
  - Isolated secondaries may be eradicated directly with external cobalt therapy but ^{131}I therapy offers the only prospect of success when metastasis are multiple.
  - Prognosis depends on invasive / non-invasive picture histologically.
    (Newer concept: Total Thyroidectomy for Follicular Ca).
- **Anaplastic carcinoma**
  - Extremely lethal tumours.
  - Survival for >6 months after presentation is most unusual.
  - An attempt at curative resection is only justified if there is no infiltration through thyroid capsule.

- Radiotherapy is given in all cases and may provide a worthwhile period of palliation.
- Tracheostomy following an isthumectomy is usually done to avoid respiratory obstruction.

- **Medullary carcinoma**
  - The tumour is not hormone dependent and does not take up radioiodine.
  - Prognosis depends principally on presence or absence of lymph node metastasis.
  - Treatment is by total thyroidectomy and resection of involved nodes (RND + MND)

- **Malignant lymphoma**
  - Difficult to differentiate it from a small cell anaplastic carcinoma
  - Good palliation may follow
  - Total thyroidectomy, irradiation and / or chemotherapy.

3. SALIVARY GLANDS

PAROTID GLAND

- H/o swelling
  - Below and behind the ear lobule
  - At the angle of mandible
  - In the retromandibular sulcus

Detailed history of the swelling has to be asked (onset, duration, progress) with special emphasis on:

- H/o unilateral / bilateral swelling
  - Parotid tumours are usually unilateral though Warthin's tumour may be bilateral
- H/o swelling appeared in the tail / body of the parotid gland.
  - Pleomorphic adenomas occur in the tail of the gland
  - Tumours mimicking a pleomorphic adenoma but present in the body of the gland:
    - Neuromas of facial nerve
    - Myxoma of masseter muscle
    - Lipomas
- H/o slow / rapid growth of the tumour
  - Benign tumours grow slowly whereas malignant tumours grow rapidly and may have associated sudden pain and facial nerve paralysis
  - Sudden increase in size is seen in:
    - Malignancy
    - Infection in a cyst
    - Haemorrhage in a cyst
    - Infection of lymphoid component of tumour
- H/o pain associated with the swelling.

Painless tumours	:	Pleomorphic adenoma
Painfull enlargement with meals	:	Stone obstructing the duct
Sudden appearance of pain	:	Malignant transformation
Severe pain	:	Abscess formation
Bilateral painful enlargement	:	Parotitis

- H/o involvement of skin and facial nerve

  It is seen in malignant parotid tumours, tuberculosis, sarcoidosis. Pressure from a benign tumour never causes facial paralysis. Facial paralysis may be due to previous surgery sacrificing the facial nerve. Parotid abscess may have associated skin inflammation

- H/o change in the size of gland

  It is seen in calculus or inflammatory disease of the gland. Change in size may be seen during meals

- H/o inability to open mouth or trismus

  It is seen in inflammation or malignant change

  Other History:
  - H/o watery discharge from a sinus in the parotid region (parotid fistula) or sweating in that region on meals (Frey's syndrome)

- H/o trauma to that region (parotid fistula, facial paralysis) or bursting of an abscess (parotid fistula)
- H/o enlargement of all salivary glands (Mikulicz's disease).
- H/o fever (parotitis, parotid abscess)
- H/o systemic illness

  Parotomegaly is seen in the following systemic illnesses:

  - Diabetes
  - Tuberculosis
  - Myxoedema
  - Gout
  - Cirrhosis
  - Cushing's disease
  - Alcoholism
  - Bulimia

  - Drugs
  - Contraceptive pills
  - Thiouracil

- H/o similar complaints in the past (Recurrent pleomorphic adenomas, recurrence seen after malignancy).
- H/o any medical / surgical treatment taken in the past.

Examination:
General examination
Look for
- Signs of systemic illness
- Anaemia, cachexia (malignancy)

Local examination
Inspection
- **Unilateral / bilateral**
- **Site:** in front, below and behind the ear lobule.

  It obliterates the retromandibular sulcus and shifts the ear lobule.
- **Extent / size, shape, surface:**
  - Mixed parotid tumours can be very large. Surface is nodular and bosselated.
  - Malignant tumours have an irregular surface. Inflamed gland bears the shape of the gland.
  - A blue or purplish hue over the skin might signify a vascular swelling.
- **Edge:**
  - Well defined in a tumour
  - Ill defined in parotitis
- **Fixity to surrounding structures:**
  - Fixity to masseter muscle shows no movement of the gland on clenching the teeth.
  - Skin fixity / infiltration is seen in malignant tumours.
- **Signs of facial paralysis:**

  They are seen in malignant tumours of the parotid gland and previous radical surgery.

Palpation
- **Temperature / tenderness**

  Rise in temperature and tenderness is seen in acute parotitis, parotid abscess
- **Surface:**

  Smooth   :   Benign swellings

  Irregular, nodular   :   Malignant swellings

- **Size, shape, edge**
- **Consistency**

  Firm   :   Pleomorphic adenoma

  Cystic   :   Warthin's tumour

                 Mucoepidermoid tumour

                 Parotid cyst

                 Pleomorphic adenoma

  Indurated: Parotitis

- **Fluctuation test:**

  It is positive in parotid cysts, abscess

- **Fixity:**

  It is tested at rest and by making the masseter taut and checking the movements of the swelling. They will be decreased if the swelling is fixed to the muscle.

- **Examination of facial nerve**
- **Movements of Temporo-mandibular joint:**

  Movements are decreased in inflammatory swellings and malignant tumours.

- A sinus, fistula or an ulcer over the gland is examined and mentioned in detail.

Examination of oral cavity and oropharynx:

Parotid duct:

The parotid duct opening lying against the upper second molar tooth is inspected for any signs of inflammation. The duct end over the masseter muscle is palpated by rolling the finger over the taut masseter muscle. Its terminal part can be palpated bimanually by placing the index finger in the mouth near its opening and the thumb over the cheek.

On pressing the parotid gland, pus or blood-stained discharge may extrude from its opening. This may be seen in suppurative parotitis and malignancy respectively.

Deep lobe of parotid gland:

The oropharynx is inspected to see if the ipsilateral tonsil and soft palate are pushed anteromedially by an enlarged deep lobe or parapharyngeal extension of a tumour. Swellings, seen both in the parotid region and the pharynx indicate a deep lobe tumour which pushes the parotid externally and the palate and fauces medially, thus extending into the parapharyngeal space. Such a swelling on bimaunal examination shows the typical sign of ballotment between the examining fingers which is absent in a pure parapharyngeal space tumour.

Palpation of the deep lobe:

Palpation of the deep lobe is done by placing one finger inside the mouth in front of the tonsil and behind the third molar and the other finger externally behind the ramus of the mandible.

Examination of regional lymph nodes:

The preauricular, parotid and submandibular group of lymph nodes get involved in parotid pathologies and are examined as per lymph node examination.

Auscultation:

A vascular hum on auscultation signifies a vascular swelling in the gland.

SUBMANDIBULAR SALIVARY GLAND

Apart from routine history of a swelling, specific points are listed below:

- H/o presence of swelling in the submandibular triangle (neck / floor of mouth)
- H/o increase in size of swelling with pain during meals / intake of food.

  (Submandibular calculi)

Examination:

Inspection:

On intraoral inspection the opening of the submandibular duct (Wharton's duct) may be inflamed. The orifices are situated on either side of the frenum linguae. A stone lying in the ampulla just below the orifice may be seen at times on careful inspection.

The patient may be given a sialagogue / lemon to suck to check for appearance of a swelling, confirming the presence of a stone obstructing the submandibular duct. Also two dry swab sticks can be placed on the orifices and each checked for salivation following some lemon juice drops on the tongue. A swab remaining dry suggests impaction by a stone.

Palpation:

The gland is palpated to confirm inspectory findings.

Pressure on the gland on palpation may lead to extrusion of pus from its orifice.

Bimanual palpation:

A gloved index finger placed on the floor of the mouth medial to the alveolus below the lateral border of the tongue is pressed as far back as possible along with an another finger placed externally just medial to the inferior margin of the mandible being pushed upwards. This method ensures palpation of both the lobes of the gland and can also determine the presence of a calculus in the duct. It is one of the most efficient ways of differentiating an enlarged gland from a submandibular lymph node swelling.

The submandibular lymph nodes are palpated as a part of routine examination.

SUBMANDIBULAR SALIVARY GLAND	SUBMANDIBULAR LYMPH NODES
• Single gland on each side	• Multiple nodes on either side
• Bimanually palpable	• Bimanually not palpable
• Smooth surface	• Nodular surface
• No other focus of infection	• Primary focus of infection / malignancy present elsewhere
• Enlarges on intake of lemon juice / sialagogues if ductal obstruction present	• No enlargement on any tests

Scheme I

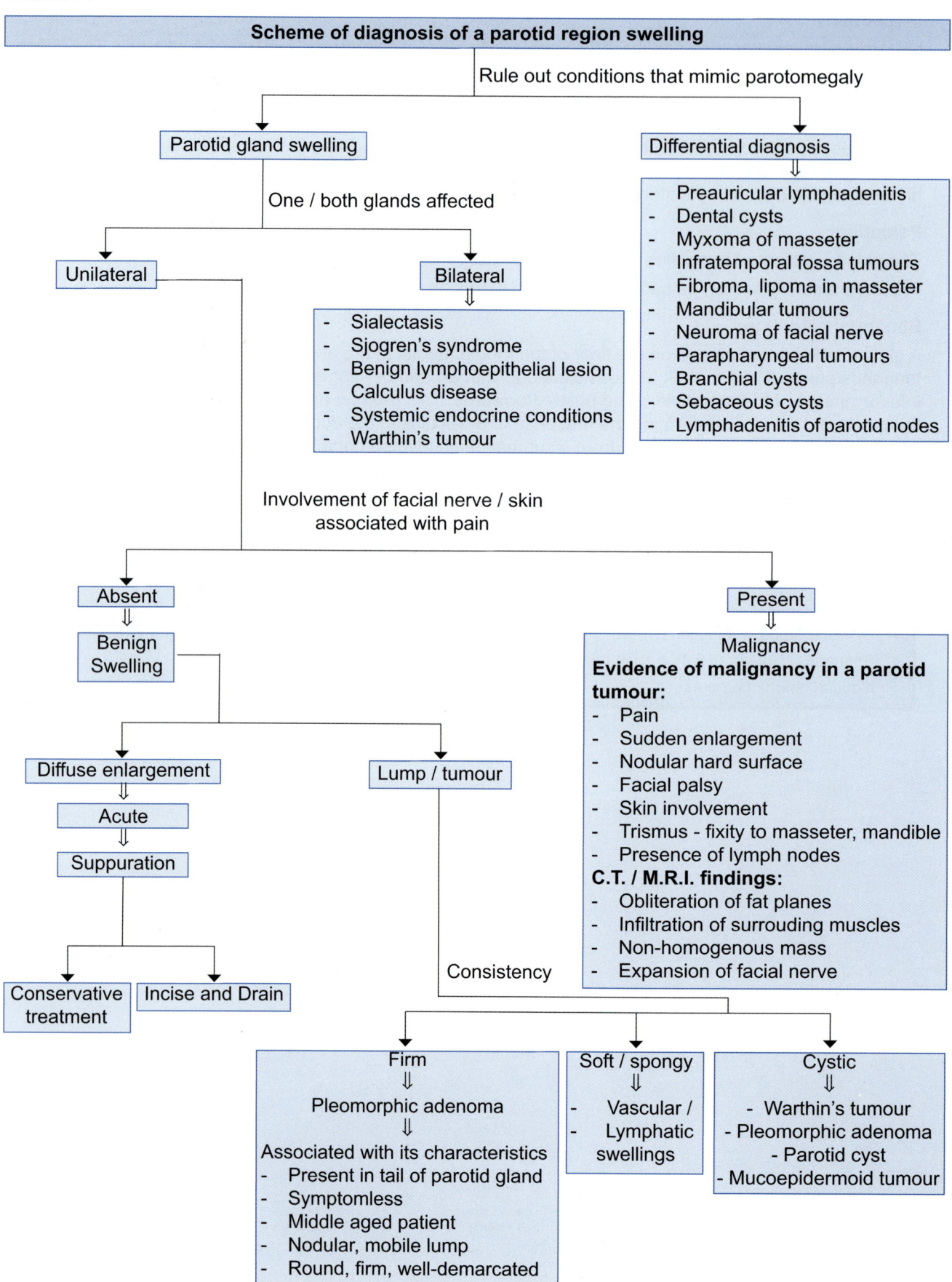

Scheme of diagnosis of a parotid region swelling

Rule out conditions that mimic parotomegaly

Parotid gland swelling

One / both glands affected

Unilateral

Bilateral
- Sialectasis
- Sjogren's syndrome
- Benign lymphoepithelial lesion
- Calculus disease
- Systemic endocrine conditions
- Warthin's tumour

Differential diagnosis
- Preauricular lymphadenitis
- Dental cysts
- Myxoma of masseter
- Infratemporal fossa tumours
- Fibroma, lipoma in masseter
- Mandibular tumours
- Neuroma of facial nerve
- Parapharyngeal tumours
- Branchial cysts
- Sebaceous cysts
- Lymphadenitis of parotid nodes

Involvement of facial nerve / skin
associated with pain

Absent

Benign Swelling

Present

Malignancy
Evidence of malignancy in a parotid tumour:
- Pain
- Sudden enlargement
- Nodular hard surface
- Facial palsy
- Skin involvement
- Trismus - fixity to masseter, mandible
- Presence of lymph nodes

C.T. / M.R.I. findings:
- Obliteration of fat planes
- Infiltration of surrouding muscles
- Non-homogenous mass
- Expansion of facial nerve

Diffuse enlargement

Acute

Suppuration

Lump / tumour

Conservative treatment

Incise and Drain

Consistency

Firm
Pleomorphic adenoma
Associated with its characteristics
- Present in tail of parotid gland
- Symptomless
- Middle aged patient
- Nodular, mobile lump
- Round, firm, well-demarcated

Soft / spongy
- Vascular /
- Lymphatic swellings

Cystic
- Warthin's tumour
- Pleomorphic adenoma
- Parotid cyst
- Mucoepidermoid tumour

Scheme II

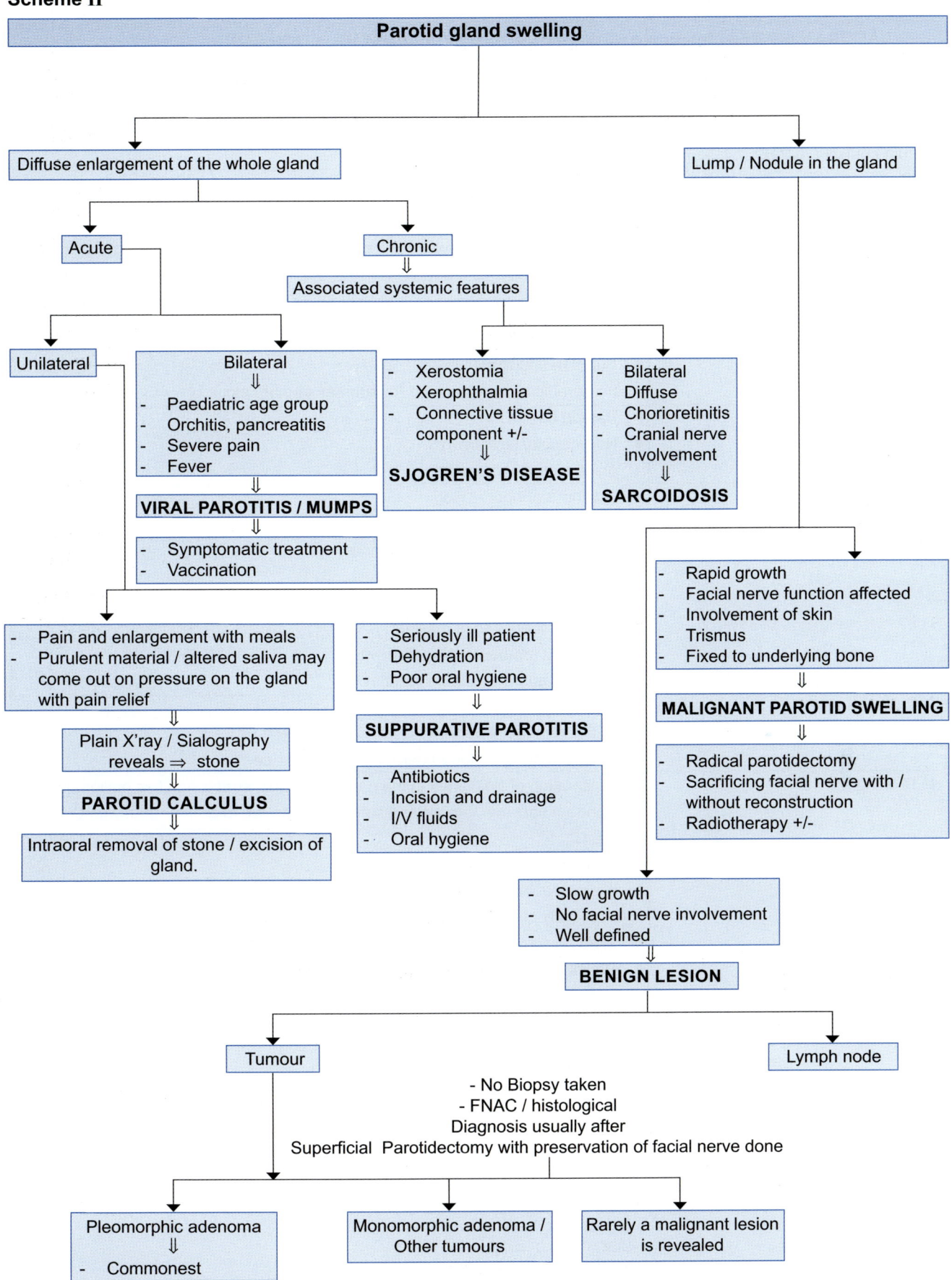

Parotid gland swelling

Diffuse enlargement of the whole gland | Lump / Nodule in the gland

Acute | Chronic ⇓

Associated systemic features

Unilateral | Bilateral ⇓
- Paediatric age group
- Orchitis, pancreatitis
- Severe pain
- Fever
⇓
VIRAL PAROTITIS / MUMPS
⇓
- Symptomatic treatment
- Vaccination

- Xerostomia
- Xerophthalmia
- Connective tissue component +/-
⇓
SJOGREN'S DISEASE

- Bilateral
- Diffuse
- Chorioretinitis
- Cranial nerve involvement
⇓
SARCOIDOSIS

- Pain and enlargement with meals
- Purulent material / altered saliva may come out on pressure on the gland with pain relief

Plain X'ray / Sialography reveals ⇒ stone
⇓
PAROTID CALCULUS
⇓
Intraoral removal of stone / excision of gland.

- Seriously ill patient
- Dehydration
- Poor oral hygiene
⇓
SUPPURATIVE PAROTITIS
⇓
- Antibiotics
- Incision and drainage
- I/V fluids
- Oral hygiene

- Rapid growth
- Facial nerve function affected
- Involvement of skin
- Trismus
- Fixed to underlying bone
⇓
MALIGNANT PAROTID SWELLING
⇓
- Radical parotidectomy
- Sacrificing facial nerve with / without reconstruction
- Radiotherapy +/-

- Slow growth
- No facial nerve involvement
- Well defined
⇓
BENIGN LESION

Tumour | Lymph node

- No Biopsy taken
- FNAC / histological Diagnosis usually after Superficial Parotidectomy with preservation of facial nerve done

Pleomorphic adenoma
⇓
- Commonest

Monomorphic adenoma / Other tumours

Rarely a malignant lesion is revealed

Investigations:

LABORATORY TESTS	COMMENT / LOOK FOR
Endocrine tests: Blood sugar Thyroid function test Serum cortisol / ACTH	 Diabetes Myxoedema Cushing's disease
ESR Protein electrophoresis Antinuclear factor	Sjogren's syndrome Sjogren's syndrome Sjogren's syndrome
Kviem test	Sarcoidosis
Collection and examination of saliva	
Radiological tests: Plain X'rays	 • Parotid calculi - usually radiolucent • Submandibular calculi - radioopaque • Intraoral films may be used for submandibular calculi
Sialography	• Parotid calculi • Non-neoplastic salivary gland disease-sialectasis
Radioisotope scanning (Technetium pertechnate)	• Warthin's tumour - "Hot" • Other tumours - "Cold"
Ultrasonography	Differentiates solid from cystic tumours • Parotid cysts - radiolucent • Warthin's tumour - cystic appearance • Other tumours - solid masses • Malignant tumours - low reflectivity • Mixed tumours - variable reflectivity
C.T. Scanning	Evaluation of Parotid tumours • Relation to facial nerve • Extension to deep lobe / parapharyngeal space
M.R. Imaging	• Obliteration of fat planes in the parapharyngeal space signifies malignancy. Contrast between tumour and surrounding tissue is greater than with C.T. scan. • Lack of Ionizing radiation.
Biopsy	• It is not recommended because of fear of implantation and recurrence especially of pleomorphic adenoma and carcinomas. • FNAC is preferred. • Obvious malignant tumour involving skin may be subjected to incisional biopsy. • Sublabial biopsy is done for Sjogren's syndrome

SALIVARY TUMOURS

BENIGN TUMOURS	SYNONYM	AGE	SEX	INCIDENCE	FEATURES	SYMPTOMS AND SIGNS

1. Pleomorphic adenoma	Mixed parotid tumour (because they were thought to have epithelial and cartilagenous elements within)	40 years	Equal Incidence	- Forms 90% of all benign tumours in parotid gland
				- Incidence of malignancy is the 6%. It depends on the duration, the tumour has been present.
				- Recurrence rate
				  ● following surgery - 5%
				  ● enucleation - 20-30%
					- Usually unilateral
					- Slow growth
					- Long quiescent periods
					- Occurs in the tail of the parotid gland followed by the retromandibular portion.
					- Can present as deep lobe / dumb-bell tumours
					- Its capsule is a false capsule formed by compressed and fibrosed surrounding parenchyma
					- Tumour grows with pseudopodal extension through the capsule
					- It is likely to undergo cystic / haemorrhagic changes.
					- It is a highly implantable tumour
					- Cut surface is greyish white and cystic.
						- Symptomless / vague discomfort
						- Lump may be seen
						- No facial nerve involvement
						- Palpation:
						  ● Smooth
						  ● Round
						  ● Mobile
						  ● Soft
						- The tumours of the submandibular gland are large, hard and nodular mimicking a carcinoma.

2. Warthin's tumour	- Papillary cystad-enoma lymphomat-sum - Adenoly-mphoma - Monom-orphic adenoma	70 years	M:F 7:1	6-8% of all salivary gland tumours	- It is a neoplastic proliferation of heterotopic parotid tissue present within the lymph nodes of the gland. - Slow growing - Commonly bilateral - Present in the tail of the gland - Never malignant - Cut surface: areas of solid whiteness (because of the lymphoid tissue) present among cystic areas containing brown mucoid-fluid. - Multiple lobules are present - It is susceptible to infection / inflammation because of the lymphoid tissue within.	- Soft, cystic - Compressible and fluctuant at times - Non-bosselated lump in the tail of the gland.

BENIGN TUMOURS	SYNONYM	AGE	SEX	INCIDENCE	FEATURES	SYMPTOMS AND SIGNS
3. Oncocytoma	Oxyphil cell adenoma	Older patients and above 50 years	Equal Incidence	< 1% of all salivary gland tumours	- Slow growth - Arise from striated duct cells - Cystic more than solid - Malignancy rarely occurs	- Painless - Slow growing
4. Vascular tumours a. Haemangioma	-	Diagnosed by 1 year of age	F>M	- Most common tumours in children - It forms more than ½ of the tumours in children	- Glandular parenchyma is replaced by vasoformative tissue with retaining of normal glandular lobulations - Types: Capillary, Cavernous, Mixed - Skin lesions may co-exit - Spontaneous regression does occur - No treatment given for about 12 yrs of age followed by surgery if required.	- Soft - Painless mass
b. Lymphangioma	-	Present at birth	F>M	-	- Types ⇒ Simple ⇒ Cavernous ⇒ Cystic hygroma - The thin-walled lymphatic spaces invade the gland and surrounding tissues but do not replace normal glandular parenchyma. - They are surgically removed if they cause cosmetic problems.	- Soft - Transilluminant - Fluctuant
5. Cysts					- Types of cysts that occur: ● Retention cyst ● Hydatid cyst ● Branchial cyst in the gland or its lymph nodes - Lipomas and pleomorphic adenomas may be cystic. Commonest cystic lesion is a Warthin's tumour	

BENIGN TUMOURS	SYNONYM	AGE	SEX	INCIDENCE	FEATURES	SYMPTOMS AND SIGNS
6. Granulomatous diseases						
a. Sarcoidosis	-	-	-	-	- Bilateral - Diffuse	● Associated with (Heerfordt's disease) - Chorioretinitis - Cranial nerve involvement - Lacrimal gland swelling
b. Tuberculosis	-	-	-	-	- Affects the lymph nodes or the gland	
c. Actinomycosis					- Follows oral trauma or tooth extraction.	

4. SINUS OR FISTULA

H/o onset - congenital eg: preauricular sinus-acquired eg: thyroglossal fistula

H/o previous swelling over the site

H/o abscess / cyst / lymph nodes which brust to form a sinus

H/o progress   -   Spreading

                   -   Healing / stationary

H/o discharge from sinus / fistula

- Quantity and quality
- Nature - serous, serosanguinous, purulent, bloody
- Colour and smell
- Duration

H/o pain -   Inflammation of tract

               -   Blockage of outer opening

H/o weight loss eg: tuberculosis

H/o any treatment taken

H/o recurrence

H/o trauma or surgery - foreign body or suture material inside

GENERAL EXAMINATION

Stigmas of tuberculosis or syphilis

- Anaemia, cachexia, malnutrition

Examination of respiratory system

- For pulmonary tuberculosis

LOCAL EXAMINATION

Inspection:

1. **Site** - determined from the position of the opening

   Preauricular sinus - roof of helix or tragus and directed upwards / backwards (because of non fusion of the ear tubercles)

   Branchial fistula - lower $\frac{1}{3}^{rd}$ of neck, infront of sternomastoid (failure of fusion of 2nd branchial arch with the fifth)

   Actinomycosis - back of the neck, foot

   Parotid fistula - parotid area

   Tuberculosis - over lymph nodes in neck

2. **Number**

   Single - parotid or lymphatic fistula following trauma to thoracic duct

   Multiple - actinomycosis

3. **Size and appearance**

   Wide opening - tuberculous sinus resembling an ulcer

Edge of tuberculous sunis is undermined while that of a malignant one is irregular.

Sprouting granulation tissue - underlying foreign body

4. **Discharge**
   - Pus - osteomyelitis
   - Serosanguinous - tuberculosis
   - Sulphur granules - actinomycosis (the sulphur granules are the colonies of actinomyces)

5. **Surrounding skin**
   - Loss of hair - tuberculosis, oesteomyelitis
   - Dermatitis and pigmentation - actinomycosis

Palpation:

1. Temperature - increases in inflammation
2. Tenderness - inflammatory process
3. Discharge on pressure
4. Wall of sinus - thickened due to fibrosis, secondary to chronic inflammation
5. Mobility / fixity - osteomyelitic sinus is fixed to the underlying bone.
6. Surrounding tissue - enlarged matted lymph nodes - tuberculous sinus thickening and irregularity of underlying bone - osteomyelitis
7. Probe examination of the sinus - The following points are noted
   - Direction and depth of the sinus
   - Presence of a foreign body inside
   - Communication with hollow viscus
   - Relation to deeper structures
   - Fresh discharge on withdrawal of probe
8. Regional lymph nodes - whether palpable or not

SINUS

A sinus is a blind tract lined by epithelium or granulation tissue from a surface epithelium into the deeper tissues.

FISTULA

- It is an abnormal communicating tract between two epithelial surfaces.
  - External fistula - between the skin surface and an internal hollow viscus.
  - Internal fistula - fistula between two internal hollow viscera.
    Both the types are lined by epithelium or granulation tissue.

INVESTIGATIONS

1. Examination of the discharge from the fistula
   - Actinomycosis - Sulphur granules
   - Salivary fistula - Ptyalin
2. Biopsy - either the edge or entire tract is excised for histopathological examination for tuberculosis or malignant change
3. X-ray chest - PA view -   For tuberculosis
4. Plain X-ray of bones   -   Osteomyelitis / sequestrum
                            -   Foreign body
5. Sinogram / Fistulogram - Injection of a radio-opaque fluid (lipiodol / hypaque) will delineate the tract

CAUSES OF PERSISTENCE OF A SINUS / FISTULA

1. Epithelisation of the tract
2. Repeated trauma to the part
3. Chronic irritation by the discharge
4. Untreated infection - tuberculosis, actinomycosis, syphilis
5. Untreated malignancy
6. Inadequate drainage - Small opening
                                - Non dependent drainage
7. Presence of foreign body or necrotic material
8. Unrelieved obstruction of lumen of a viscus distal to fistula
9. Dense fibrosis which prevents contraction and healing
10. Persistent mobility of the part

Exuberant granulation tissue / Proud flesh

It is seen in

- Pyogenic granuloma
- Sinus
- Fistula

  It is due to the persistence of the source of infection.

Treatment:

1. Excision of excessive granulation tissue
2. Use of acriflavin in the dressing
3. Removal of source of irritation / foreign body
4. Excision of sinus / fistula tract

SALIVARY FISTULA

Salivary fistula more commonly arise from the parotid gland than the submandibular gland.

The fistula may be

- External   :   Opening on skin surface
- Internal   :   Opening in the oral cavity
- Ductal   :   Arising from the main duct system
- Glandular   :   Arising from the gland substance
- Congenital   :   Since birth, arising from aberrant salivary tissue or as a part of branchial cleft anomalies.
- Acquired   :   Following - partial parotidectomy, trauma and sepsis / infection. Ductal fistulas leak profusely, the discharge being saliva with a high amylase content. Major ductal fistulas causing skin excoriation need operative treatment for closure.

Treatment:

1. Conservative

   Decrease in production of saliva can be achieved by:
   - Drugs: Probanthine bromide
   - Irradiation
2. Operative:
   - Denervation: Tympanic neurectomy, auriculotemporal neurectomy
   - Excision of the fistula tract

- Reconstruction of the duct: Newmann and Seabrook's operation
- Diversion into mouth: Conversion to internal fistula
- Removal of the gland eg: - Submandibular gland.

  Ideally salivary fistulae should be avoided by dividing the duct most distally and then ligating it, followed by tight pressure dressing post-operatively.

SECTION - II
INSTRUMENTS

EAR

EAR

1. AURAL SYRINGE

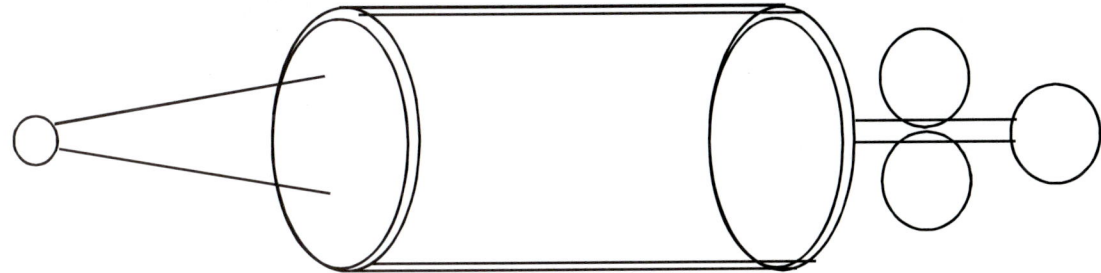

Fig. 1.1 AURAL SYRINGE

It is a metallic syringe with a cylinder and a well fitting piston and nozzle.

Uses:

- To remove softened wax.
- To remove (non-hygroscopic) foreign body eg: buttons
- To remove contents of external auditory canal, mostly dust / debri, to inspect the tympanic membrane.

Syringing

It is a procedure in which the contents of external auditory canal usually wax, foreign body etc. are syringed / removed by the force of water.

Indications:

Refer uses above.

Contraindications:

- Hygroscopic foreign body.
- Perforation of tympanic membrane.
- CSF otorrhoea.
- Otitis externa
- Avoided in patients with previous ear surgery.

Procedure

It is done in a sitting position with the head turned to the opposite side of the ear to be syringed. Children are to be held firmly by their attendants by positioning the child's legs between their's and holding the childs crossed arms. The corresponding arm is draped with a cloth and a kidney tray is held below the ear.

The syringe is held in the right hand and its filled to its full capacity with water. A 4 ounce syringe with the capacity of 120 ml is commonly used. The water should preferably be sterile and at body temperature to avoid stimulation of the labyrinth. The thumb fits in the middle ring and the index and the ring finger in the other two rings of the syringe. The tight fit of the nozzle is checked and the water jet is injected directing it to the postero-superior canal wall. This direction allows the water to get behind the mass. It may be required to pull the pinna upwards and backwards in adults and downwards and backward in children, to maintain the direction. Care should be taken to avoid pointing the nozzle directly on the eardrum to protect it from inadvertant injury and to avoid the full force of the water jet striking the drum. The washed out material is collected in a kidney tray and inspected. Syringing may be repeated if required. The canal is mopped dry with a swab stick to prevent otomycosis.

Complications:

1. Trauma to the external auditory canal and eardrum. It may cause bleeding and lead to otitis externa.
2. Vertigo can occur due to stimulation of the labyrinth.
3. Otitis externa can occur due to trauma or use of unsterilized water.
4. Otomycosis can result because of persistent dampness in the external auditory canal.
5. Exacerbation of otitis media occurs if syringing is performed on a ruptured ear drum.
6. Vaso vagal attack.

Essentials of syringing:

- Firm holding of the child.
- Sterile water at body temperature to be used.
- Greased syringe with a well fitting nozzle has to be directed postero-superiorly.
- Examination and mopping of external auditory canal is required after the procedure.

WAX

Wax is the external secretion of the ceruminous and pilosebaceous glands of the external auditory canal along with dust, debri and squamous epithelium. Ceruminous glands are specialised glands with apocrine and eccrine function situated deep within the skin of the outer two-third of the external auditory canal. Wax is assisted in expulsion by the natural movements of the jaw.

Contents of wax :

- Fatty acids
- Amino acids
- Lysozymes
- Immunoglobulins
- Bactericidal agents
- Squamous epithelium
- Dust / debri

Types:

- **Dry**   :   Grey, granular and brittle seen in Mongoloids.
- **Wet**   :   White, brown coloured seen in Caucasians, Negroes.

Features of wax impaction:

- Earache
- Deafness
- Itching
- Fullness in the ear.
- Tinnitus
- Reflex cough (through auricular branch of vagus nerve).
- Giddiness.
- Obscuring of eardrum.
- May precipitate otitis externa.

    Water jet directed on hard impacted wax impacts if further. It has to be either softened before removal or a chink has to be made in it with a hook before removal.

Treatment

Removal of wax by means of:

1. Hooking   :   Wax hook / vectis passed beyond the wax.
2. Suction   :   Sucking out under direct vision.
3. Syringing   :   Refer above.
4. Ceruminolytics :   These are agents which dissolve the wax and assist its removal. They should ideally not cause any chemical irritation. Some agents only soften wax, do not dissolve it.

Agents incorporated in ceruminolytics:

AGENT	PROPERTY
Choline salicylate	Analgesic Anti-inflammatory
Glycerine	Emolient
Polyoxypropylene glycol	Cerumen softener,
Olive oil, almond oil	Organic solvents (can cause irritation of skin)

FOREIGN BODY IN EAR

Foreign bodies:

TYPES		
LIVING	**NON-LIVING**	
Insects, flies, maggots	**Hygroscopic**	**Non-Hygroscopic**
	Nuts, peas, flour, vegetable matter.	Metals, stones, tubes, plastics, beads, button batteries, silicone material.

The foreign body enters the ear through the external auditory canal and generally lodges at the isthmus, the narrowest part of the canal about 5 mm lateral to the tympanic membrane. If present for a short time, it may not cause any problems, but longer duration foreign bodies may induce an inflammatory reaction of the external auditory canal by blocking the clearance of cerumen, releasing toxins, becoming oedematous and swelling up thereby damaging squamous epithelium, if hygroscopic in nature.

A foreign body can perforate the tympanic membrane, enter the middle ear and rarely cause bacterial labyrinthitis. Button batteries can leak an alkaline electrolyte solution and cause extensive liquefactive necrosis.

Clinical features:

- No symptoms or
- H/o foreign body in ear.
- H/o trauma.
- H/o pain, bleeding (because of instrumentation or scratching)
- H/o deafness
- Signs of otitis externa obscuring the foreign body.

Treatment:

Removal by means of a:

- Hook
- Forceps
- Syringing - for non hygroscopic objects

- Suction aspiration :   -   For vegetable matter to avoid breaking it into pieces.
                        -   For spherical objects as it is difficult to probe beyond these objects.

Removal under general anaesthesia may be required for impacted foreign bodies with otitis externa along with medical line of treatment for the infection.

2. JOBSON HORNE'S PROBE AND RING CURETTE

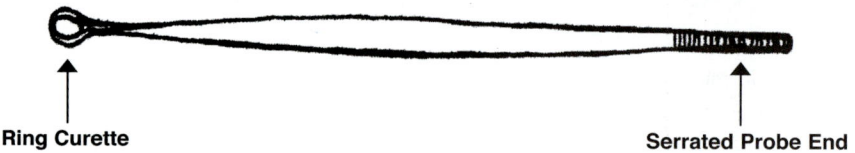

Ring Curette   Serrated Probe End

Fig. 2.1 JOBSON HORNE'S PROBE AND RING CURETTE

Uses:

- **Curette**
  - Removal of wax
  - Removal of foreign body
  - Removal of granulations from external auditory canal
- **Probe**
  - Probing of polyp in ear.
  - For aural toilet, to clean aural discharge as a cotton swab carrier
  - To trace a sinus track
  - To apply medications in external auditory canal.

TYPES OF AURAL POLYP	PASSING OF PROBE ALL AROUND THE POLYP
1. External ear	1. Can pass all around
2. Middle ear	2. Cannot pass all around

3. TUNING FORK

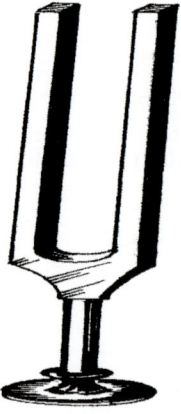

Parts of tuning fork
● Prongs
● Shoulder
● Base
● Stem
● Foot Piece

Fig. 3.1 TUNING FORK

Uses:

- To know type of hearing loss
- Degree of hearing loss

The following frequency tuning forks are used in clinical practice.

FREQUENCY Hz	COMMENT
128	• Neurologists use it to test vibration sense • To detect degree of hearing loss • May be more sensitive to detect air-bone gap
256	• Produces more overtones • May enhance perception by vibration sense
512	• Ideal for use • Falls in mid speech frequency range. • Overtones are minimal • Mild hearing loss can be detected • Sounds last longer • Sound is more auditory than vibratory. • Tone decay is optimal
1024	• To detect degree of hearing loss • Tone decay is very fast

Tuning fork is struck at the junction of upper $\frac{1}{3}^{rd}$ with lower $\frac{2}{3}^{rd;}$ of the prongs, to minimize overtones. Distance between tuning fork and auricle is 2.5 cms.

Audible frequency :   20-20,000 Hz

Speech frequency :   87-1175 Hz

Overtones   :   Frequency above fundamental frequency

They are present if the vibrations of the tuning fork are felt by the examiner's hands in the stem of the fork.

4. POLITZER BAG

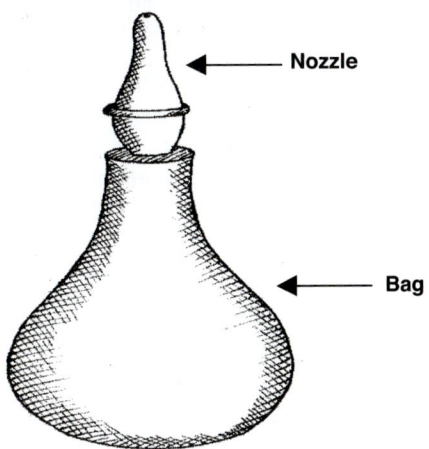

Fig. 4.1 POLITZER BAG

Use:

To perform politzerisation to test eustachian tube patency.

Politzerisation

The nozzle of the bag is inserted in one nostril and the other nostril is blocked by pressing with fingers against the septum. The patient is asked to say 'K' while the bag is pressed. This manoeuvre increases nasopharyngeal pressure and opens up the eustachain tubes and air gushes inside the middle ear.

5. SIEGLE'S PNEUMATIC SPECULUM

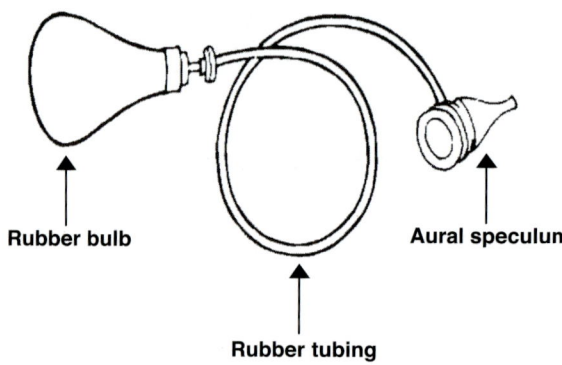

Fig. 5.1 SIEGLE'S PNEUMATIC SPECULUM

It consists of an aural speculum attached to a rubber bulb by a hollow rubber tubing. The aural speculum is placed in the external auditory canal and the rubber bulb is squeezed to alter pressure in the canal. The drum is simultaneously visualized through the speculum with the help of a head mirror and lamp.

Uses:

Diagnostic

- To examine external auditory canal and tympanic membrane with magnification.
- To assess mobility of tympanic membrane
- To elicit fistula sign.
- To assess eustachian tube patency by seeing mobility of drum on Valsalva's manoeuvre.
- To differentiate between healed perforation and adhesive otitits media.

Difference between healed perforation and adhesive otitis media on seigalization

Healed perforation	Adhesive otitis media
Thin drum moves	Strong adhesions to middle ear prevent drum from moving

Therapeutic

- To instill medication / powder in chronic suppurative otitis media
- To suck discharge from deep recesses
- To cause mobility of the drum to break adhesions between drum and middle ear mucosa.

Magnification : 2X.

Power   : 10 diopter

6. EUSTACHIAN TUBE CATHETER

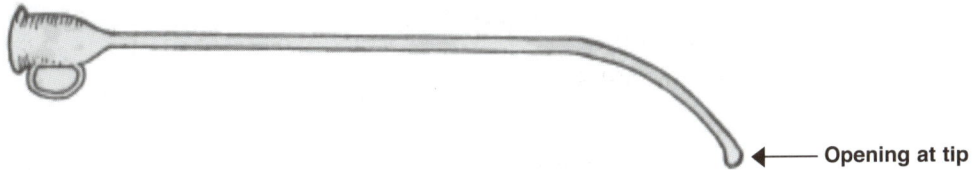

◄— Opening at tip

Fig. 6.1 EUSTACHIAN TUBE CATHETER

Uses:

Diagnostic

- To assess patency of eustachian tube by catheterization

Therapeutic

- To clear eustachian tube block
- As a suction cannula for nasal cavity
- For removal of nasal foreign bodies.

Methods to test Eustachian tube patency

1.	Valsalva's manoeuvre	Forced expiration on a closed glottis
2.	Frenzel's manoeuvre	Voluntary contraction of floor of mouth
3.	Toynbee's manoeuvre	Swallowing with mouth and nose closed
4.	Tympanometry	Change in middle ear pressure on respiration.
5.	Politzerisation	Air insufflation into the eustachian tube
6.	Instillation of agents in presence of tympanic membrane perforation	
	a. Sterile sweet / sugar solution.	Sweet taste in mouth if tube is patent
	b. Radio-opaque substance	Eustachian tube and passage of substance visualized radiologically.
	c. Ligature material	Studying the ease of passage of material intraoperatively and also seeing it in the nasopharynx.

Types of eustachian tube block:

1.	Anatomical	Obstruction of lumen of tube by mass effect eg: tumour
2.	Physiological	Defect in mucociliary clearance leading to failure in drainage of secretions from ear to nasopharynx. Stagnation of secretions occurs leading to a block. No mass lesion obstructing the lumen.

7. EAR SPECULUM

TOYNBEE'S AURAL SPECULUM

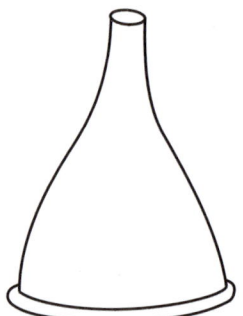

Fig. 7.1 EAR SPECULUM

The speculum is gently inserted into the ear canal by a rotatory motion; (after ruling out otitis externa). It is inserted only upto the cartilagenous meatus, not touching the bony meatus as it is very sensitive and can be painful. The pinna is pulled backwards, laterally and upwards in adults and backwards, laterally and downwards in children to straighten the canal for easy insertion of the speculum.

Uses

- Examination of external auditory canal and tympanic membrane for

EAC	TM
Wax: examination and removal	Chronic otitis media
Foreign body	Adhesive otitis media
Otomycosis	Retraction pocket
	Acute otitis media
	Granular myringitis
	Grommet

- In operative procedures:
  - Myringotomy
  - Grommet insertion
  - Polypectomy
  - Foreign body removal under anesthesia
  - Granuloma removal
  - A black (carbon coated) speculum is used to take an endomeatal incision for Stapedectomy and Tympanic neurectomy. Black colour of the speculum prevents reflection of light to the surgeon's eye from the operating microscope.

8. LEMPERT'S ENDAURAL SPECULUM

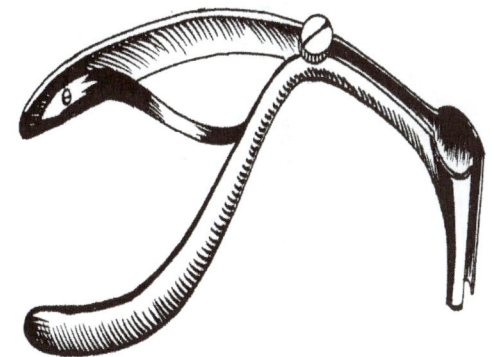

Indications for an endaural incision:
- Myringoplasty
- Tympanoplasty
- Stapedectomy
- Atticotomy
- Foreign body removal.

Fig. 8.1 LEMPERT'S ENDAURAL SPECULUM

Use:

- To take an endaural incision.

9. MYRINGOTOME (DAGGET'S MYRINGOTOME)

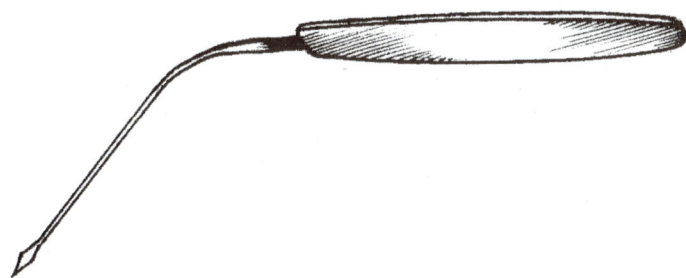

Fig. 9.1 MYRINGOTOME (DAGGET'S MYRINGOTOME)

Use:

To puncture tympanic membrane for insertion of a grommet. (Myringotomy).

Myringotomy

A radial incision is made on the tympanic membrane in the appropriate quadrant and a ventilating tube is inserted if indicated.

INDICATION	DURATION	SITE OF PUNCTURE
Otitis media with effusion	Short or medium term	Antero-inferior quadrant
	Long term	Antero-superior quadrant
Acute otitis media		Postero inferior quadrant

MYRINGOTOMY INCISIONS

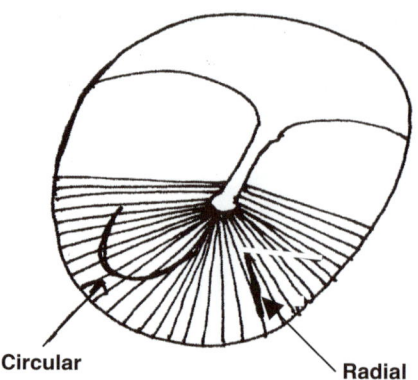

Circular   Radial

Fig. 9.2 MYRINGOTOMY INCISIONS

INCISION	RADIAL	CIRCULAR
Relation to tympanic membrane fibres	Along tympanic membrane fibres	Cuts across the fibres
Blood supply from annulus	Does not hamper it	It gets cut off.
Edge	Less chance of inward edges	Edges get curled inwards
Healing on grommet extrusion / removal	Takes less time to heal	More time to heal May not heal leading to a small perforation
Character	More physiological / anatomical	Less physiological / anatomical

Treatment of otitis media with effusion

Medical

- Valsalva's manoeuvre
- Anti-inflammatory drugs
- Antibiotics
- Mucolytics
- Decongestants
- Enzymes

Surgical

- Aspiration of the effusion
- Myringotomy
- Myringotomy with uni / bilateral ventilating tube insertion
- Adenoidectomy combined with the above
- Cortical mastoidectomy

10. MOLLISON'S SELF-RETAINING HAEMOSTATIC MASTOID RETRACTOR

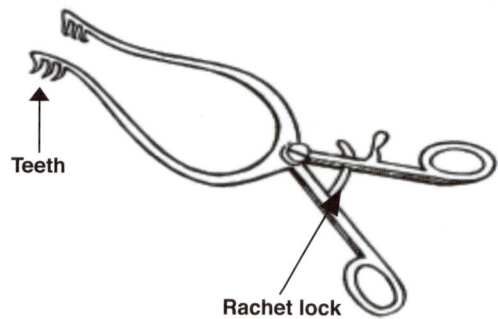

Teeth

Rachet lock

Fig. 10.1 MOLLISON'S SELF-RETAINING HAEMOSTATIC MASTOID RETRACTOR

Uses:

- To retract skin edges and deeper tissues after aural incisions.
- To remove temporalis fascia graft in ear operations like
  - Mastoidectomy
  - Tympanoplasty
  - Facial nerve decompression.
- To retract cartilagenous or bony edges / incision edges in
  - Laryngofissure
  - Burr hole operation
  - Craniotomy
  - External ethmoidectomy
  - Optic nerve decompression

Advantages

- Self-retaining, no help is required to hold the incision edges
- Haemostasis is well achieved by the pressure exerted by the teeth of the retractor on the tissues
- It retracts away from the field of vision

11. FARABEUF'S PERIOSTEAL ELEVATOR

It has a broad end and a thumb rest.

Broad end ⟶

Fig. 11.1 FARABEUF'S PERIOSTEAL ELEVATOR

Uses:

- To elevate periosteum over mastoid bone in Mastoidectomy.
- To elevate periosteum over the antrum in Caldwell-Luc operation
- To elevate periosteum over bony surfaces in head and neck surgeries eg: Maxillectomy, External fronto ethmoidectomy
- To elevate soft tissues

12. BALANCE'S AURAL SNARE

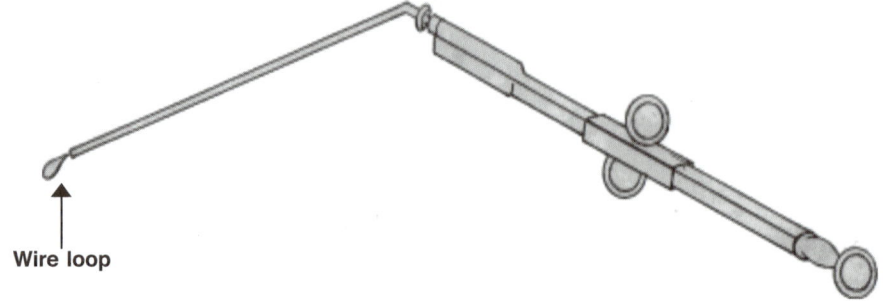

Wire loop

Fig. 12.1 BALANCE'S AURAL SNARE

It is the smallest of all the snares used in ENT.

Use:

- For aural polypectomy. It is performed via the external auditory canal. Aural polyp should never be avulsed (pulled) as it may be attached to important structures like the facial nerve, ossicles and labyrinth. Avulsion can cause damage to these structures.

Advantage of using a snare:

- It crushes and cuts the pedicle of an aural polyp.

13. LEMPERT'S MASTOID SCOOP

Fig. 13.1 LEMPERT'S MASTOID SCOOP

> **Contribution of Lempert:**
> - Lempert's endaural speculum
> - Lempert's endural incision
> - Lempert's mastoid scoop.
> - Lempert's malleus head nipper
> - Lempert's periosteal elevator.

Uses:

- In Mastoidectomy
    - Removal / scooping of bone and mastoid air cells (diseased bone is softer)
    - Scoop out granulation tissue.
- In Stapedectomy
    - To curette posterior superior meatal wall till pyramidal process is seen.

14. MACEWEN'S CELL SEEKER WITH SCOOP

Uses:

Seeker

● To seek the antrum and mastoid air cells.

● To seek aditus ad antrum.

Scoop

● To curette bony prominences

● To curette posterior superior bony wall.

● To curette anterior, posterior buttresses.

● To scoop diseased air cells.

15. MALLET

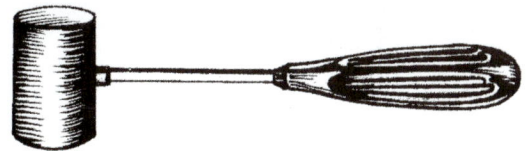

Fig. 15.1 MALLET

Uses:

To hammer bone for its removal

TO HAMMER	SURGERIES
● Bone chips / cortical bone	Mastoidectomy
● Spurs	Septoplasty
● Nasal bones	Rhinoplasty
● Antral walls	Caldwell – Luc operation, Maxillectomy
● Mandible parts	Mandibulectomy

Disadvantages

● Slow and tedious process

● Difficult to assess depth of breaking

● Damage to facial nerve, sigmoid sinus, lateral sinus, labyrinth, dural plate and ossicles is likely to occur at mastoidectomy

16. CHISEL

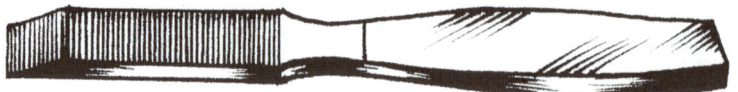

Fig. 16.1 CHISEL

17. JENKIN'S MASTOID GOUGE

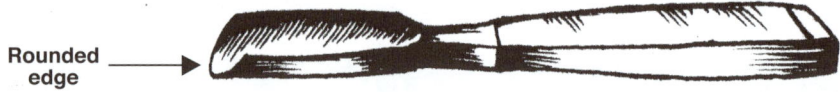

Fig. 17.1 JENKIN'S MASTOID GOUGE

Uses:

- In Mastoidectomy
  - To remove bone
  - To explore antrum and air cells
  - To lower facial bridge in radical operations (chisel)
- To remove bone (along with mallet / hammer) in
  - Caldwell – Luc operation
  - Rhinoplasty
  - Septoplasty
  - Head and neck surgeries.
- To remove exostosis, osteomas from external auditory canal.

CHISEL	GOUGE	OSTEOTOME
Straight edge	Curved rounded edge	Straight edge
Single bevel	No bevel	Double bevel
	Bone removal is done parallel to the structure exposed	
	A gouge is more preferred as bone removal is easier because of its edge	

18. DRILL AND BURR

The drill bears a motor to which the hand piece is connected. Burrs are connected to the hand piece.

Motor

Types:

- Hanging type
- Stand type

- Table top - 12,000 – 20,000 rpm
- Micro motor - 30,000 – 40,000 rpm.

Hand piece

Types:

- Straight: Ordinary burrs are used with it.
- Curved / cotrangular: Gear fitting burrs are needed for this kind of handpiece

Burr

Types:

- Cutting
- Diamond
- Polishing

Tungsten carbide is used as the cutting edge in all the burrs. Each variety is available in sizes 1 to 10 mm. The shape of the burr is usually round.

BURR	USE
1. Cutting	1. Cutting bone-work
2. Polishing	2. Smoothening the cavity
3. Diamond	3. Used near structures like facial nerve, dura, sinus

The hand piece is held like a pen and the side of the burr is used for cutting bone. While using burrs, continuous irrigation is essential to prevent overheating and clogging of burrs. Ringer lactate can be used as the irrigating fluid. The burrs and hand-pieces are cleaned thoroughly after use. They are then lubricated with oil and stored. They are sterilized by formalin vapour.

Advantages of using drill and burr

- Bone cutting is very fast
- Bone is cut smoothly and more precisely
- No irregular cavity or bone chips are left behind
- Damage to ossicles, facial nerve, dura etc. is minimized
- Shaping of ossicles is easier
- Depth of bone cutting can be adequately judged
- Less time-consuming.

19. SICKLE KNIFE

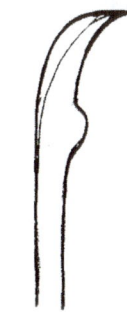

Fig. 19.1 SICKLE KNIFE

Uses:

1. To make a myringotomy incision
2. To freshen the edge of the perforation in myringoplasty, tympanoplasty.
3. To elevate tympanomeatal flap and annulus from tympanic sulcus
4. To tuck graft in myringoplasty, tympanoplasty, mastoidectomy and other aural surgeries
5. To put and remove gelfoam in aural surgeries
6. To manoeuvre ossicles in ossiculoplasty
7. To dislocate incudo-stapedial joint
8. To downfracture stapedial crura in stapedectomy
9. To break middle ear adhesions (between ossicles, tympanic membrane and promontory)
10. To cut stapedius tendon and tensor tympani tendon
11. To cut facial nerve sheath in facial nerve decompression.
12. To dissect out granulations in tympanoplasty, mastoidectomy.
13. To remove cholesteatoma matrix

20. SIDE KNIFE

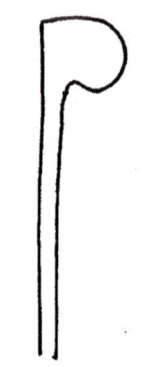

Fig. 20.1 SIDE KNIFE

It is a microsurgical instrument, also known as the **flag knife** or **Plester's first incision knife**.

Uses:

1. To elevate tympanomeatal flap from posterior meatal wall in aural surgeries like myringoplasty, tympanoplasty, mastoidectomy, stapedectomy etc.
2. To take 6 and 12 O'clock incisions before elevation of tympanomeatal flap.
3. To elevate chordatympani nerve and the annulus
4. To peel off cholesteatoma matrix.

21. CIRCULAR KNIFE

It is a microsurgical instrument, also known as **Rosen's knife**.

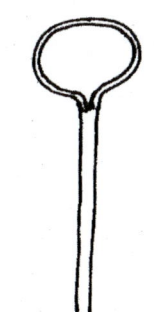

Samuel Rosen
• Stapes mobilisation
• Transtympanic stapedectomy

Fig. 21.1 CIRCULAR KNIFE

Uses:

1. Freshening the edge and undersurface of the perforation in myringoplasty and tympanoplasty.
2. Elevation of tympano-meatal flap from the posterior meatal wall and annulus from the tympanic sulcus
3. Breaking of adhesions between handle of malleus and promontory
4. To clear sinus tympani and hypotympanum of cholesteatoma

22. PICKS

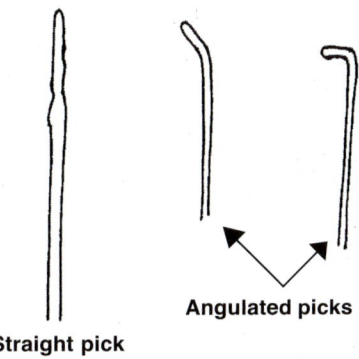

Angulated picks

Straight pick

Fig. 22.1 PICKS

Types:

1. Straight
2. Angulated.

Uses:

Straight

1. To clear cholesteatoma matrix from footplate area, sinus tympani and ossicles.
2. To put graft and manoeuvre ossicles
3. To elevate tympanomeatal flap and chordatympani nerve
4. To manoeuvre grommet and teflon piston.

Angulated

1. To remove part of footplate in stapedectomy.
2. To dislocate incudostapedial joint.

23. ANTRUM CELL SEEKER / BALL-POINT

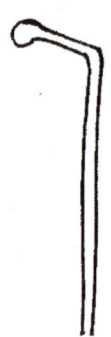

Fig. 23.1 ANTRUM CELL SEEKER / BALL-POINT

It is a blunt angulated microsurgical instrument. It is also called as a ball-point instrument by some. It is an atraumatic instrument.

Uses:

1. To seek the antrum and aditus during a mastoidectomy
2. To probe sinus plate, sinus, dural plate and dura.
3. To probe retraction -pockets.
4. For dislocation or mobilization of necrosed ossicle
5. To check for dehiscence of facial nerve
6. To remove cholesteatoma from eustachian tube area, over labyrinthine fistula and over dehiscent facial nerve
7. To check graft position and middle ear air pocket
8. To peel off granulations
9. To peel off squamous epithelium over promontory in Grade IV atelectasis.

24. CURETTE

Uses:

1. To curette posterior superior bony meatal wall in stapedectomy, ossiculoplasty, tympanoplasty.
2. To curette anterior and posterior buttress in mastoidectomy

Methods to remove postero-superior bony overhang:

1. Use of hammer and chisel
2. Drilling
3. Curettage

25. HOUSE'S MEASURING ROD

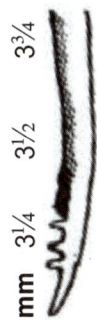

Fig. 25.1 HOUSE'S MEASURING ROD

Uses:

- To measure length from footplate to undersurface of incus in stapedectomy

  There are three markings present at a distance of 3¼, 3½ and 3¾ mm. from the lower end of the rod.

  The length of the teflon piston to be inserted is decided by adding 0.5 mm to the length from footplate to undersurface of incus, measured with the help of the markings.

26. JIG

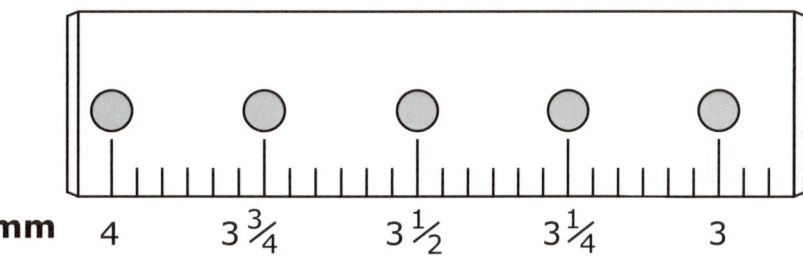

Fig. 26.1 JIG

It is an instrument like a measuring scale. It has markings and perforations on the scale. The Teflon piston is to be inserted in the perforation corresponding to the marking which denotes the decided length of the piston to be put. The excess length of the piston is cut.

27. PERFORATOR

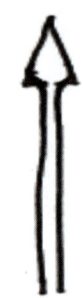

Fig. 27.1 PERFORATOR

It is a slender microsurgical instrument with a guard little away from its tip to avoid excessive penetration through the footplate.

Causse's method of stapedectomy
In this method, the stapedial tendon is cut near the stapes and it is then attached to the new prosthesis

Methods to perforate stapes footplate
• With a perforator
• Use of Portmann's perforator
• With a laser beam

Use

• To perforate stapes footplate in stapedectomy

28. MICROSURGICAL SCISSORS

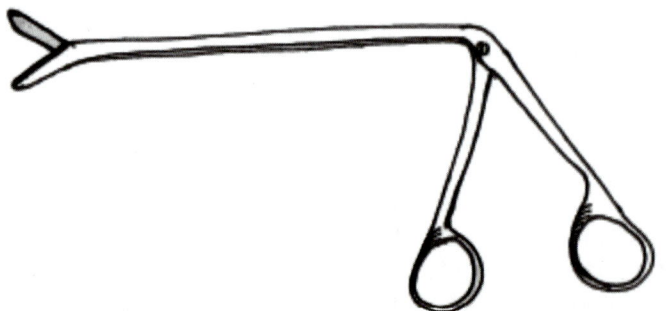

Fig. 28.1 MICROSURGICAL SCISSORS (BALUCHI SCISSORS)

Use

1. To cut stapedius tendon, tensor tympani tendon
2. To cut adhesions
3. To cut pedicle of a polyp.

29. CROCODILE FORCEPS

Fig. 29.1 CROCODILE FORCEPS

Uses:

1. To hold graft material and put in the tympanic / mastoid cavity
2. To put and remove cotton pledgets and gelfoam
3. To put and remove ossicles.
4. To put teflon piston. (Some use special piston holding forceps).
5. To hold and put grommet or prosthesis
6. To achieve haemostasis by pressure with adrenaline soaked cotton pledgets.

30. POLYPECTOMY FORCEPS

Fig. 30.1 POLYPECTOMY FORCEPS

Use

1. To hold an aural polyp and cut its pedicle
2. To remove granulations
3. As an alternative to crocodile forceps.

31. MALLEUS HEAD NIPPER FORCEPS

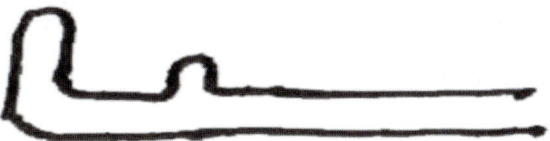

Fig. 31.1 MALLEUS HEAD NIPPER FORCEPS

Use:

To remove head of malleus for access to area medial to it and to remove cholesteatoma matrix, granulations etc.

32. MICROSCOPE

Uses:

- For all ear operations
- Nasal surgeries
  - Trans-sphenoid approaches
  - Hypophysectomy
- Microlaryngoscopy
- Head and neck surgery where minute work is required.

Parts of the microscope

I. Optical system

- Controls distance between lens and object
- Controls magnification

The optical system has the following parts:

1. Binocular assembly	Eye pieces	**Magnification:** • 10x • 12.5 x (commonly used) • 16 x • 20 x **Diopter scale** • - 5 to + 5
2. Magnification changer	Knobs on the side of the head of the microscope (turette)	**Magnification** • 6 • 10-Routine ear work • 16-Finer ear work • 25-Structure identification • 40
3. Objective lens	Fitted at the bottom of the head of the microscope Focal length is the distance between the object and the lens	Surgery : Focal length Ear : 200 mm Nose : 300 mm Laryngeal : 400 mm

II. Lighting

Source:

- Incandescent lamp of 6V, 30V, 50V
- Halogen lamp
- Fibre optic light system.

  The light should give good illumination and not cause a glare.

III. Stand

The microscope is fitted on the stand and can be moved in any direction with the number of knobs and arms present.

Advantages of an operating microscope:

- Magnification
- Illumination
- Identification
- Depth perception

33. MIDDLE EAR TELESCOPE

Uses:

To examine middle ear through a perforation or a surgically made puncture.

34. OTOSCOPE

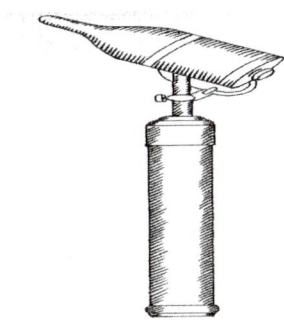

Fig. 34.1 OTOSCOPE

It is an instrument used to examine the tympanic membrane and external auditory canal

It has a fibreoptic light built in system. Various specula can be attached to the end used for otoscopy.

Uses:

- Examination of tympanic membrane and external auditory canal
- To perform seigalization

Advantages

- Magnified (2X) view of tympanic membrane is obtained
- Better assessment and diagnosis of pathology
- Direct vision
- Easy to carry / portable instrument
- Easy to handle
- Strong illumination
- Battery operated
- Various size of the specula can be attached to the otoscope
- Seigle's pneumatic speculum can be attached to it to perform seigalization.

NOSE

NOSE

1. THUDICUMS NASAL SPECULUM

Named after Johann Ludurig Wilhelm Thudicum

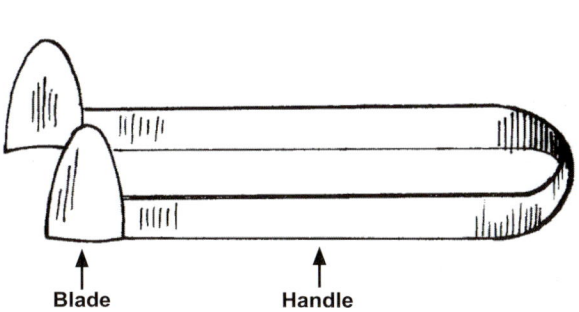

Blade   Handle

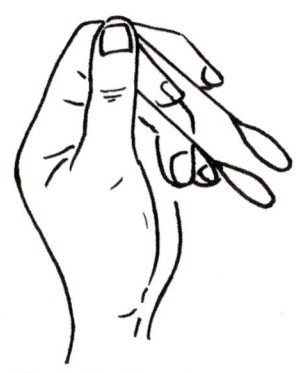

Method of holding the speculum

Fig. 1.1 THUDICUMS NASAL SPECULUM

It is held in the left hand. The index finger and the thumb hold the junction of the two handles and the ring and middle finger control the movement of the handles.

Before anterior rhinoscopy, the tip of the nose should be elevated to examine the nasal vestibule as the blades of the speculum do not permit visualization of the vestibule and an ulcer, furuncle or mild caudal deviation could be missed.

Uses :

Diagnostic

For Anterior rhinoscopy to examine :

- Little's area
- Nasal septum and its deviations
- Lateral wall of nose
- Anterior ends of inferior and middle turbinates
- Floor
- Pus in middle meatus
- Rhinolith, foreign body, polyps
- Septal perforation
- Nasal masses

Therapeutic

- Removal of foreign bodies
- Antral puncture
- Nasal packing (insertion and removal)
- Cauterization
- Application of medications

- Nasal surgeries
  - Sub mucous resection
  - Septoplasty
  - Polypectomy
- Infiltration of local anaesthesia

2. ST. CLAIR THOMPSON'S LONG BLADED NASAL SPECULUM

It is used only after the patient is anaesthetized, otherwise it can cause pain and reflex sneezing

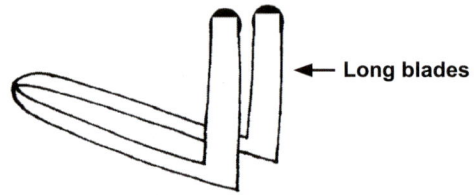

← Long blades

Fig. 2.1 ST. CLAIR THOMPSON'S LONG BLADED NASAL SPECULUM

Uses :
- To retract mucoperichondrial and mucoperiosteal flaps in SMR / Septoplasty. The long blades protect the flaps against injury
- To examine deeper structures in the nasal cavity for any pathologies
- To retract lateral wall of nose away for polypectomy, probing of nasal masses, biopsy taking

Advantages :
- Allows visualization of deeper structures
- Decreases chances of septal perforation or damage to flaps

| **Contribution of St. Clair Thompson :** |
| • Long bladed nasal speculum |
| • Posterior rhinoscopy mirror |
| • Adenoid curette |

3. KILLIAN'S SELF-RETAINING NASAL SPECULUM

It is a long-bladed self-retaining instrument. The blades are available in different sizes. The distance between the blades can be adjusted and fixed with the screw.

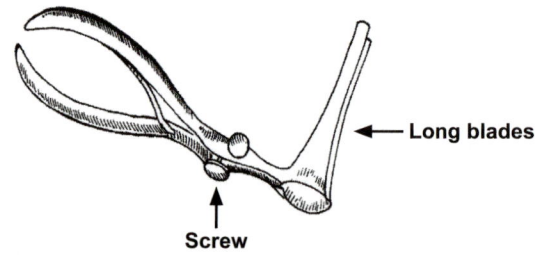

← Long blades

Screw

Fig. 3.1 KILLIAN'S SELF-RETAINING NASAL SPECULUM

Uses :

- SMR / septoplasty
- Nasal polypectomy
- Biopsy taking

Advantages

- Self retaining
- Blades can be adjusted
- Allows visualization of deeper structures
- Decreases chances of mucosal damage or septal perforation

Other nasal specula

- Cottle's speculum
- Palmer self-retaining nasal speculum
- Lenox-Browne's nasal speculum

Killian's contribution
- Killian's mucoperichondrial elevator
- Killian's nasal speculum
- Killian's incision for SMR
- Killian's SMR
- Killian's polyp (AC polyp)
- Killian's dehiscence (pharyngeal diverticulum)
- Killians nasal gouge

---

4. ST. CLAIR THOMPSON POSTERIOR RHINOSCOPY MIRROR

This instrument has a bayonet shaped handle (to differentiate it from indirect laryngoscopy mirror), so that examiner's hands do not block the vision. The mirror should be of an appropriate size so as to pass behind the soft palate and also reflect enough light for the image to be seen. The size (written on the back of the mirror) is selected seeing the intertonsillar distance on tongue depression. It is available in sizes 0 to 5.

It has a plane mirror without any magnification.

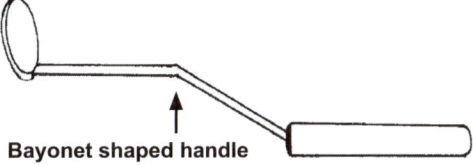

Bayonet shaped handle

Fig. 4.1 ST. CLAIR THOMPSON POSTERIOR RHINOSCOPY MIRROR

Used for posterior rhinoscopy

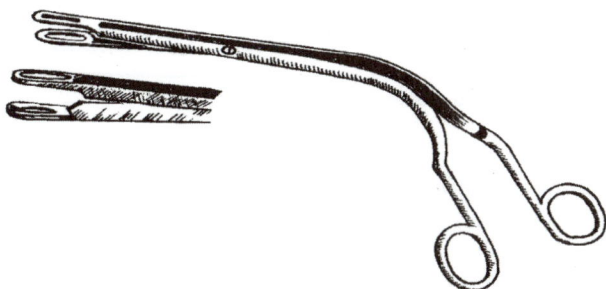

Fig. 5.1 LUC'S FORCEPS

This forceps has a screw joint and 2 fenestrated sharp ended blades which provide a secure grip on the tissue held. The tissues bulge through the fenestra and are therefore not crushed.

Uses :

- SMR / septoplasty : removal of cartilage or bone
- Caldwell-Luc operation / nasal polypectomy : removal of polyp
- Punch biopsy from oral cavity and oropharynx
- Substitute to tonsil holding forceps in tonsillectomy
- Turbinectomy
- Removal of adenoid tags

6. GLEGG'S NASAL SNARE

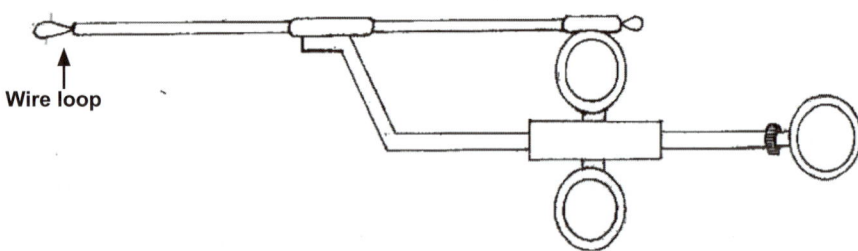

Fig. 6.1 GLEGG'S NASAL SNARE

It is used for nasal polypectomy.It removes polyp by the mechanism of avulsion. The steel wire of the snare does not withdraw completely on closure. This prevents cutting of the polyp and instead pulls it out gently (avulsion)

Snare	Gauge of wire
Aural	32
Nasal	30
Tonsillar	28

7. KILLIAN'S MUCOPERICHONDRIAL / PERIOSTEAL ELEVATOR

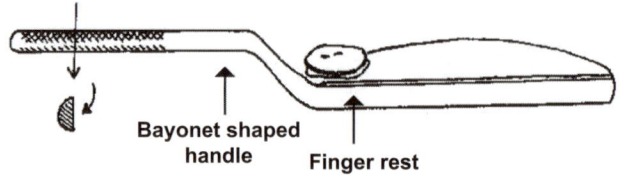

Fig. 7.1 KILLIAN'S MUCOPERICHONDRIAL / PERIOSTEAL ELEVATOR

This instrument is bayonet shaped and has a finger rest. One side of the elevator is flat and the other is convex. The flat side faces the septum, and the convex side faces the mucoperiosteal flap.

8. FREER'S MUCOPERICHONDRIAL ELEVATOR

Fig. 8.1 FREER'S MUCOPERICHONDRIAL ELEVATOR

Uses

- To elevate mucoperichondrium / osteum flaps in SMR / septoplasty operation. The plane of elevation is the submucoperichondrial plane
- Septal perforation repair
- Harvesting cartilage for rhinoplasty, tympanoplasty
- For fracturing of turbinates
- To displace inferior turbinate in antrostomy operation
- To remove maxillary crest is SMR

9. BALLENGER SWIVEL KNIFE

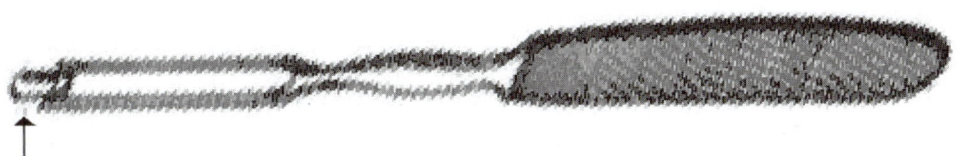

Fig. 9.1 BALLENGER SWIVEL KNIFE

This knife can rotate around for 360^0. It can cut without rotating or reintroducing the whole instrument (only the knife rotates) being advantageous in the small nasal cavity. It is called a swivel knife since the cutting blade can revolve around the two bars.

Uses :

- To remove cartilage in SMR. The movement of the instrument is backwards, downwards and forwards
- To harvest cartilage for
  - Rhinoplasty
  - Tympanoplasty

Advantages of a swivel knife

- Cartilage can be removed in one piece
- Left-over cartilage has smooth edges

10. KILLIAN'S NASAL GOUGE

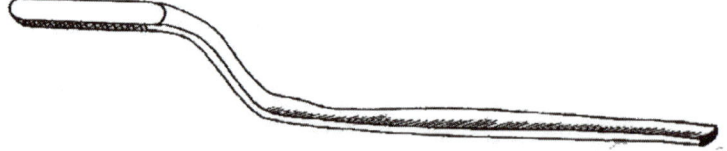

Fig. 10.1 KILLIAN'S NASAL GOUGE

This gouge is bayonet shaped to allow adequate visualization inside the nasal cavity. Its edge is rounded, concave or 'V' shaped for a better grip on the bone. It is to be used with a mallet or a hammer.

Uses :

- Removal of spurs in SMR / septoplasty
- Removal of maxillary crest
- Opening the bone of the canine fossa in antral surgeries / Caldwell-Luc operation

11. HENCKEL TILLEY'S PUNCH FORCEPS

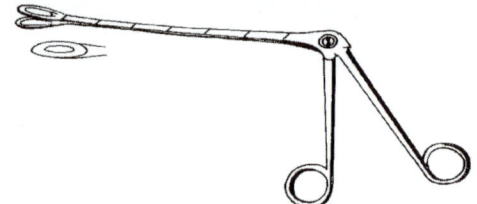

Fig. 11.1 HENCKEL TILLEY'S PUNCH FORCEPS

It is a nasal forceps with markings on the upper surface to estimate the depth, the instrument has reached and the region underneath. It is an ethmoid punch forceps and the markings help to prevent damage to important surrounding structures.

Uses :

- Intranasal ethmoidectomy
- Frontoethmoidectomy
- Punch biopsy from nasal cavity

12. CITELLI'S PUNCH FORCEPS

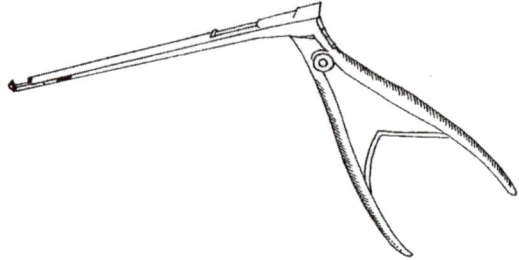

Fig. 12.1 CITELLI'S PUNCH FORCEPS

It is a stout instrument with no markings

Uses :

- To remove or punch bone in
  - Caldwell-Luc operation
  - External frontoethmoidectomy
  - Intranasal antrostomy
  - Sphenoidectomy

13. TILLEY'S ANTRAL HARPOON

It is an instrument used to make an opening in the maxillary antrum. It is held like a dagger in one hand and the index finger and thumb of the other hand are used for an adequate fulcrum.

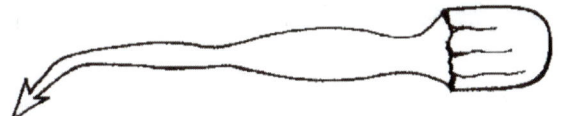

Fig. 13.1 TILLEY'S ANTRAL HARPOON

Uses :

- For intranasal antrostomy

  The puncture is made just below the genu of inferior turbinate, where the bone is the thinnest. The opening made is large, of the size of 2 x 1.5 cms. A large opening remains patent for a longer time

Intranasal antrostomy indications

- For additional drainage of maxillary sinus
- As an adjunct to Caldwell-Luc operation
- In children, where Caldwell-Luc operation is contraindicated
- Chronic sinusitis not responding to conservative measures.

14. MYLE'S NASO ANTRAL PERFORATOR

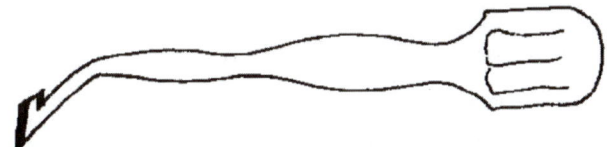

Fig. 14.1 MYLE'S NASO ANTRAL PERFORATOR

This instrument has an antegrade and a retrograde cutting edge.

Uses :

- It is used to enlarge an antrostomy opening. The opening is enlarged to the size of 2 x 1.5 cm. It is not enlarged posteriorly to avoid damage to sphenopalatine artery and its branches.

15. TILLEY'S ANTRAL BURR

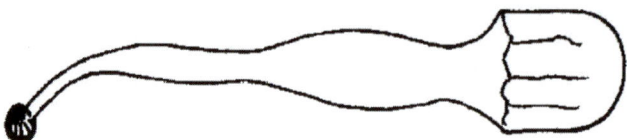

Fig. 15.1 TILLEY'S ANTRAL BURR

Uses :

- It is used to smoothen the edges of an antrostomy opening.

16. OSTROM'S ANTRAL PUNCH FORCEPS

Uses :

- To enlarge maxillary ostium anteriorly

  The ostium is widened posteriorly with Luc's forceps or Erwin Moore's forceps.

17. TILLEY LITCHWITZ ANTRAL TROCAR AND CANNULA

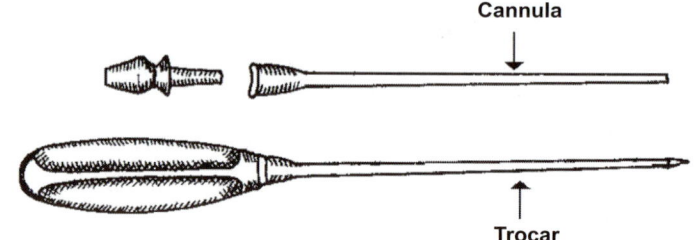

Fig. 17.1 TILLEY LITCHWITZ ANTRAL TROCAR AND CANNULA

Uses :

- To puncture maxillary antrum for antral wash. The site of puncture is just the below the genu of inferior turbinate in the inferior meatus as the bone is the thinnest here.

18. HIGGINSON'S RUBBER SYRINGE

Uses :

- Antral wash following antral puncture
- Antral wash after antrostomy
- Nasal douching in atrophic rhinitis post - operatively.

  It is made up of a red rubber bulb with tubing on both the sides. One end has a one-way valve and the other a nozzle to which an antral trocar and cannula is attached. The capacity of the syringe is about 90 ml (3 oz). The one-way valve allows only inflow of fluid into the syringe.

19. ROSE'S ANTRAL WASHING CANNULA

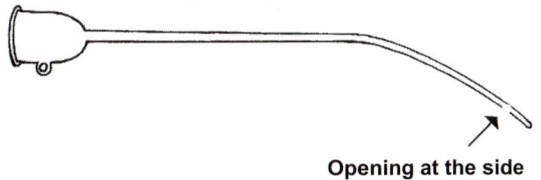

Opening at the side

Fig. 19.1 ROSE'S ANTRAL WASHING CANULA

It looks similar to the Eustachian tube catheter.

	ET CATHETER	ROSE'S ANTRAL WASHING CANNULA
Length	Longer	Shorter
Opening	At tip	Side of catheter

It has an opening at the side to prevent blockage by antral mucosa on entering the antrum.

Uses :

- For antral wash after an antrostomy is made. It is used with a Higginson's syringe

20. JENSON MIDDLETON'S DOUBLE-ACTION BONE PUNCH

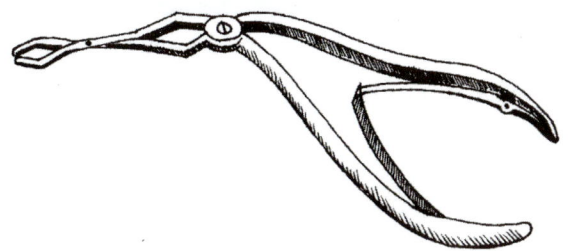

Fig. 20.1 JENSON MIDDLETON'S DOUBLE-ACTION BONE PUNCH

This instrument is called a double action punch since it has four joints with double lever system to allow the punch to open and close to a limited extent. This is useful in a narrow deep cavity. The double lever system allows greater amount of force to be exerted at the tip of the instrument.

Uses :

- Removal of bony spurs during septal surgery

Advantage

- It crushes bone while removing it, thus achieving haemostasis

21. RONGEUR

- **GLASGOW PATTERN**   **- KERRISON**

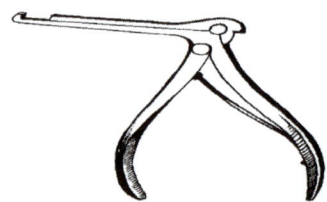   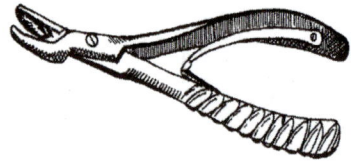

Fig. 21.1 RONGEUR

Uses : For

- Maxillectomy
- Mandibulectomy

Types of mandibulectomy :

- Mandibulectomy
  - Median
  - Paramedian
- Marginal mandibulectomy
- Segmental mandibulectomy
- Hemimandibulectomy

Osteotomies in maxillectomy :

- Palatal
- Zygomatic
- Pterygoid process
- Frontal process of maxilla

22. BLAKESLEY UPWARDS CURVED FORCEPS

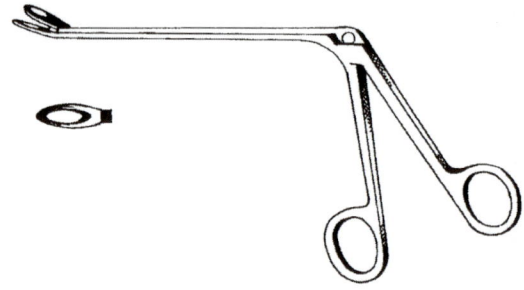

Fig. 22.1 BLAKESLEY UPWARDS CURVED FORCEPS

23. COTTLE'S ALAR RETRACTOR

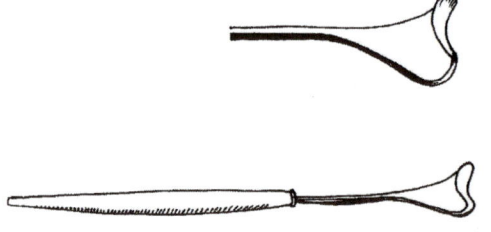

Fig. 23.1 COTTLE'S ALAR RETRACTOR

Uses :

- To retract nasal alae in
  - Rhinoplasty
  - Vestibuloplasty for
    - Atrophic rhinitis
    - Vestibular stenosis

24. HILDYARD POST NASAL BIOPSY FORCEPS

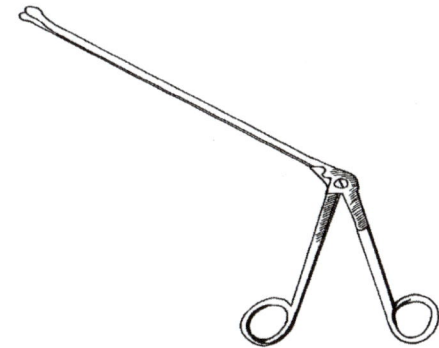

Fig. 24.1 HILDYARD POST NASAL BIOPSY FORCEPS

Uses :

- To take biopsy from post-nasal space

Advantages

- Small tumours can also be biopsied
- The scope is away from the biopsy site, vision through it is not obscured by bleeding

Routes of nasopharyngeal biopsy
● Transnasal
● Transoral

25. HARTMANN'S FORCEPS

It is a bent instrument with a diamond or olive shaped tip. The tip has a groove in the centre

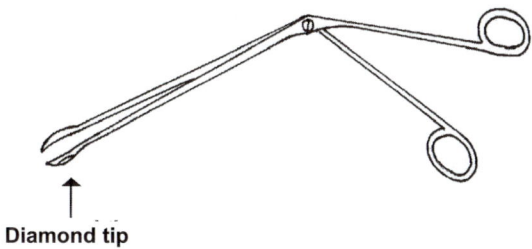

Diamond tip

Fig. 25.1 HARTMANN'S FORCEPS

Uses :

- Removal of anterior nasal packs.
- Removal of packs (medicated), cotton pledgets from external auditory canal
- Removal of nasal foreign body

- Removal of bone chips, pieces of cartilage in nasal surgeries.
- Introduction of cotton pledgets in nose for local anaesthesia.

  Its olive tip may entangle packs, hence not used for nasal packing.

26. TILLEY'S FORCEPS

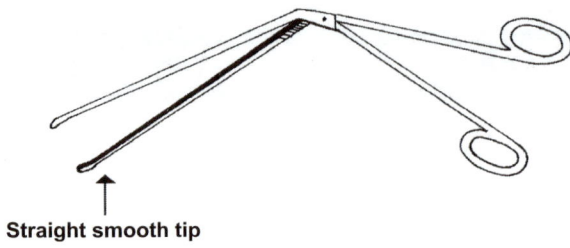

Straight smooth tip

Fig. 26.1 TILLEY'S FORCEPS

This is an angled instrument with a straight smooth tip with serrations at the end.

Uses :

- For anterior nasal packing
    - Post operatively for haemostasis
    - In epistaxis
    - In fracture nasal bones for fixation.
- Introduction of cotton pledgets for local anaesthesia.

  Its smooth tip does not entangle packs on removal of the instrument (unlike the Hartmann's dressing forceps). It is therefore used to insert packs rather than to remove them.

27. TURBINECTOMY SCISSORS

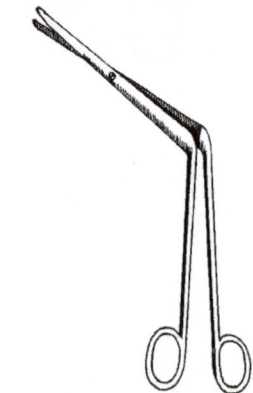

Fig. 27.1 TURBINECTOMY SCISSORS

Procedures on the turbinate

- Injection treatment
    - Corticosteroids

- Fracture of turbinates
- Cautery treatment
  - Electrocautery
  - Chemical : silver nitrate
- Cryosurgery
- Laser / Radiofrequency / Coblation application
- Partial turbinectomy
- Total turbinectomy

Complications of turbinectomy

- Crusting
- Haemorrhage
- Atrophic rhinitis

28. HAJEK'S CHEEK RETRACTOR

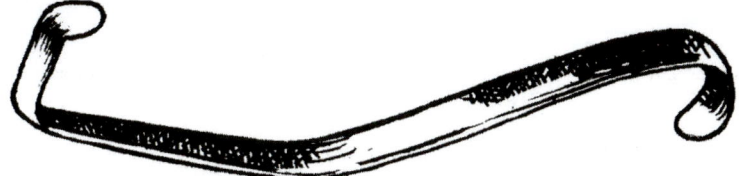

Fig. 28.1 HAJEK'S CHEEK RETRACTOR

Uses :

To retract cheek in :

- Caldwell-Luc operation
- Maxillectomy
- Repair of oro-antral fistula
- Trans-antral ligation of maxillary artery
- Vidian neurectomy

29. WALSHAM'S FORCEPS

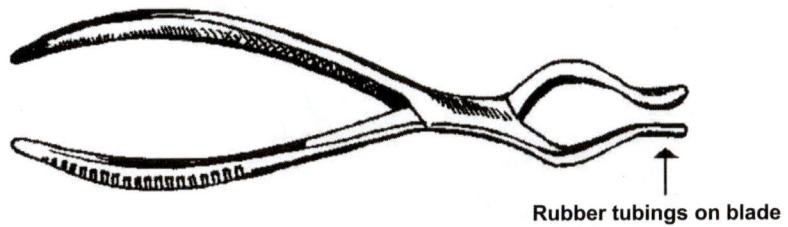

Rubber tubings on blade

Fig. 29.1 WALSHAM'S FORCEPS

It has two blades, the outer blade is covered with a rubber tubing. This outer blade lies against the skin and the rubber tubing makes it atraumatic for the skin. The other blade is introduced in the nasal cavity under the nasal bone.

Uses :

The forceps are used to refracture and disimpact fractured nasal bones. This is followed by realignment.

30. ASCH'S FORCEPS

This instrument has two blades, which when closed have a gap in between to enable to hold the septum without traumatizing it.

There is a wider gap proximally to accommodate the columella and prevent damage to it. It does not have any rubber tubing.

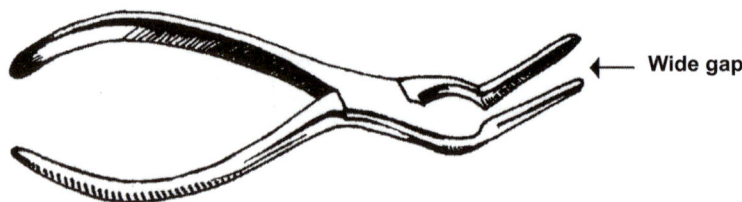
← Wide gap

Fig. 30.1 ASCH'S FORCEPS

Uses :

- It is used to elevate and straighten the septum

WALSHAM'S FORCEPS	ASCH'S FORCEPS
Straight forceps	Minimally angled forceps
Rubber tubings on blade	No rubber tubings
No gap on approximation	Gap on approximation of blades
Used to refracture and disimpact nasal bones	Used to elevate and straighten the septum

31. YANKAUER'S NASOPHARYNGEAL SPECULUM

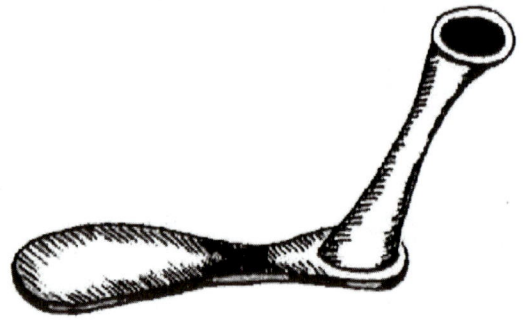

Fig. 31.1 YANKAUER'S NASOPHARYNGEAL SPECULUM

Uses :

- To visualize the nasopharynx and obtain biopsy

Methods to visualize the nasopharynx :

- Posterior rhinoscopy
- Yankauer's nasopharyngeal speculum
- Rigid nasopharyngoscopy
- Flexible nasopharyngoscopy
- Digital palpation under local or general anaesthesia
- Lifting of soft palate with retractors or rubber catheters passed through the nose under anaesthesia
- Retracting the palate with the curved end of two Lack's tongue depressors

THROAT

THROAT

1. DOYEN'S SELF RETAINING MOUTH GAG

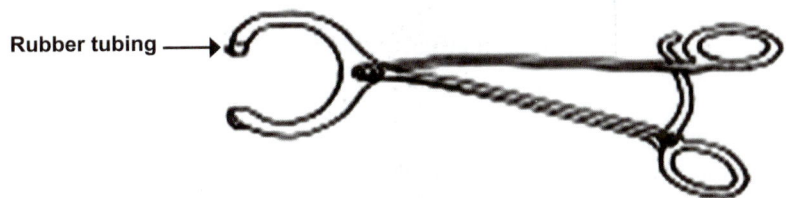

Rubber tubing →

Fig. 1.1 DOYEN'S SELF RETAINING MOUTH GAG

This mouth gag has two blades which are covered with rubber tubing. They are set against the second premolars or molars (as they are teeth bearing two roots and can withstand the pressure of an open mouth.) and then opened. The rubber tubing provides atraumatic coverage over enamel of teeth and gums.

It can be used only under general anaesthesia.

Uses:

- **To open mouth in intra-oral surgeries:**
    - Glossectomies
    - Palatal surgeries
    - Tongue-tie release
    - Dental surgery
    - Marsupialization of salivary cysts
    - Removal of calculus from salivary ducts
    - Removal of benign tumours, submucous cysts
    - Laser surgery for benign swellings
    - Excision of ranula

- **To open mouth in:**
    - Unconscious patients for oral toilet and to prevent airway obstruction
    - Temporomandibular joint fibrosis / ankylosis
    - Forcible opening in submucous fibrosis, under anaesthesia.
    - Before a rigid nasopharyngoscope is introduced.
    - In poisoning cases.

Advantages

- Self-retaining
- Avoids the use of a tongue depressor
- Atraumatic

Disadvantages

- Cannot be used in edentulous patients since it fulcrums on the teeth.

2. JENING'S MOUTH GAG

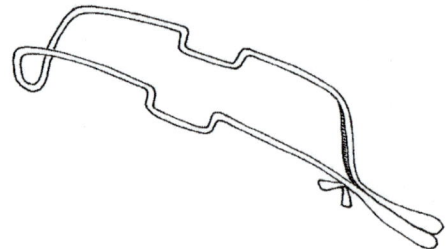

Fig. 2.1 JENING'S MOUTH GAG

It is a mouth gag which can be used in edentulous patients. Its blades open on closing and close on opening. The blades rest on the alveolar margin. It is a self-retaining instrument.

Uses:

As for DOYEN'S MOUTH GAG.

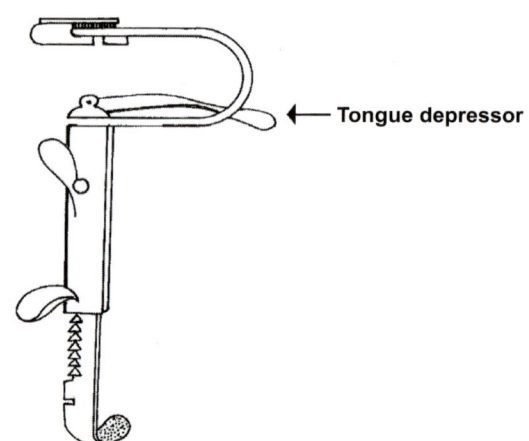

← **Tongue depressor**

Fig. 3.1 BOYLE DAVIS MOUTH GAG

This is a self-retaining mouth gag used with Draffin's bipods. It has Boyle's blade and Davis's gag. The tongue depressor is inbuilt in the gag. It is introduced in the closed position after depressing the lower jaw. The mouth gag is then gradually opened and the rachet lock makes it self-retaining. The whole assembly can be lifted up and maintained in that position by using Draffin bipods.

Parts:

- Jaw piece
- Tongue plate / depressor

Uses:

To open jaws in:

- Tonsillectomy

- Adenoidectomy
- Palatal surgery-for cleft plate, submucous cleft
- Operations on the nasopharynx, oropharynx.
- Operations in cranio-vertebral anomalies.

Disadvantages

- Swelling of lips and palate can occur
- Injury to incisor teeth.
- Can be used under general anaesthesia only.

Advantages

- Can perform operations / tonsillectomy from head end of patient in sitting position.
- In-built tongue depressor, obviates the need for an assistant
- Can be used for various surgeries.

4. DINGMAN'S MOUTH GAG

This instrument has a tongue depressor, cheek retractors and a wire spring on all sides which help to fix the palatal flaps with stay sutures.

Uses:

Other mouth gags
• Doyen Collin
• Davis Meyer
• Whitehead

- Repair of cleft palate / palatoplasty
- Pharyngoplasty
- Uvulopalatopharyngoplasty
- Palatal fenestration
- Operations on the nasopharynx
- Nasopharyngeal biopsy
- Surgery for choanal atresia
- Transpalatal operations
  - Sphenoidectomy
  - Hypophysectomy
  - Vidian neurectomy
- Can be used for Tonsillectomy.

5. DRAFFIN BIPODS

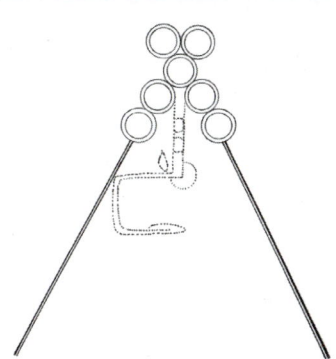

Fig. 5.1 DRAFFIN BIPODS

It is a bipod metallic stand. It comprises of 2 stands with multiple rings in a row to fix the Boyle Davis mouth gag. The stand lies on either side of the patient's head with the neck extended in supine position.

Use:

To fix Boyle-Davis mouth gag for oral or oropharyngeal surgeries. It is mainly used for tonsillectomy, not for adenoidectomy.

6. LACK'S TONGUE DEPRESSOR

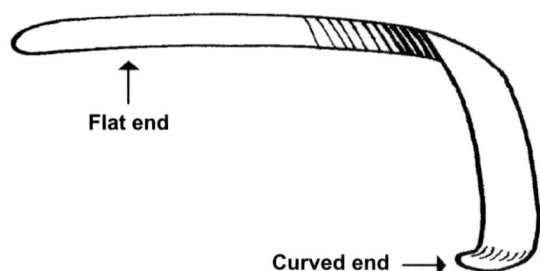

Fig. 6.1 LACK'S TONGUE DEPRESSOR

It has one flat end and another slightly curved end. The flat end is placed over the anterior ⅔ʳᵈ of the tongue to depress it. It should not touch the posterior ⅓ʳᵈ, to prevent gagging.

Uses:
- Examination of oral cavity and oropharynx for:
  - Ulceromembranous conditions of oral cavity
  - Cysts
  - Openings of submandibular ducts
  - Dental caries
  - Bifid uvula
  - Tonsils
  - Posterior pharyngeal wall
  - Submucous cleft etc.
- To retract lips and cheek
- To squeeze tonsils to detect pus within
- To test gag reflex
- "Spatula test": To test for spasm of masseter muscle is a suspected case of tetanus.
- In posterior rhinoscopy along with its mirror
- Test air blast from the nostrils / **"Cold Spatula Test"**. The tongue depressor is held in front of both the nostrils and the misting / fogging area on it is seen from the exhaled air.
- Examine nasopharynx: The soft palate is lifted up by the curved end of two tongue depressors
- Dental caries: Sensitivity of the tooth is tested by rubbing the depressor over the affected tooth.
- In oral cavity procedures like
  - Injection of steroids in the pillars
  - Biopsy taking from oral / oropharyngeal mass.
  - Excision of cysts.
  - Surgeries on submandibular ducts

Tongue depressors:
• Hartmann (fenestrated handle)
• Davis Meyer

- Operations like tonsillectomy, when a mouth gag with no tongue blade is used. In dissection method, the tongue is depressed enough to make the anterior pillar taut and an incision is then taken.
- Nasal surgeries like SMR / Septoplasty in which oral suction is required.
- Quinsey drainage
- Removal of foreign body from throat
- To check post operative post nasal bleeding

7. YANKAUER'S OROPHARYNGEAL SUCTION

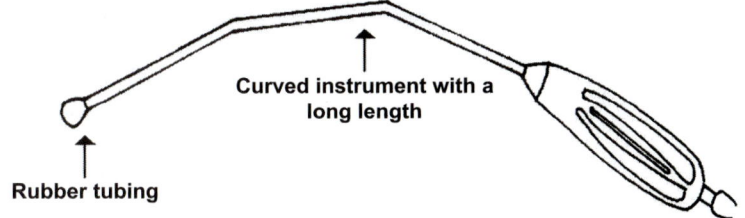

Curved instrument with a long length

Rubber tubing

Fig. 7.1 YANKAUER'S OROPHARYNGEAL SUCTION

Uses:
- To suck out oropharyngeal secretions or blood in
  - Tonsillectomy
  - Adenoidectomy
  - Palatal surgeries
  - Laryngectomy
  - Other oral surgeries
  - Nasal surgeries

Advantages:
- The rubber coating at the tip makes it atraumatic for the oropharyngeal mucosa
- Curve of the instrument helps to suck without obstructing view
- Its long length and the large handle help to suck from a distance. The operating field is therefore not obscured by the hand of the surgeon
- Multiple openings on the tip prevent blockage of the suction. (If one opening gets blocked, others still function)

8. BALLENGER'S GUILLOTINE

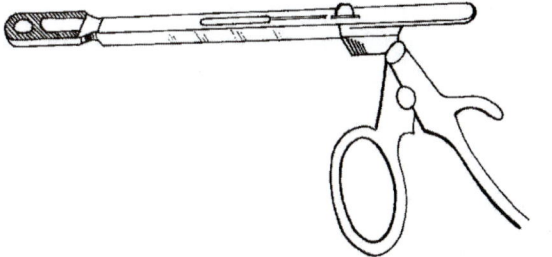

Fig. 8.1 BALLENGER'S GUILLOTINE

Uses:

- For Guillotine method of tonsillectomy.

Guillotine method

- Tonsil is engaged in the Guillotine
- Tonsil is cut by one slide of the fenestrated blade.

GUILLOTINE METHOD	DISSECTION METHOD
• Fast procedure	• Slow procedure
• Incomplete removal of tonsils is likely	• Complete removal of tonsils occur
• More bleeding	• Less bleeding
• Damage to surrounding structures is more	• Less chance of damage
• Ghastly or crude method	• This method follows the principles of surgery
• Difficult to remove non-hypertrophied tonsils	• Non-hypertrophied tonsils can also be removed.

Disadvantages of guillotine:

- More bleeding.
- Difficult to achieve haemostasis
- Incomplete removal is likely.
- Only hypertrophied tonsils can be properly removed.
- Damage to surrounding structures can occur

Methods of tonsillectomy
- Dissection and snare method
- Guillotine method
- Cryosurgery
- Electrocautery
- Laser surgery

Tonsillar hypertrophy:

GRADES	% OF OROPHARYNGEAL REGION OCCUPIED BY BOTH THE TONSILS
0	Tonsil in fossa
1	- <25%
2	- 25-50%
3	- 50-75%
4	- >75%

This grading takes into account the medial to lateral space occupied by the tonsils, not the anterior to posterior space.

9. TONSIL KNIFE

It has a no: 12 'J' shaped blade attached to a Bard Parker handle

Uses:

- To take inverted 'J' shaped submucosal incision on the anterior pillar in tonsillectomy.

Advantage

- The 'J' shaped blade helps to take a superficial submucosal incision. The incision therefore does not go deep and cause bleeding by cutting across a wrong plane or the substance of the tonsil.

10. MOLLISON'S BLUNT TONSILLAR DISSECTOR AND PILLAR RETRACTOR

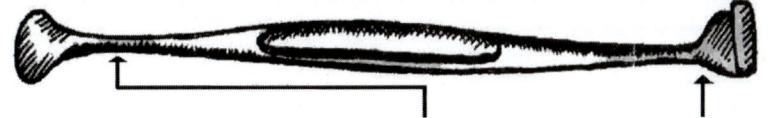

Fig. 10.1 MOLLISON'S BLUNT TONSILLAR DISSECTOR AND PILLAR RETRACTOR

Uses:

Dissector

- To separate tonsillar capsule from its bed.

Retractor

- To retract the anterior pillar:
  - Postoperatively to look for bleeding points
  - To look for tonsillar tags in the fossa
  - To look for retained gauze pieces
- To cross clamp and ligate bleeders.

11. DENNIS BROWN TONSIL HOLDING FORCEPS

LUC'S FORCEP	DENNIS BROWN TONSIL HOLDING FORCEP
Cutting edge	No cutting edge
Traumatic	Atraumatic
Box joint	No box joint

Uses:

- To hold the tonsil during dissection tonsillectomy
- To hold medial tip of anterior pillar after incision for tonsillectomy.

This instrument is similar to a Luc's forcep but it does not have a cutting edge. Hence it is atraumatic.

12. EVE'S TONSILLAR SNARE

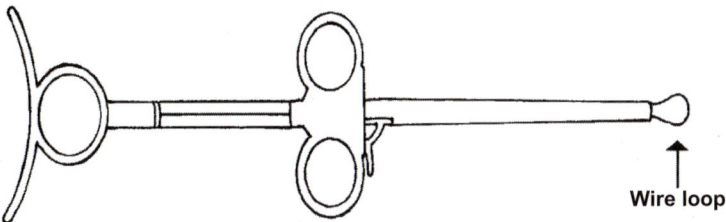

Wire loop

Fig. 12.1 EVE'S TONSILLAR SNARE

Uses:

- To remove the tonsil by snaring the lower pole after dissection. By snaring the tonsil, cutting and crushing of the lower pole is achieved.

  The lower pole is snared since tonsillar blood vessels enter and leave from this pole. On crushing, thromboplastin is released which causes vasoconstriction and platelet aggregation. This helps in haemostasis.

Blood loss in routine tonsillectomy: 50 ml

The snare has a stainless steel wire which is 3 inches long and a thickness of 28 gauge. The middle and index fingers are inserted into the two rings provided on the outer tube. The thumb is inserted in the single ring provided at the distal end of the central movable slide. The tonsil is engaged in the loop and then snared by withdrawing the wire totally inside the tube by bringing the thumb and index and ring fingers together.

13. TONSILLAR HAEMOSTAT

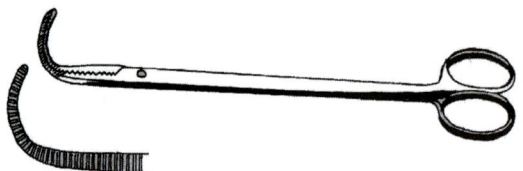

Fig. 13.1 TONSILLAR HAEMOSTAT

It is a long and slender instrument used to catch bleeders at a depth and to avoid catching soft tissues along with the bleeders.

Uses:

- To clamp and ligate bleeders during tonsillectomy

Blood supply of tonsil:

Arterial supply

Upper pole:

- Ascending palatine branch of facial artery
- Tonsillar branch of dorsal lingual artery
- Tonsillar branch of facial artery

Lower pole:

- Ascending pharyngeal artery
- Lesser palatine artery.
- Contributions from
  - Internal carotid artery
  - Vertebral artery

Venous Drainage

- Mainly to the Paratonsillar vein (Dennis Brown Vein)

14. NEGUS LIGATURE SLIPPER OR KNOT TIER

Uses:

To slip the ligature over the tip of the tonsillar haemostat during ligation of blood vessels following tonsillectomy. It is a long instrument with a blunt forked end.

15. VALSELLUM_

Use:

- To hold tonsil and pull it medially during dissection.

16. TONSILLAR PUNCH FORCEPS

Uses:

- For biopsy of the tonsil. Biopsy is usually taken in suspected carcinoma cases.

> **Unilateral enlargement of tonsil**
> - Carcinomatous
>   - Squamous cell carcinoma.
>   - Lymphoma
> - Peritonsillar abscess
> - Tonsillolith
> - Tonsillar cyst
> - Tonsillar foreign body
> - Parapharyngeal mass pushing tonsil medially
> - Carotid aneurysm pushing tonsil medially.

17. THILENIUS QUINSEY DRAINING FORCEPS

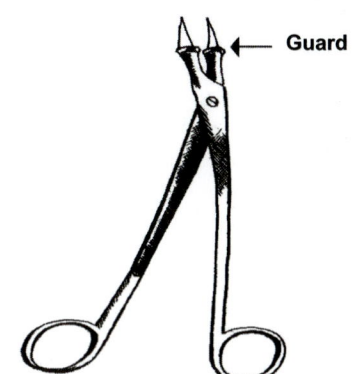

← Guard

Fig. 17.1 THILENIUS QUINSEY DRAINING FORCEPS

Uses:

- Drainage of peritonsillar abscess.

Advantages

- It has a guard at some distance from its tip, preventing more deeper penetration and avoiding complications.

18. ST. CLAIR THOMSON ADENOID CURETTE WITH / WITHOUT CAGE

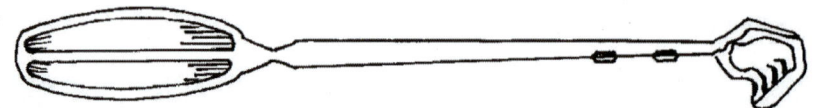

Fig. 18.1 ST. CLAIR THOMSON ADENOID CURETTE WITH / WITHOUT CAGE

It is an instrument used to remove the adenoids. The curette, first held like a pen, is introduced into the oral cavity beyond the soft palate with the blades facing down. It is then rotated by 180⁰ and positioned against the posterior superior part of the nasopharyngeal wall in the midline against the posterior end of nasal septum. The grip is then changed to that of a dagger and with a single sweeping movement, the adenoids are curetted out.

Uses of the cage

- It prevents slipping of tissue and aspiration into lower respiratory tract.
- It ensures complete removal of adenoids.

Curette without cage

- To remove remnants of adenoid tissue.
- To remove tubal tonsils without damaging eustachian tube openings, since without cage, the instrument becomes relatively atraumatic.

Adenoidectomy
Removal of adenoids by

- Natural finger nail (obsolete now)
- Steel nail
- Laforce adenotome
- St. Clair Thomson adenoid curette

Adenoids hypertrophy
Grading:

GRADE	OBSTRUCTION OF CHOANA
I	Upto $\frac{1}{3}^{rd}$
II	$\frac{1}{3}^{rd}$ to $\frac{2}{3}^{rd}$
III	$>\frac{2}{3}^{rd}$
IV	Complete obstruction of choana

Differential diagnosis of adenoids

- Adenoids
- Thornwald's cyst
- Chordoma
- Juvenile nasopharyngeal angiofibroma
- Antrochoanal polyp
- Craniopharyngioma
- Meningioma

19. TROUSSEAU'S TRACHEAL DILATOR

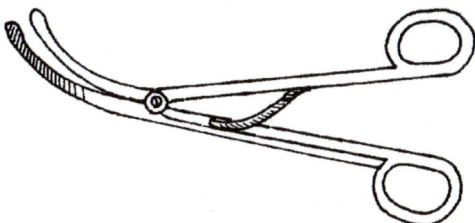

Fig. 19.1 TROUSSEAU'S TRACHEAL DILATOR

It is an instrument used to dilate the opening made on the anterior tracheal wall at tracheostomy. On closing the handle of the forceps, the dilator end opens. It does not have a catch and there are no serrations at the tip.

Uses:

To dilate tracheal opening for

- Introduction of tracheostomy tube
- Changing of tracheostomy tube.

Advantages

- Allows easier introduction of tracheostomy tube
- Less chances of a false passage.

20. DOUBLE HOOK RETRACTOR

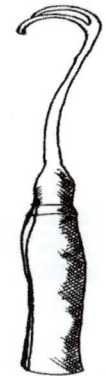

Fig. 20.1 DOUBLE HOOK RETRACTOR

It is a blunt instrument with two hooks.

Uses:

- To retract pretracheal layers or strap muscles in the neck during tracheostomy. It is used to retract skin, subcutaneous tissue, strap muscles on both sides of the incision.

21. SINGLE HOOK RETRACTOR

SHARP / CRICOID HOOK

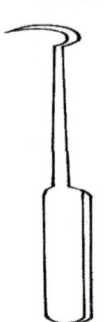

Fig. 21.1 SINGLE HOOK RETRACTOR

Use:

To retract cricoid cartilage superiorly and to stabilize trachea prior to tracheal incision in tracheostomy.

22. BLUNT / ISTHMUS HOOK

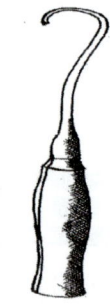

Fig. 22.1 BLUNT / ISTHMUS HOOK

Use:

To retract soft tissues / isthmus of thyroid gland superiorly in tracheostomy.

23a. TRACHEOSTOMY TUBES

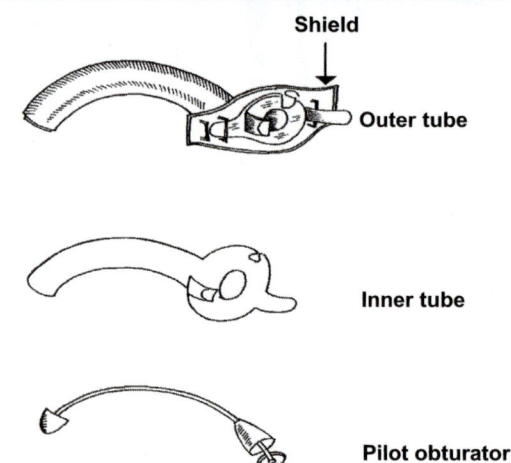

Fig. 23a.1 CHEVALIER JACKSON'S TRACHEOSTOMY TUBE

The Chevalier Jackson's metallic tube consists of an outer tube, an inner tube and a pilot obturator

Parts

- Outer tube : Fits into tracheostomy tract
- Inner tube : Protrudes beyond the outer tube for 2-3 mm.
- Pilot obturator : Blunt ended curved obturator
- Shield : It is attached to the proximal end of the outer tube. It has holes on its sides through which linen thread is passed to fix the tracheostomy tube to the neck
- Luer lock : It is fitted to the shield and fixes the inner tube to the outer one.

The inner tube is longer than the outer tube to prevent blockage by dried secretion / crusts. The inner tube is removed when blocked and then cleaned and reinserted. Metallic tubes are thus more suited for permanent tracheostomy. Luer lock helps in fixing the tube and retains it during excessive coughing. The pilot obturator allows smooth insertion and acts as a tracheal dilator. It is made of German silver which is a non-irritant. The outer tube with the obturator is passed through the tracheostomy opening. Once in the trachea, the pilot is withdrawn and the inner tube is inserted and then locked.

23b. FULLER'S BIVALVED TUBE

The bivalve acts as a dilator and helps in introduction of tube. There is an opening present on the postero superior wall of the inner tube which helps to determine the air-flow and hence the time of decannulation. Decannulation can be carried out if normal air flow is established on blocking the tracheostomy tube.

23c. PORTEX TRACHEOSTOMY TUBE

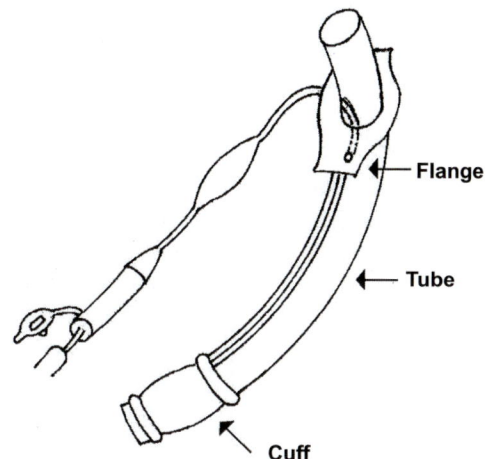

Fig. 23c.1 PORTEX TRACHEOSTOMY TUBE

Parts

1. Single tube: It may be cuffed or non-cuffed
2. Pilot
3. Flanges : The flanges are attached to the tube through which ribbon tapes are passed which are tied around the neck for fixing the tube.
4. Cuff : - low volume high pressure cuff
   - high volume low pressure cuff

5. Blue radio opaque line impregnated with barium salt is present throughout the tube for radiological evidence of the site of the tube.

Advantages of a cuffed tube

- Prevents aspiration
- Can use it for intermittent positive pressure ventilation
- Makes it partly self-retaining

Advantages of a portex tube

- Less irritant
- Can be used for intermittent positive pressure ventilation
- Can be used in radiotherapy patients
- Prevents aspiration
- Used to give general anaesthesia. Cuff prevents leakage of anaesthetic gases

24. INDIRECT LARYNGOSCOPY MIRROR

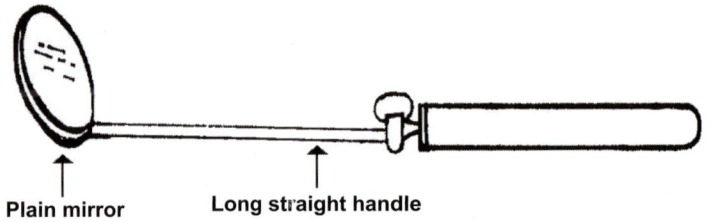

Plain mirror   Long straight handle

Fig. 24.1 INDIRECT LARYNGOSCOPY MIRROR

It has a long straight handle with a plane mirror without magnification.

Uses:

- It is used to perform indirect laryngoscopy
- To remove foreign bodies from oropharynx (eg: fish bone)
- Superior laryngeal nerve block for direct laryngoscopy under local anaesthesia.

Ways of heating the mirror_

- Spirit lamp
- Rubbing against the buccal mucosa.
- Dipping in hot water.

Indirect laryngoscopy

Advantages

- Simple procedure
- Out patients procedure

Disadvantages

- Mirror image is an anterior-posterior reversal of structures
- Vocal cords appear flat.
- Size of lesions at the anterior commissure appear smaller due to angulation of the mirror.
- Overhanging epiglottis may hide lesion.

> **Structures not seen on IDL**
> - Post cricoid region
> - Apex of pyriform fossa
> - Anterior commissure (difficult to see)
> - Ventricles
> - Laryngeal surface of epiglottis.

- Ventricle of larynx cannot be seen.
- Foreshortening of antero-posterior diameter to $\frac{1}{3}^{rd}$.
- Vocal cords appear white.
- Difficult to see anterior commissure
- Depth appears less than actual
- Ventricular bands appear at the level of vocal cords like flat bands.
- Patient co-operation is required.

25. TONSIL NEEDLE

It is a curved needle on a long handle.

Uses:

To suture anterior pillars together for control of post-tonsillectomy bleeding.

Methods to control post-tonsillectomy bleeding:

- Pressure packing
- Cross clamping and ligation of vessels
- Haematinics, vitamin K, coagulants etc.
- Control of blood pressure, antibiotics
- Hydrogen peroxide gargles
- Dislodging of clot
- Tincture benzoin cauterization
- Pillar suturing
- Resuscitation, blood transfusion
- External carotid artery ligation

SCOPE

SCOPES

1. DIRECT LARYNGOSCOPE

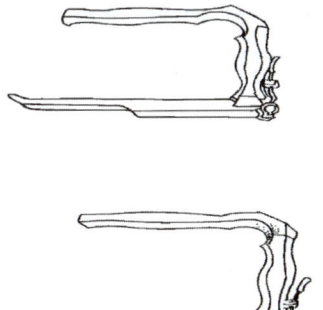

Fig. 1.1 DIRECT LARYNGOSCOPE

The direct laryngoscope is 'U' shaped and is made up of German silver. The illumination is by fibreoptic light system. There is no magnification.

Types:

CHEVALIER JACKSON	NEGUS
Distal illumination	Proximal illumination

Uses:

- To examine hypopharynx and larynx
- Removal of foreign body from hypopharynx and larynx
- To take biopsy from suspected lesions.
- To remove benign tumours / nodule from vocal cord
- For introduction of bronchoscope, (laryngoscope with a detachable blade is of use)

2. KLEINSASSER'S MICROLARYNGOSCOPE

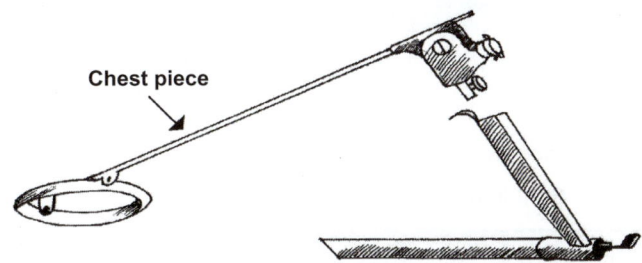

Chest piece

Fig. 2.1 KLEINSASSER'S MICROLARYNGOSCOPE

It is a stainless steel scope consisting of a wider proximal aperture and a narrower distal one. It is made self-retaining with the help of a chest piece fixed to the laryngoscope on one hand and the patient's chest on the other. Microlaryngoscopy is performed with the help of an operating microscope with a 400 mm lens.

1. **Surgical laryngoscope**
   - Proximal end having wide flat plane surface which lies in apposition to the teeth
   - Distal oval end.
   - The greatest diameter of the tube lies oblique to the longitudinal axis of the handle.
   - The broad flat proximal end of the laryngoscope evenly distributes pressure and prevents dental trauma.
   - The inner surface is roughened to avoid reflections during photography
   - The illumination is provided by a simple low voltage bulb affixed to a rod

2. **Chest holder (Riecker's)**
   - Easy to handle and very stable
   - Holds laryngoscope in place.
   - Has a wide pressure plate / plastic plate covered with foam rubber to be placed under the chest holder to avoid pain and undesirable pressure spots.

Use:

For microlaryngoscopy.

Advantages

- Wider proximal aperture / broad lumen: allows good visualization, use and manipulation of wider instruments.
- Self-retaining: surgeon's hands are free for instrumentation
- Can be used with operating microscope, so magnification is possible for various procedures.
- Flat bottom allows good stabilization of scope
- Photography and videography of endolarynx is possible
- Biopsy can be taken
- Therapeutic procedures like stripping of vocal cords, laser surgery can be coupled with ML scopy.
- Ideally the scope should be matt black to prevent glare and reflection of light from the microscope.
- Flat lower surface on the patient's teeth allows even distribution of force.

Types:

- Anterior commissure laryngoscopes
- Hollingers: anterior curved lips are present to visualize anterior commissure.
- Negus

3. CRICOPHARYNGOSCOPE / HYPOPHARYNGOSCOPE / OESOPHAGEAL SPECULUM / UPPER END OESOPHAGO-SCOPE

It is same as an oesophagoscope but shorter in length (length = 29 cms.).

Uses:

- To remove foreign body from cricopharynx / hypopharynx
- Biopsy from post-cricoid region malignancy.

> Most common site of foreign body: Cricopharynx in upper aerodigestive tract

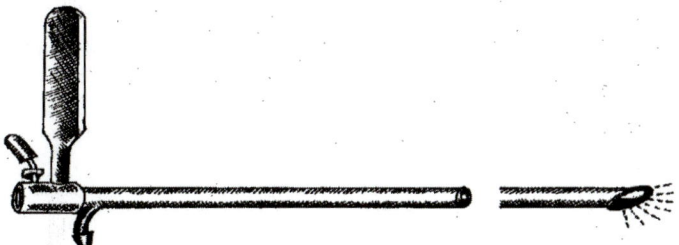

Fig. 3.1 CRICOPHARYNGOSCOPE / HYPOPHARYNGOSCOPE / OESOPHAGEAL SPECULUM / UPPER END OE-SOPHAGOSCOPE

4. BRONCHOSCOPE

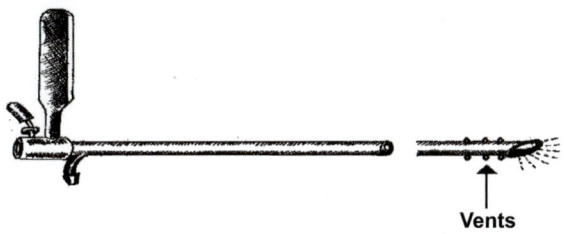

Vents

Fig. 4.1 BRONCHOSCOPE

(Bronchios = Wind pipe

Skopos = Inspect)

It is a hollow metallic instrument with distal illumination. A fibreoptic light source is used. A ventilating broncho-scope has vents on its distal end. They are so placed that few of them remain above the level of the carina to ventilate the remaining lung when the scope in introduced in one of the major bronchus.

Parts

- Shaft
- Handle
- Light source
- Eye piece
- Suction connection
- Ventilation connection

GENERAL INSTRUMENTS

GENERAL INSTRUMENTS

1. BULL'S EYE LAMP

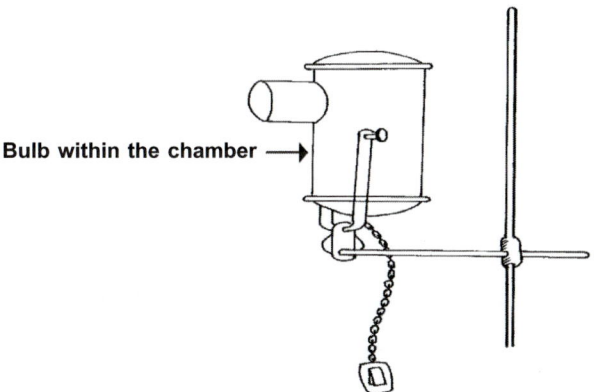

Bulb within the chamber →

Fig. 1.1 BULL'S EYE LAMP

It is the light source used for outpatient's examination. It has a 100 watt white frosted bulb in a chamber which is dark or black from within. A convex lens is attached to the chamber which allows dispersion of light from the bulb. The rays of light fall on the head mirror used by the examiner.

2. HEAD MIRROR

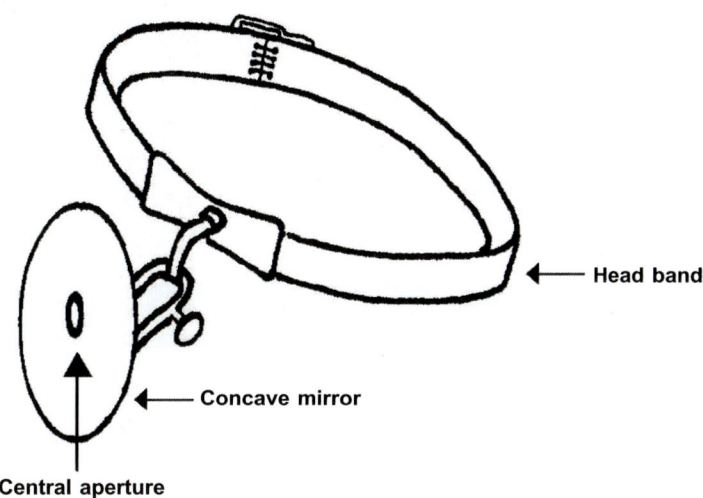

← Head band

← Concave mirror

Central aperture

Fig. 2.1 HEAD MIRROR

It consists of an adjustable head band to which a concave mirror is attached

MIRROR	DIMENSIONS
1. Focal length	1. 23.6 cm
2. Diameter	2. 9 cm
3. Central circular aperture	3. 2 cm

Use :

For routine ear, nose, throat examination. The light from the light source / Bull's lamp is reflected on the head mirror to the examined area. The head mirror is adjusted with the central aperture over right eye.

Advantages of using eye lamp with head mirror

● Binocular vision is retained

● Part under vision is brilliantly illuminated and clearly seen as the circular aperture coincides with the right eye pupil. The examiner's gaze is parallel to the reflected beam of light.

● Both hands are free to carry out procedures eg : aural syringing.

3. SPONGE HOLDING FORCEPS

It is a long straight instrument with round fenestrated ends, which bear transverse serrations. The adequate length of the instrument ensures that antiseptics can be applied to the part from a distance. The rachet lock allows a secure grip.

Uses :

● Preparation of the operative site.

● Haemostasis by pressure of a swab.

● To dry operative field by application of a dry swab.

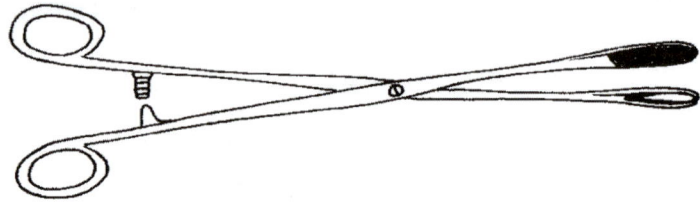

Fig. 3.1 SPONGE HOLDING FORCEPS

4. TOWEL CLIP

Doyen's towel clip - short instrument with curved ends that end in sharp points with handles joined at the proximal ends so that when pressed the tips open and vice-versa.

Mayo's towel clip - shaped like a haemostat but has tips like those of a towel clip. The ratchet catch achieves a secure grip.

Uses :

● To fix the draping towels in position.

● To fix the suction tube to the draping sheet.

- To hold the tongue during intra-oral operations like tongue-tie release
- To fix faciomaxillary fractures.

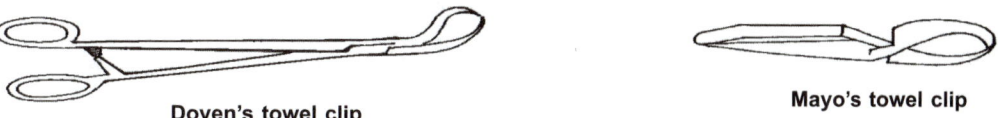

Doyen's towel clip   Mayo's towel clip

Fig. 4.1 TOWEL CLIP

5. SCALPEL

A scalpel is a sharp cutting instrument. It is basically a knife, but in surgical practice, a knife refers to an amputation or skin grafting knife, hence the term scalpel.

The combined handle and blade type are not used but instead, Bard-Parker handles with disposable blades are used. The blades are sterilised by gamma irradiation and are packed in aluminium foils. The handles are sterilised by autoclaving or boiling.

Ideal scalpel :
- It is light in weight.
- It has a sharp cutting edge
- It has a good grip.
- It is easy to sterilise.
- Different types of blades should fit to the same handle.

Diagram of Blades

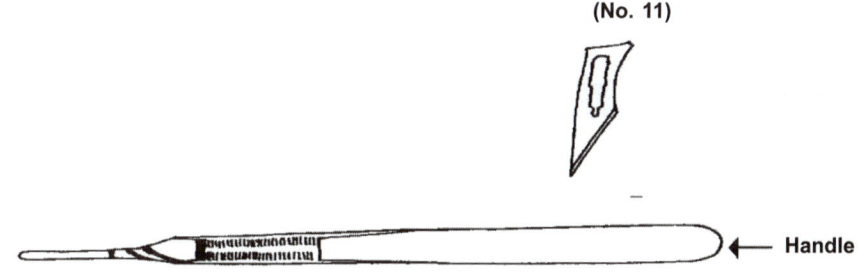

(No. 11)

← Handle

Fig. 5.1 SCALPEL

6. DISSECTING FORCEPS

Plain or nontoothed forceps have no teeth but have transverse serrations on the inner surface of the blades near the tip for a secure but nontraumatic grip on the structures held.

Toothed forceps have 1 or 2 teeth for a secure grip on the structures held. The joint has a spring action.

- Plain forceps are used to hold soft and friable tissues which may be traumatised by toothed forceps.
- Tough structures like fascia and muscles are held with toothed forceps.

- Small and fine forceps (**Adson's**) are used in microsurgery.

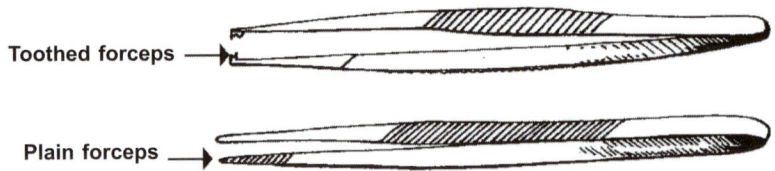

Toothed forceps →

Plain forceps →

Fig. 6.1 DISSECTING FORCEPS

7. SCISSORS

Scissors are sharp cutting instruments; small, medium or large in size, straight or curved at the end.

Curved scissors are used for dissection, by both, division of connective tissue fibres and insertion of closed scissors into a tissue plane and then opening the blades.

Straight scissors are usually used to cut sutures. Steeli's or Metzenbaum's scissors are long, curved or flat, fine scissors used for fine dissection.

Uses :

- Temporalis fascia graft harvesting in ear operations (small scissors).
- Tissue dissection e.g. : in thyroid operations.
- To cut sutures and ligatures during surgery.
- Suture removal (fine, sharp, pointed scissors).
- Cutting bandages.
- Venesection.

8. HAEMOSTAT

A haemostat is an instrument designed for haemostasis by catching bleeding vessels. Since it is used to catch both arteries and veins, it is better to use the term 'haemostat'.

It may be long or short, straight or curved.

Its blades have transverse serrations either throughout their entire extent (pedicle clamp) or only in their distal halves (haemostat).

Mechanism of Haemostasis :

The serrations permit a secure grip on the structures held and also crush it. It achieves haemostasis by occlusion of the lumen of the blood vessel. Crushing of the intima causes a blot clot formation which also promotes haemostasis. The ratchet catch helps to maintain a grip on the tissues held.

Uses :

- To catch bleeding vessels for haemostasis.
- As a pedicle clamp.
- To hold the cut edges of the fascia during dissection and while suturing them.
- As sinus forceps to open abscess cavity.
- To hold the ends of the ligature.
- To hold 'peanuts' for blunt dissection : (a 'Peanut' is a small ball of gauze with cotton inside, about 3-4 mm in diameter).

- To clamp a catheter / tubing / suction drain - it is preferable to use the portion between the hinge and ratchet catch as it is less traumatic.

  A good haemostat does not permit one to see through the approximated blades on locking the ratchet once.

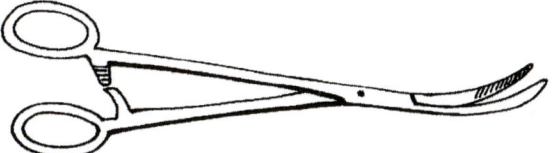

Fig. 8.1 HAEMOSTAT

9. MOSQUITO FORCEPS

Mosquito forceps is a fine curved short haemostat. It is known as mosquito forceps because its tip is said to be so fine as to be able to catch the proboscis of a mosquito.

Uses :

- To catch fine bleeding vessels.
- To hold the ends of fine sutures.
- For tissue dissection.

10. BABCOCKS FORCEPS

It is a **nontraumatic** instrument with 2 finger grips, a ratchet catch and fenestrated curved blades. They are useful for holding soft tissues and delicate structures.

Uses :

- To hold lymph nodes during lymph node biopsy.
- To hold cysts and lumps during dissection.

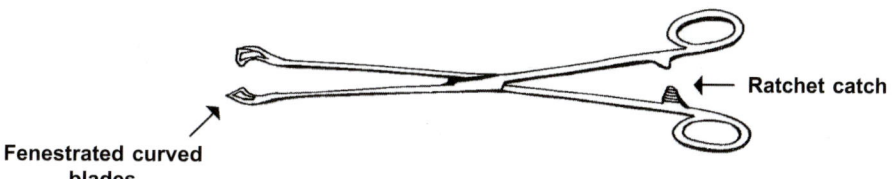

Ratchet catch

Fenestrated curved blades

Fig. 10.1 BABCOCKS FORCEPS

11. ALLIS FORCEPS

It has 2 finger grips, a ratchet catch and tips which are flattened, curved inwards a little and with fine teeth on the distal edges for a secure grip on the structures held. It cannot be used to hold delicate structures, since its teeth are traumatic.

Uses :

- To hold fascia tissue and aponeurosis.
- To hold fibrous capsule of various structures.

● To hold subcutaneous tissue just under the skin..

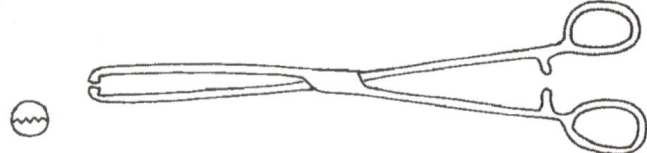

Fig. 11.1 ALLIS FORCEPS

12. SINUS FORCEPS

Sinus forceps are long, straight with slightly expanded tips but no ratchet catch on the handles.

Uses :

● Incision and drainage of an abscess - to explore the abscess cavity and break all the septae within by Hilton's method to drain the pus inside.
● To remove foreign bodies from wounds or sinuses.
● To place a drain in an abscess or sinus cavity.
● To pack an abscess cavity.
● To drain a haematoma.

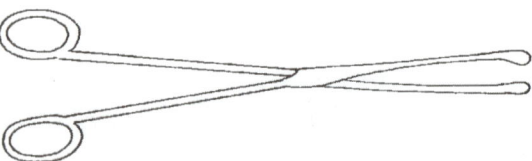

Fig. 12.1 SINUS FORCEPS

13. NEEDLE HOLDER

A needle holder is available in different sizes - small medium and large. It has two finger grips, ratchet catch and small blades. The ratio of lengths of the handle to blades is 4:1. Thus the grip is strong.

The inner surface of blades have criss-cross serrations for a secure grip on the needle held. Each blade has a longitudinal groove on its inner surface, which makes the grip on the needle stronger and stabilises it during use.

Uses :

● A needle holder is used to hold a curved needle for suturing.

   It is held at the tip of the instrument, at the junction of proximal ⅓rd and distal ⅔rd of the needle.

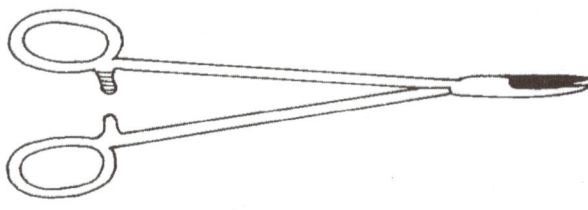

Fig. 13.1 NEEDLE HOLDER

14. SUTURE NEEDLES

Anatomic parts of a needle :

- Eye
- Body
- Point

Types :

1. Cutting
2. Round bodied

Cutting needle :

These have sharp edges, often triangular in section.

A cutting needle is triangular in cross - section, the apex of the needle directed upwards. The cutting force is maximum at the apex of the tract cut in the tissues, which increases the risk of the ligature cutting through the tissues when a knot is tied.

A reverse cutting needle is also triangular in cross - section, but the apex is directed downwards. The force of cutting is spread over the base of the tract cut in the tissues which decreases the risk of the ligature cutting through when a knot is tied.

Round bodied needle :

These needles have pointed tips. They do not cut tissues but puncture them and the punctures close very easily afterwards. These are used for suturing delicate tissues like serosa, mucous membranes etc.

Suture needles may be straight, curved, half circle, five-eights of a circle or of any special shapes.

CLEFT PALATE AND RHINOPLASTY INSTRUMENTS

- Dr. Uday Bhatt

CLEFT PALATE AND RHINOPLASTY INSTRUMENTS

CLEFT PALATE INSTRUMENTS

1. Dingman's mouth gag
2. Mucoperiosteal elevator
3. Periosteal elevator
4. Howarth periosteal elevator
5. Mitchel periosteal elevator
6. Detachable blade for Dingman's gag with groove to accommodate the endotracheal tube
7. Long BP handle.

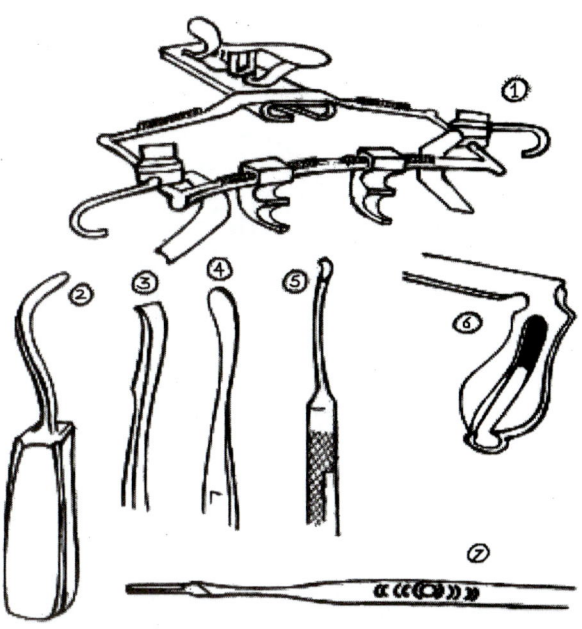

RHINOPLASTY

1. Nasal Aesthetics
   A. 1. Nasofrontal angle
       2. Tip columellar angle
       3. Naso (columellar) labial angle
       4. Soft Triangle
   B. 1. Bony dorsum
       2. Cartilagenous
       3. Supratip area
       4. Light reflex point
       5. Tip
       6. Columella
       7. Ala
       8. Alar-facial junction

C. 1. Soft triangle
    2. Nostril sill
    3. Nostril floor
    4. Medial crura foot plates
    5. Nares

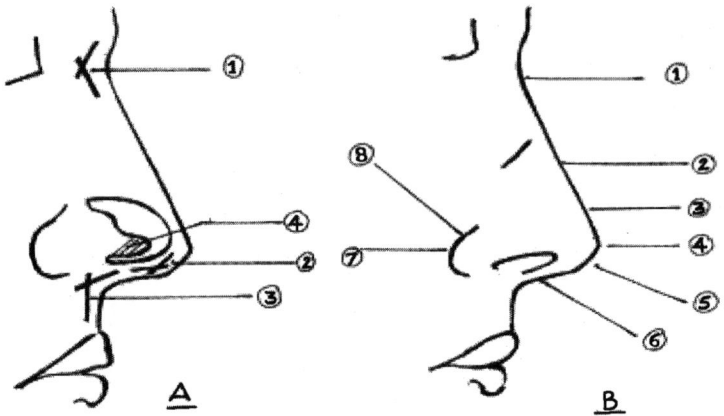

NASAL AESTHETICS

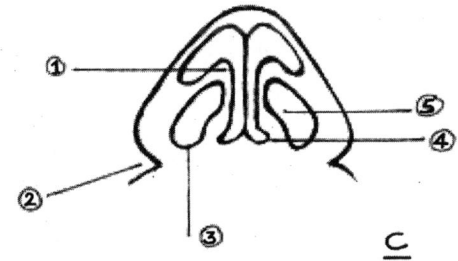

2. Osteocartilagenous Framework
    1. Nasal bone
    2. Lateral cartilage
    3. Alar cartilage
    4. Septal cartilage

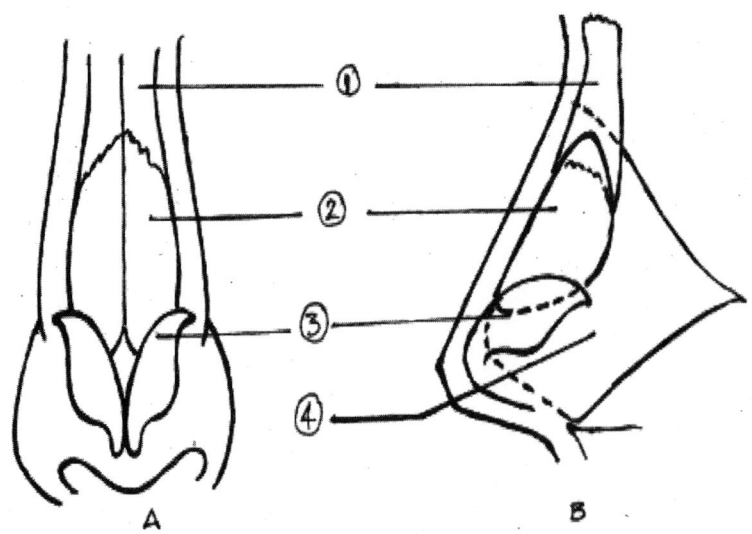

OSTEOCARTILAGENOUS FRAMEWORK

Rhinoplasty Instruments
1. 2 mm Osteotome
2. 2 mm Osteotome with guard
3. 10 mm Osteotome
4. 10 mm Osteotome with guard
5. Walsham's nasal forceps
6. Mallet
7. Cartilage scissors

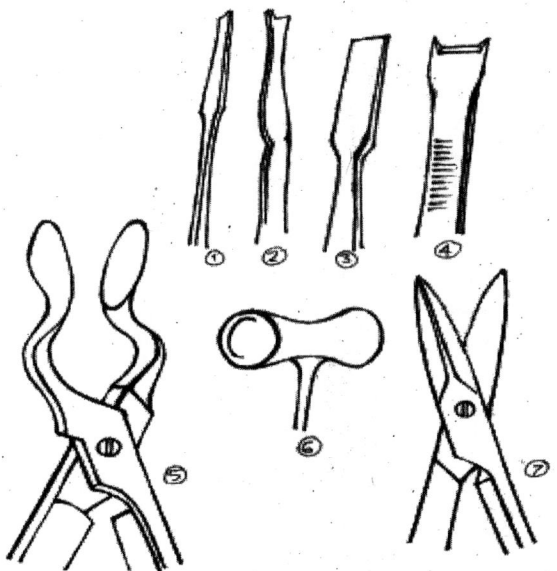

Incisions and Osteotomies
1. Medial Osteotomy
2. Lateral Osteotomy
3. Intercartilagenous incision
4. Intracartilagenous incision
5. Rim incision
6. Transfixion incision

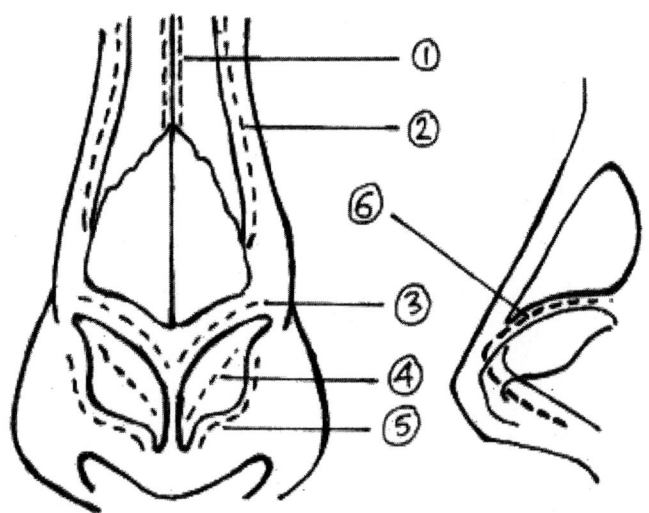

INCISIONS AND OSTEOTOMIES

Rhinoplasty instruments
1. Aufritch retractor
2. Kilian's ala retractor
3. Push rasp
4. Pull rasp
5. Joseph saw

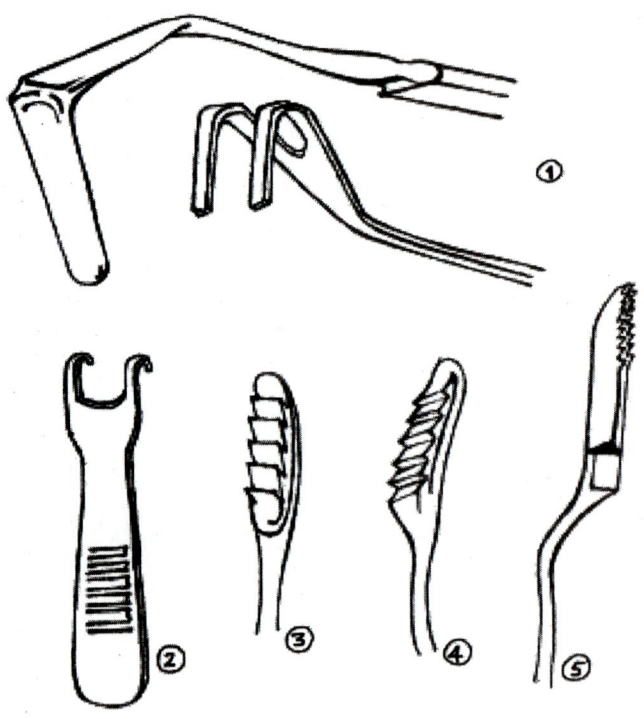

SECTION - III
OPERATIVE SURGERY

1. MYRINGOPLASTY

It is an operation performed to repair or reconstruct the tympanic membrane (without disturbing the middle ear ossicular chain).

INDICATION

It is indicated in benign type of chronic suppurative otitis media ie; tubotympanic type of disease with a dry central perforation and no ossicular or middle ear pathology.

CONTRAINDICATIONS

1. Active stage of chronic suppurative otitis media
2. Eustachian tube malfunction
3. Ossicular chain pathology
4. Squamous epithelium lining the middle ear.

PREREQUISITES

1. Ear should ideally be dry for atleast six weeks preoperatively ie; a dry central perforation.
2. Patent and functioning eustachian tube
3. Tuning fork tests and pure tone audiometry showing conductive hearing loss.
4. No ossicular chain pathology
5. No squamous epithelium lining the middle ear.
6. No focus of infection in the nose, paranasal sinuses and the nasopharynx.

PREOPERATIVE

ANAESTHESIA

Local or General anaesthesia

Local anaesthesia is preferrable as it causes less bleeding, making of an air-pocket medial to the graft is easier and hearing can also be tested on table if required. General anaesthesia is used in children and uncooperative adults.

POSITION

Supine position with affected ear up.

INCISION

A postaural, endaural or an endomeatal incision can be taken. The incision is deepened upto the mastoid mucoperiosteum.

PROCEDURE

After the incision is deepened, its edges are retracted with self-retaining mastoid retractors.

A temporalis fascia graft is harvested. Temporalis fascia is the fascia covering the temporalis muscle. Via the same incision, all the layers above the fascia are separated with an artery forceps and then held up by a retractor. An incision is taken on the fascia according to the amount of graft material required. The fascia is elevated from the underlying muscle and the graft is removed.

Injection of a little amount of saline underneath the graft helps in easy separation of the graft from the underlying muscle. The graft is spread on a glass slide and then covered with another slide.

A semicircular or 'Y' shaped incision is made on the mastoid mucoperiosteum. The mucoperiosteum is elevated with a periosteal elevator. A meatotomy is made in the elevated flap at the level of the spine of Henle, to enter the external auditory canal from behind. The external auditory canal is cleaned and the perforation is inspected.

The perforation is made raw by removing the edges with a sickle knife. A tympanosclerotic plaque abutting the edge needs to be removed. The undersurface of the edge is made raw with a circular knife till the edge becomes thin.

Once the perforation is made raw, the canal skin lying on the posterior canal wall ie; the tympanomeatal flap is elevated from the canal wall. A 6 O'clock and 12 O'clock incision is taken on the canal skin deep down to the bone upto the annulus. The flap is then raised including the annulus. The middle ear is entered after raising the flap and the ossicles are inspected.

The flap is abutted to the anterior canal wall and thorough cleaning and suction is carried out to prepare the ear to lay out the graft. The graft is either put wet or dry like parchment paper.

It is spread on the canal wall and then underlaid (beneath all the layers of the tympanic membrane) with the help of a sickle knife and suction. The edges of the graft are tucked properly under the remnants of the tympanic membrane. There should be an adequate air-pocket medial to the graft. The tympanomeatal flap is replaced on the posterior canal wall. Small pieces of gelfoam are placed over the tucked edges of the graft to secure it in place. The external auditory canal is filled with gelfoam and the wound is closed in layers.

Anterior tucking:

It is the procedure done when the anterior remnant of the tympanic membrane is insufficient to hold the graft. A small tympanomeatal flap is raised from the anterior canal wall and the edge of the graft is tucked beneath it.

POSTOPERATIVE

- Oral antibiotics
- Anti inflammatory analgesics.
- Decongestants
- Local antibiotic ear drops once the external canal gelfoam gets dissolved (at around three weeks).
- Valsalva's manoeuvre from second day to enable better contact between the graft and its bed if underlay technique has been used.

2. CORTICAL MASTOIDECTOMY

SYNONYM : Simple mastoidectomy

Schwartz operation

Definition : It is an operation in which complete exenteration of all accessible mastoid air cells is carried out, keeping the posterior canal wall intact.

INDICATIONS

1. Coalescent mastoiditis
2. Subperiosteal mastoid abscess or fistula.
3. Masked mastoiditis
4. As an approach to:
   - Labyrinthectomy
   - Endolymphatic sac decompression
   - Facial nerve decompression
   - Vestibulo-cochlear nerve section
   - Acoustic neuroma excision
   - Petrosectomy

PREOPERATIVE

X'ray mastoid is essential for: - Delineation of mastoid air cell system.

- Position of dura, sinus plate.

POSITION

Supine position with head turned to opposite side.

ANAESTHESIA

General anaesthesia: for

- Children
- Uncooperative adults
- Patients with intracranial complications.

INCISION

Post auricular incision: A curved incision few milimeters behind and parallel to the postauricular groove.

OPERATION

1. The incision is deepened onto the mastoid periosteum
2. **Exposure of mastoid cortex**

   The mastoid mucoperiosteum is elevated in all directions with the help of a Lemperts mucoperiosteal elevator. The limits are as follows:

   - Superiorly : To the level of upper attachment of pinna.
   - Anteriorly / Forwards : Lateral end of posterior bony meatal wall.

- Posteriorly / Backwards : A few millimeters.

Adequate haemostasis is achieved. The elevated mucoperiosteum is kept retracted with the help of Mollison's self retaining haemostatic mastoid retractor.

3. **Exposure of mastoid antrum**

The mastoid antrum is first located as it is the most consistent and largest air cell.

MacEwen's triangle boundaries

- Superiorly   : Supramastoid crest
- Anteroinferiorly : Posterior margin of external canal which cuts the suprameatal crest.

    Posteroinferiorly: A tangent to external canal which cuts the suprameatal crest.

> **Mastoid Antrum Landmarks:**
> - MacEwen's Triangle-surface marking
> - Depth of 15 mm from the triangle in an adult
> - Depth of few mm in an infant / child.

In the adult the antrum lies 1.5 cm deep to the supra-meatal triangle. A first straight cut with the burr is made along the supramastoid crest starting from anterior part of MacEvens triangle, extending towards the sino-dural angle. A second straight cut is made posterior to posterior meatal wall starting from anterior part of MacEwen's triangle extending towards mastoid tip. Cortex removal with good saucerization is necessary before, deeper penetration into the antrum.

It is better to open the antrum at a higher rather than a lower level to avoid injury to lateral semicircular canal or facial nerve.

To confirm that the antrum has reached

- Pass a Dundas Grant probe / Antral cell seeker into the aditus.
- Lateral canal dome can be seen on its medial wall.
- Judge the adequacy of the aditus.

> **Antrum:**
> - Largest mastoid air cell
> - Aditus in its anterior wall
> - Smooth white dome of horizontal semicircular canal on its medial wall.

The above manoeuvres are performed with great caution to avoid dislodging the short process of incus from the fossa incudis. The aditus may be enlarged with a bone curette if required for adequate drainage. If pus is encountered on opening the antrum, a swab may be collected for culture.

Air cell exenteration

After identifying the antrum, the air cell tracts are slowly drilled from the antrum outwards in all directions

It is important to clear the following air-cell groups:

- Sino-dural angle cells
- Root of zygoma cells in a well-pneumatized bone
- Mastoid tip cells
- Peri labyrinthine cells
- Cells in relation to the vertical facial nerve
- Removal of mastoid tip if it is necrotic, in cases of Bezold's abscess.

TEMPORAL AIR-CELL GROUPS / TRACTS: (ALLAM'S CLASSIFICATION)				
Middle ear:	Mastoid:	Perilabyrinthine	Petrous:	• Zygomatic
• Epitympanum	• Mastoid antrum	• Supralabyrinthine	• Peritubal	• Occipital
• Mesotympanum	• Tegmental / Dural	• Infralabyrinthine	• Apical	• Styloid
• Hypotympanum	• Sinodural		Accessory:	• Squamous
• Protympanum	• Sinal			
• Posterior tympanic	• Facial			
	• Tip cells.			

The air cell tracts are then removed one by one and a bony cavity results. After complete removal of air-cell tracts, the surgeon should be able to see the following boundaries:

Boundaries of a cortical mastoidectomy cavity:		
Superiorly	:	Dural plate
Inferiorly	:	Digastric ridge
Anteriorly	:	Bony meatal wall, Aditus.
Posteriorly	:	Sinus plate
Depth	:	Lateral semicircular canal at the deepest point.

Special cases:

The following techniques are followed in special cases:

CASE	ALTERATION IN TECHNIQUE
1. Extradural abscess	• Part of dural plate is removed • Middle fossa dura is exposed • Check for granulations, pus collection / extradural abscess • If present, the pus is evacuated and exposure is continued till healthy dura is reached
2. Lateral sinus thrombophlebitis	• Part of sinus plate is removed • Sinus is exposed • Fibrosed / organised clot if present is not touched • Unorganised clot is aspirated with wide bore needle.

Smoothening of cavity:

The cavity thus created should have bevelled edges and is to be smoothened with the help of diamond burrs. It is then washed with an antibiotic solution.

Closure of wound:

The mastoid mucoperiosteum is reposited. Some surgeons advocate the use of a drain, inserted into the antrum and brought out from the mastoid tip. The cavity heals by formation of bony granulation tissue and fibrosis. Closure of skin is achieved and a tight mastoid drressing is given.

POSTOPERATIVE

1. Antibiotics, Decongestants
2. Drain removal after discharge stops.
3. Suture removal on seventh day.

COMPLICATIONS

1. Damage to structures	

a. Dural plate	● No treatment is required or
	● Bridge the edges with a graft
	    - Temporalis fascia
	    - Temporalis muscle.

b. Dura	● CSF leak:
	● Repair the tear with temporalis muscle / fascia graft with post-operative:
	    - Head high position
	    - Avoid straining / coughing
	    - Antibiotics

c. Lateral sinus	● Massive bleeding occurs which is treated as follows:
	    - Pressure pack the site
	    - Arrest haemorrhage with surgicel
	    - Bridge the gap in sinus plate with bone wax.
	    - Pack the mastoid cavity with an antibiotic soaked roller gauze which is removed partially everyday.

d. Lateral semicircular canal	● Cover the fistula with bone plate' (bone dust + blood) over which a tissue graft is put.

e. Facial nerve	● Partial cut: suture
	● Complete cut without a gap: suture
	● Complete cut with a gap:
	    - Nerve graft
	    - Rerouting

2. Dislocation of Incus	- Pure tone audiogram: Persistent post-operative conductive hearing loss. - Impedance audiogram : Disruption of ossicular chain. - Reconstruction of ossicular chain may be required.

3. Persistent otorrhoea	Causes of persistent otorrhoea are:
	● Incomplete exenteration of infected cells
	● Infection of residual cells.
	Treatment:
	    - Reopening of mastoid and exenteration.
	    - Antibiotic therapy

3. SEPTAL SURGERY

HISTORY OF SEPTAL SURGERY

SURGEON	OPERATION	PRINCIPLE
Metzenbaum (1929)	Devised the operation for caudal dislocation of the septum	• He compared caudal deviation of the septum to a swinging door, with a hinge on one side and free edges on the rest • In the Metzenbaum operation, the hinge was produced by an incision at the level of the deviation
Peer (1937)	Operation for caudal deviation of the septum.	• Devised the principle of cartilage excision followed by cartilage replacement • Excised the deviated caudal segment and inserted it / other grafting material as a free graft
Galloway (1946)	Extended Peer's principle to the septum	• Removal of entire nasal cartilage and replacing the anterior septum with the free cut cartilage
Fomon (1948) Rees (1986)	Septal removal followed by septal replacement	• Use of small autografts
Cottle (1958)	Septoplasty	• Mobilization and repositioning of septal cartilage
Rubin (1983)	Cartilage morselization	• Deviated septum is crushed with a morselizer • New flattened cartilage may remain on a permanent basis

4. SUBMUCOUS RESECTION OF THE SEPTUM (SMR)

DEFINITION

It is an operation in which the deviated cartilage is removed submucosally. It is done for deviations posterior to the Cottle's Line.

INDICATIONS

1. Symptomatic deviated nasal septum (headache, nasal obstruction, epistaxis) All septal deviations posterior to the imaginary line joining nasal process of frontal bone to nasal spine of maxilla are treated by SMR.

> **Cottle's Line**
> It is a vertical line joining nasal process of frontal bone to nasal process of maxillary bone

2. Complications of deviated nasal septum like recurrent sinusitis, headache, middle ear infections etc.

3. As an approach to the sphenoid sinus, pituitary gland and vidian nerve.

4. To obtain graft material (nasal cartilage, vomerine bone) for rhinoplasty, plastic surgery of ear etc.

5. As a treatment for heriditary telangiectasia. Here the mucoperichondrial flaps are elevated and repositioned to cause fibrosis and prevent epistaxis.

6. For closure of septal perforation

7. As an access for endoscopic sinus surgery

8. As an access for removing polypii

9. As an access for ethmoidectomy

10. As a part of septorhinoplasty

11. Before palatoplasty

CONTRAINDICATIONS

I   Absolute

1. Bleeding disorders
2. Age less than 18 years as
   - Ossification of vomer is not complete and
   - Development of face is incomplete till then

II Relative

1. Acute rhinitis
2. Acute sinusitis
3. Lower respiratory tract infection
4. Hypertension
5. Diabetes mellitus
6. Tuberculosis

PREOPERATIVE

ANAESTHESIA

Local anaesthesia is used as it is performed in adults mainly

Advantages of local anaesthesia :

a) Patient is conscious.

b) Bleeding is less

c) Air blast or relief of nasal obstruction can be checked on table after correction of deformity.

Patient is sedated with 1ml of Fortwin with 1ml of Phenergan diluted to 10 ml given intravenously slowly. The nose is packed with gauze strips dipped in 4% lignocaine with 1:1,00,000 adrenaline for ten minutes prior to surgery.

In the operation theatre, the packs are removed followed by infiltration of the submucoperichondrial plane and nasal floor with 2% lignocaine with 1:1,00,000 adrenaline solution.

Advantages of infiltration

1. It creates a plane submucoperichondrially
2. Tissue planes are thus easily elevated
3. Bleeding is less
4. Provides local anaesthesia.

General anaesthesia with endotracheal intubation and throat packing is done for uncooperative adults and in indicated children. It is useful if rhinoplasty needs to be carried out.

POSITION

Supine position with the head minimally extended.

INCISION

An incision is made 5mm behind the anterior free edge of the nasal septum **(Killian's incision)**. It is preferably made on the concave side of the nasal septum for better visualisation and more operative space.

The mucoperichondrial flap on the side of the incision is elevated with the help of a Freer's elevator. The plane of elevation is the submucoperichondrial plane. It is a relatively white avascular plane. If elevation is made in the correct plane, there is minimal bleeding and elevation is smooth.

An incision is then made on the cartilage through its entire thickness leaving a caudal strip of the septum. The mucoperichondrium on the opposite side should not be incised. Through this incision, the mucoperichondrial flap on the opposite side is elevated. The mucoperiosteal flaps over the bony septum and the maxillary crest are elevated on both the sides. A Killian's self-retaining nasal speculum is inserted on the sides of the septum. A small nick is made on the edge of the septal cartilage 2-3mm below the roof of the nose. The blade of the Ballenger swivel knife is inserted in this nick and the knife is moved backwards, downwards and forwards. The septal cartilage gets separated in one piece and is removed with Luc's forceps.

The Killian's nasal speculum is removed and the flaps are brought to the midline. The incision in the mucoperichondrial flap is sutured with 3-0 chromic catgut. The nasal air blast can be checked on table on a tongue depressor.

Advantages of using Ballenger swivel knife
• Cartilage comes out in one piece
• The cut edges of the cartilage are smooth.

Both the nostrils are packed with roller gauze dipped in liquid paraffin.

POSTOPERATIVE

- Antibiotics
- Anti-inflammatory analgesics
- Tincture benzoin inhalation four times a day to humidify air breathed in through the mouth
- Condy's gargles to prevent halitosis.
- Nasal pack removal after 48 hours.
- Liquid paraffin nasal drops four times a day to loosen crusts after pack removal.

COMPLICATIONS

I.	Immediate	
	a. Primary haemorrhage	This occurs from maxillary crest area. It is controlled by adrenaline packs, electro-cautery or use of bone wax
	b. Trauma to surrounding structures	Damage to mucosa, mucoperichondrial flaps and turbinates can occur.
	c. Anaesthetic complications	Cardiac arrhythmias, hypertension, sensitivity to Xylocaine.
II.	Delayed	
	a. Reactionary haemorrhage	It occurs by 48 hours of surgery. Causes : ● Effect of adrenaline wearing off ● Rise in blood pressure after coming out of general anaesthesia (if given). It is treated by tight anterior nasal packing.
	b. Secondary haemorrhage	It occurs 48 hours after surgery and is caused by infection. Treatment ● Repacking of nose ● Change of antibiotics
	c. Septal haematoma	It is accumulation of blood between the two mucoperichondrial flaps. Excessive accumulation of blood can cause pressure necrosis of the underlying cartilage as it is depleted of its nutrition from the perichondrium. It is treated by drainage of the haematoma by making a nick in one of the mucoperichondrial flaps followed by insertion of a long wick in the space and anterior nasal packing.
	d. Septal abscess	It is collection of pus in between the flaps and is due to infection of the haematoma. It can give rise to fever, severe throbbing pain, nasal obstruction and intracranial complications, if untreated. It is treated with urgent incision and drainage, putting a wick in the space and intravenous antibiotics and analgesics.
	e. Septal perforation	It occurs if both the mucoperichondrial flaps are torn at the same site
	f. Flapping septum	This condition occurs if excessive nasal mucosa is left behind after removal of a grossly deviated septum. The mucosa sags on one side on lying down and makes a flapping sound on respiration.
	g. Infection	Infection of the nose or paranasal sinuses can occur if the packs are kept longer than 48 hours or if drainage of the sinuses suffer.
	h. Synechiae and adhesions	These develop between the septum and lateral nasal wall resulting in nasal obstruction. They are cut and a silastic sheet is inserted in between the raw areas.
	i. External nasal deformity	The operation can result in a saddle nose deformity, columellar retraction etc. if the cartilage at the roof and the caudal strip are not preserved.

5. SEPTOPLASTY

DEFINITION

It is an operative procedure in which the deviated part of the septum is corrected by removal of bony and/or cartilagenous septum. It is carried out for deviations anterior to the Cottle's line.

INDICATIONS

1. Symptomatic deviated nasal septum
2. Complications of deviated nasal septum like recurrent sinusitis, epistaxis, headache, upper respiratory tract infection.
3. As a part of septorhinoplasty.

CONTRAINDICATIONS

I Absolute

1. Bleeding disorders
2. Age less than 18 years as
   - Ossification of vomer is not complete and
   - Development of face is incomplete till then

II Relative

1. Acute rhinitis
2. Acute sinusitis
3. Lower respiratory tract infection
4. Hypertension
5. Diabetes mellitus
6. Tuberculosis

PREOPERATIVE

ANAESTHESIA

It is usually done under local anaesthesia. In uncooperative patients, in children and in cases where a rhinoplasty would be carried out, it is done under general anaesthesia.

POSITION

Supine position with minimal head extension.

INCISION

Freer's incision: A unilateral hemitransfixation incision is made at the lower border of the septal cartilage.

Advantages of the incision:

1. The incision is in a relatively avascular plane
2. Mucosal edges are thick and tough, therefore less chances of a tear
3. It provides good access to the whole of the septum, caudal border, anterior nasal spine and the premaxillary crest.
4. The incision can be extended to the opposite side producing a full transfixation incision, which can be used for a rhinoplasty.

The incision is deepened, including the perichondrium. Elevation of the submucoperichondrial plane is done with a Freer's elevator.

Exposure

The subperichondrial plane is elevated to expose the cartilagenous and bony septum. The mucosal flap is elevated on one side only ie; usually the concave side. The opposite mucoperichondrial flap is maintained.

Advantages of elevation of a unilateral mucoperichondrial flap:

1. It ensures the viability of the cartilage
2. It reduces the chances of
   - Septal perforation
   - Septal abscess
   - Septal haematoma
   - Overriding of segments of cartilage.

Difficult flap elevation

- It is encountered in cases with variation of anatomy.
- It occurs at junction of septal cartilage above, anterior nasal spine, premaxillary crest and vomer below.
- Most iatrogenic perforations occur along the chondrovomerine suture.

PROCEDURE

After elevating the mucoperichondrial flap from the concave side, the cartilagenous and bony septal junction is identified and punctured with a Freer's elevator. The posterior edge of the cartilage is separated from the bony septum and the inferior edge is separated from the maxillary crest on the concave side. Once the cartilage is free, the opposite side mucoperiosteum is separated from the bony septum and the deviations of the bony septum are removed with Luc's forceps. The deviations of the cartilage if any, are corrected by resection or cross-hatching of the cartilage. The maxillary crest is then removed. The mucoperichondrial flap is repositioned and the incision is sutured with 3-0 chromic catgut sutures. Both the nostrils are packed with roller gauze dipped in liquid paraffin.

POSTOPERATIVE

- Antibiotics
- Anti-inflammatory analgesics
- Tincture benzoin inhalation four times a day to humidify air breathed in through the mouth
- Condy's gargles to prevent halitosis.
- Nasal pack removal after 48 hours.
- Liquid paraffin nasal drops four times a day to loosen dry crusts after pack removal.

COMPLICATIONS

- Anaesthetic complications
- Haemorrhage: primary, reactionary or secondary
- Trauma to surrounding structures
- Synechiae formation
- Persistence of nasal obstruction.

SUBMUCOUS RESECTION	SEPTOPLASTY
• Usually cartilage is removed in this operation	• Usually bone is removed.
• Flaps are elevated on both sides of the septum	• Flap is elevated on one side of the septum.
• Risk of septal perforation is higher	• Chance of perforation is less.
• Septal haematoma and abscess can occur	• Chance of haematoma and abscess formation is less.
• Cosmetic complications like supratip deformity, columellar retraction and saddle nose deformity are more	• These cosmetic complications are less.
• Cannot be combined with rhinoplasty	• Can be combined with septorhinoplasty.
• Revision surgery is difficult	• Revision surgery is relatively less difficult.

6. ANTRAL PUNCTURE

It is a procedure in which lavage of the maxillary sinus is carried out with a trocar and cannula inserted through the inferior meatus.

INDICATIONS

Diagnostic

1. To confirm diagnosis of chronic maxillary sinusitis.
2. To examine the returning fluid for bacterial culture, antibiotic sensitivity and malignant cells.

Therapeutic

1. Lavage in chronic maxillary sinusitis
2. Acute maxillary sinusitis not responding to conservative measures
3. Atrophic rhinitis causing sinusitis.

CONTRAINDICATIONS

1. Age : It is not indicated in children under 3 yrs. of age as the sinus is very small.
2. Acute maxillary sinusitis : If performed in acute cases, it results in flaring up of inflammation, osteomyelitis and increase bleeding.
3. Systemic conditions like
   - Hypertension
   - Diabetes mellitus
   - Bleeding disorders

PREOPERATIVE

- Nil by mouth for 4 hours before the procedure
- Injection Atropine 0.6mg intramuscularly ½ hour before the procedure to prevent vasovagal attack
- Injection Tetanus toxoid 0.5 ml intramuscularly before the procedure.
- Written informed valid consent

ANAESTHESIA

Local anaesthesia

It is given using three swab sticks dipped in 4% Lignocaine with adrenaline (1:2,00,000) placed at the following sites for ten minutes :

a) Inferior meatus - for anaesthesia of superior alveolar nerve
b) Middle meatus - for anaesthesia of sphenopataline ganglion and its branches
c) Roof of nose - for anaesthesia of anterior ethmoidal nerve.

General anaesthesia

It may be required in children under 12 yrs. of age and in uncooperative nervous adults. The endotracheal tube is passed through the mouth.

POSITION

Supine position

The Tilley-Lichwitz trocar and cannula and the Higginson's syringe are inspected. The trocar should be sharp and its tip should project 3mm. beyond the cannula. The trocar should easily slide in and out of the cannula.

The patient's head is steadied and the trocar and cannula are held in the left hand for a left antral puncture. The site of puncture in the inferior meatus is visualised with a Thudicum's nasal speculum. The trocar and cannula (the cannula covering the point of the trocar) are then inserted in the inferior meatus along its lateral wall, nearer to the roof than the floor.

The tip is pointed in the direction of the tragus of the ipsilateral ear. With a gentle boring motion and moderate pressure after withdrawing the cannula so that the trocar protrudes out, the trocar is made to pierce the medial wall of the antrum. There is a sudden feeling of give-way as the trocar and cannula enter the antrum. In the adult, the ideal point of entry is 3.5cm posterior to the lateral edge of the vestibule. This point lies behind the nasolacrimal duct and pierces the thinnest area of the bony wall of the meatus (Robsmith). A properly positioned cannula moves in all directions and does not fall back.

A Higginson's syringe filled with sterile normal saline at 37^{0}C is attached to the cannula. The patient is asked to bend forwards, flex his neck and breathe through his open mouth. The antral washout is carried out by compressing the syringe. The fluid from the syringe passes through the cannula to the antrum. It flows out from the natural ostium into the anterior nares, from where it is collected in a kidney tray. The washing is continued till the returning fluid is clear. Thereafter the cannula is removed and the nostril is packed with a cotton pledget to prevent oozing of blood. The returning fluid is sent for bacteriological/required examination. The same procedure is repeated on the opposite side if indicated.

POSTOPERATIVE

- Oral antibiotics depending on the character of the returning fluid.
- Anti inflammatory analgesic drugs.
- Nasal decongestants

COMPLICATIONS

1. **Anaesthetic**
   - Vasovagal attack
   - Hypotension
   - Cardiac arrest
2. **Surgical**
   - **Haemorrhage**
   - **False passage into the cheek or orbit**. Bulging of cheek or proptosis results when a false passage is created and water/air enter in.
   - **Air embolism** if air enters a ruptured vein accidently from the antrum
   - **Infection**.

Difficulties that may be encountered at antral puncture :

1. **Inability to pierce bone with trocar and cannula**

   Reasons

   a) Blunt trocar

   b) Thickened bony wall in
      - Chronic sinusitis
      - Atrophic rhinitis

2. **No returning fluid**

   Reasons

   a) Blockage of cannula leads to difficult introduction of fluid itself.

b) Blockage of natural ostium of the maxillary sinus. A second cannula can be introduced besides the first to enable drainage from the sinus

c) Cannula may abut against the wall of the antrum preventing fluid from entering into the antrum.

It is withdrawn a little and then fluid can flow in smoothly.

d) A false passage may have been created in the cheek or the eye. Introduction of water results in proptosis or swelling of the cheek. The cannula is withdrawn in such cases. It is again correctly put in required cases or the procedure may be abandoned.

7. CALDWELL-LUC OPERATION

It is an operation in which an opening is made in the anterior wall of the maxillary sinus through the canine fossa to visualise and remove disease from the sinus.

It was described by Caldwell from NewYork and Luc from France.

PRINCIPLES

1. Removal of unhealthy irreversibly damaged mucosa of the sinus.
2. To facilitate aeration and drainage of the sinus by creating an antrostomy.

INDICATIONS

1. Intractable infection in the antrum
2. Non-resolution of chronic sinusitis following intranasal antrostomy.
3. Antrochoanal polyp in the antrum
4. Osteonecrosis, to clear debri
5. Foreign body in antrum (especially root of molar/premolar teeth)
6. Fracture maxilla reduction
7. Removal of dental cyst involving the antrum
8. Oroantral fistula excision
9. Fungal sinusitis
10. As an approach
    a) To pterygomaxillary fissure and sphenopalatine fossa for Internal maxillary artery ligation and vidian neurectomy.
    b) To sphenoid sinus/pituitary for hypophysectomy.
11. Treatment of atrophic rhinitis :

    Raghav Sharan operation : Implantation of maxillary sinus mucosa into nasal cavity

    Whittmack's operation : Implantation of Stenson's duct into nasal cavity.
12. Orbital decompression for malignant exophthalmos
13. Jenson Horgan operation : Transantral ethmoidectomy
14. Implantation of radioactive needles into the antrum for carcinoma of maxilla
15. Elevation and stabilization of fracture of orbital floor by intra antral packing. It is useful for reduction of blow-out fracture of the orbit.

CONTRAINDICATIONS

1. Age below 12 years

   Damage to second dentition results in hypoplasia of maxilla
2. Acute sinusitis

   Operation on inflamed sinus leads to excessive bleeding, dissemination of infection and osteomyelitis.
3. Diabetes mellitus
4. Hypertension
5. Bleeding disorders

PREOPERATIVE

ANAESTHESIA

General anaesthesia/Local anaesthesia

Local anaesthesia   :   Surface anaesthesia is given with 4% Xylocaine with adrenaline soaked cotton pledgets placed in both nostrils above and below the inferior turbinate.

Infiltration anaesthesia :   2% Xylocaine with adrenaline is injected along the gingivobuccal sulcus in the region of the canine fossa. The injection is continued superiorly to include the infraorbital nerve.

General anaesthesia   :   Endotracheal tube either orally or nasally is passed from the unaffected side. Adequate pharyngeal packing is required.

POSITION

Supine position with 15^0 head high.

INCISION

A transverse incision is made along the gingivobuccal sulcus well (3 mm) above the roots of the teeth. It extends from the level of the lateral border of lateral incisor to the second molar. The incision runs for around 3.5-4 cms, parallel to the teeth.

PROCEDURE

The incision is deepened down to the bone ie; through the mucous membrane and the periosteum. The periosteum is then elevated from the canine fossa upwards 5 mm short of the infraorbital canal with an elevator or with a chisel and gauze piece. The elevation is made as atraumatic as possible to prevent injury to the infraorbital nerve. Two retractors, one placed superomedially and the other superolaterally are used to avoid damaging the infraorbital nerve. Gentle retraction is essential. The anterior wall of the antrum is thus exposed.

Perforation of canine fossa :

The canine fossa can be fenestrated with a gouge and hammer, rotating burr or curette. Whatever method is used, a fracture has to be avoided to prevent damage to infraorbital nerve or a tooth root. The opening is enlarged with a bone punch, a burr or Kerrison bone-cutting forceps. Lateral and inferior extension of the opening is avoided to prevent damage to the branches of sphenopalatine artery and roots of the teeth respectively. Bleeding may occur from the bone margin which can be controlled by using Kerrison forceps. The entire contents of the antrum are inspected.

Inspection of the antrum :

- Irreversibly diseased lining   :   Removed with elevators, forceps, curette
- Cysts and benign tumours   :   Removed with elevators and forceps

Care has to be taken while dissecting mucosa from the roof as the nerve may not have a bony canal. Bleeding stops once all the diseased mucosa is removed. After inspecting and removing disease from the antrum, an intranasal antrostomy is performed.

Intranasal antrostomy :

An opening in the inferior meatus of the size of 1.5 cm is made with Tilley's antral harpoon. It can be enlarged anteriorly by Kerrison forceps. The lower end of the opening should be at the level of the antral floor and the anterior end upto the anterior end of inferior turbinate. Enlarging posteriorly can cause bleeding from greater palatine artery.

Following the antrostomy, the antrum is packed with an antibiotic ointment (BIPP) soaked roller gauze to achieve haemostasis and asepsis. The pack is brought out via the antrostomy opening and taped to the cheek. The incision in the gingivobuccal sulcus is closed. Good approximation preserves the sulcus which helps in denture fitting. The antral pack is removed after 24 hours. An ice pack is kept over the cheek postoperatively to prevent oedema and haematoma formation. Antibiotics are indicated if purulent secretions are encountered in the antrum. The nose is also packed.

COMPLICATIONS

Immediate

1. Soft tissue swelling : Oedema of cheek and upper lip. It is avoided by gentle retraction throughout the procedure.
2. Haemorrhage
3. Pain
4. Damage to teeth
5. Paraesthesias over cheek (damage to infraorbital nerve)
6. Damage to orbital floor
7. Osteomyelitis of maxillary bone.

Delayed

1. Infraorbital neuralgia
2. Dental neuralgia
3. Oroantral fistula
4. Devitalisation of teeth
5. Recurrent sinusitis

MODIFICATIONS OF CALDWELL-LUC OPERATION

1. **Denker's operation (1906).**

   The incision is similar to Caldwell-Luc operation except that it extends more medially upto the frenum ie; approximately to the midpoint of upper lip.

   Elevation of soft tissues reveals the anterior bony pyramid of the maxilla.

   A triangular piece of bone from lateral wall of nose and the front of antrum is removed with removal of nasal and antral mucosa.

   This procedure thus creates a window for inspection of the antrum and an anteriorly-placed antrostomy.

2. **Canfield's operation (1908)**

   In this operation, an incision is made behind the nasal vestibule. Periosteum is elevated to expose the canine fossa through the incision. Anterior angle of maxillary sinus (anteromedially) is chiselled off to expose the sinus contents. The same opening is continued posteriorly into an intranasal antrostomy.

3. **Mcneill maxillary sinus obliteration (1966)**

   In this operation, the maxillary sinus is obliterated with abdominal fat after its mucous membrane lining is completely removed. The incision, antral opening and closure is similar to Caldwell-Luc operation.

CALDWELL-LUC OPERATION
- Sublabial gingivobuccal incision
- Elevation of soft tissues including periosteum
- Exposure of anterior wall of the antrum
- An opening made in the anterior wall in the region of the canine fossa.
- Inspection of antrum
- Removal of diseased mucosa or procedure carried out as per the indication
- Creation of inferior antrostomy
- Haemostasis
- Closure
- Gentle retraction and protection of infraorbital nerve is maintained throughout the procedure.

8. FUNCTIONAL ENDOSCOPIC SINUS SURGERY

This procedure is a recent advance in sinus surgery in which blockage of the ostio-meatal unit is cleared to establish drainage and ventilation of the paranasal sinuses.

PRINCIPLE

Messerklinger's Principle: It states that chronic sinus disease is primarily due to disease in the ethmoidal air cells blocking the natural ostia in the middle meatus leading to impaired drainage of the sinuses; predisposing them to recurrent infection.

Therefore if the ostium of the diseased sinus is unblocked surgically by removal of diseased ethmoidal air cells, normal drainage and ventilation of the sinus is re-established and diseased mucosa comes back to normal. There is no need to remove all diseased mucosa as was thought earlier.

The mucociliary transport in the paranasal sinuses occurs in a genetically predetermined definite pattern, transporting the mucus always towards the natural ostium. Thus a dependent opening made as in maxillary sinus inferior antrostomy, does not result in adequate drainage as the secretions circumvent the antrostomy opening and get transported towards the natural ostium. By way of functional endoscopic sinus surgery, the middle meatus area which is the key drainage site of the paranasal sinuses is visualised and its blockage by diseased ethmoidal air cells is removed by removal of the air cells, and ventilation and drainage of the frontal and maxillary sinus is re-established. For the sphenoid sinus, disease in the sphenoethmoidal recess is similarly removed.

PATHOLOGY IN CHRONIC SINUSITIS

Disease in ethmoidal air cells

⇓

Blockage of middle meatus ostia ⇐

⇓

Stagnation of secretions in sinuses

⇓   ⇑

Secondary Infection ⇒ Loss of mucociliary clearance

⇓

Mucosal oedema   Further blocking

⇓

Polypus formation

AIM

1. To re-establish drainage through the natural ostia
2. To restore ventilation
3. To restore mucociliary clearance

INDICATIONS OF ENDOSCOPIC SINUS SURGERY

1. Chronic sinusitis
2. Recurrent sinusitis
3. Chronic sinusitis with orbital cellulitis
4. Nasal polyposis
5. Mild fungal sinusitis

> Nasal polyposis and chronic sinusitis not responding to medical line of treatment are classic indications for FESS.

6. Concha bullosa – excision
7. Partial turbinectomy
8. Interior turbinate – bipolar cautery
9. Synechae release
10. Epistaxis – cauterization
11. Dacryocystorhinostomy
12. Optic nerve decompression
13. CSF rhinorrhoea
14. Mucocoele removal
15. Pyocoele removal
16. Meningocoele removal
17. Osteoma removal
18. Inverted papilloma excision
19. Rhinosporidiosis
20. Hypophysectomy
21. Vidian neurectomy
22. Adenoidectomy
23. Sphenopalatine ganglion block
24. Nasopharyngeal biopsy
25. Endoscopic septal resection
26. Facial recess examination
27. Orbital decompression
28. Congenital choanal atresia surgery
29. Foreign body sinuses
30. Blow-out fracture repair
31. Biopsy of tumours (postero lateral wall of maxilla)
32. Inspection of post-operative cavities (maxillectomy, craniofacial resection)
33. Removal of small nasopharyngeal angiofibromas.

CONTRAINDICATIONS

1. Aggressive fungal sinusitis (Mucormycosis)
2. Sinusitis with intracranial complications
3. Stenosed frontonasal duct
4. Osteomyelitis of sinuses

PROCEDURE

Pre-requisites

C.T. scan of paranasal sinuses

- Axial and coronal views
- To study anatomical landmarks before surgery
- To study anatomical variations

> **Anatomical variations**
> - Concha bullosa
> - Enlarged ethmoidal bulla
> - Everted uncinate process
> - Paradoxical middle turbinate
> - Agger nasi cells
> - Haller cells

PREOPERATIVE

Anaesthesia

Local anaesthesia/General anaesthesia

Advantages of local anaesthesia:

1. Bleeding is less
2. Pain during surgery is recognized

   Undue pain at surgery is seen when:
   - Dura is touched
   - Orbital periosteum is breached

Nasal cavity is sprayed with 4% Xylocaine and packed with ribbon gauze soaked in Xylocaine lotion. 2% Xylocaine with 1:2,00,000 adrenaline infiltration is carried out into the lateral wall of nose and the uncinate process. Sublabial infiltration is carried out if the canine fossa is to be punctured.

OPERATION

Thorough endoscopic examination of the nose

A thorough endoscopic examination of the nasal cavity is done with a 30⁰ endoscope. The endoscope is first passed between the nasal septum and the inferior turbinate examining the whole cavity upto the choana. On reaching the choana, the eustachian tube openings; and the nasopharynx are visualised **(First pass)**. The endoscope is then passed along the middle meatus to examine any pathology there **(Second pass)**. It is then passed between the superior turbinate and the septum upto the anterior wall of the sphenoid sinus **(Third pass)**.

Uncinectomy with Infundibulectomy

An incision is given circumferentially just anterior to the uncinate process with a sickle knife using Hopkins O⁰ telescope passed through the nose. Mucosa is elevated and the uncinate process is carefully grasped with a Blakesley forceps and removed by a twisting movement, exposing the infundibulum. This procedure is known as infundibulotomy. Alternatively, the uncinate process can be straight away grasped with a reverse cutting forceps and then removed. When the whole process is completely removed, the upper part exposes the frontal recess area. The maxillary sinus ostium may now be visible in the lower part.

Anterior Ethmoidectomy and Middle Meatus Antrostomy

The bulla ethmoidalis – the largest of the ethmoidal air cells is now removed with Blakesley forceps. Ethmoid air cell exenteration is carried out within the said limits:

Superiorly   :   Upto the roof where the anterior ethmoidal artery is identified.

Laterally   :   Lamina papyracea (medial wall of the orbit)

Medially   :   Cribriform plate.

Posteriorly   :   Ground lamella-posterior bony attachment of middle turbinate, which separates the middle from the posterior ethmoidal cells

Ethmoid cell exenteration has to be done within the said limits otherwise laterally the orbit may be entered breaching the lamina papyracea and superiorly the cribriform plate with the dura can get damaged leading to CSF leaks.

The maxillary ostium if stenosed is enlarged anteriorly by using backbiting forceps.

Posterior enlargement is avoided to prevent damage to branches of sphenopalatine artery.

> **Stankwicz Sign**
> Pressure on the eyeball transmits movements of periorbital tissue or fat to the nasal cavity if the **lamina papyracea** is breached.

Exploration of the Frontal Recess

The frontal recess is explored after removal of the anterior ethmodial cells, agger nasi cells with a 30⁰ telescope and upward biting forceps.

After removing anterior cells the opening of the frontonasal duct is seen which is cleared by removing the diseased mucosa around it.

The frontal sinus is clearly visible only after removal of the cranial extension of the uncinate process.

Some surgeons prefer to keep the bulla intact, clear the frontal recess first followed by an anterior ethmoidectomy.

Posterior Ethmoidectomy and Sphenoidectomy

The posterior ethmoids can be reached after opening the ground lamella with the tip of Blakesley's forceps. The course of the ground lamella is followed with the endoscope and part of it is removed.

The bulge of the sphenoid is evident in the infero-medial aspect of the most posterior ethmoid cell and is opened. Any pathology in the sphenoid sinus is removed under direct vision because of the close relationship of the nerve and internal carotid artery to its lateral wall. The sphenoid sinus can also be approached from the posterior end of the superior turbinate where its ostium lies.

Direct visualization of maxillary sinus

The canine fossa is punctured with a trocar puncture and a 30^0 or 70^0 telescope is used for visualization.

The maxillary sinus can also be visualised through its widened ostium.

The ethmoid cavities are packed with gelfoam.

The nasal cavities may be packed if required with a BIPP or merocel pack, to be removed after 2 days.

Nasal douches are given after removal of packs to remove any crusts.

POSTOPERATIVE

- Antibiotics
- Anti-inflammatory analgesic drugs.
- Pack/merocel removal after 48 hours
- Nasal washes to remove crusts and prevent adhesions.
- Intranasal steroid sprays for indicated cases.
- Follow-up nasal endoscopy.

Nasal endoscopy is done post-operatively

1. To check healing of the ethmoid cavity
2. To remove any secretions and blood clots
3. To break any synechiae

COMPLICATIONS

- Haemorrhage
- Cerebrospinal fluid leak
- Blindness (damage to optic nerve)
- Diplopia
- Orbital haematoma (damage to anterior ethmoidal artery and retraction into the orbit)
- Orbital surgical emphysema
- Injury to internal carotid artery
- Injury to nasolacrimal duct/Epiphora
- Synechiae
- Antrostomy closure
- Toothache
- Intracranial haemorrhage
- Pneumoencephalus
- Brain abscess/Meningitis

DEGREES OF ENDOSCOPIC SURGERY	
1st	Ciliary activity present. Widening of ostio meatal unit
2nd	Associated Ethmoidal polypi. Intranasal Ethmoidectomy. Widening of ostia
3rd	Frontal sinus involvement also. The frontoethmoidal and maxillary sinus are converted to one cavity.
4th	Sphenoid sinus involvement also. Sphenoid sinus connected to the frontoethmoid and maxillary cavities.

9. RHINOPLASTY

Rhinoplasty: To mould the nose in an aesthetically pleasing shape.

Septoplasty: To change the shape of the septum to achieve functional improvement.

INDICATIONS

The basic indication is the patient's desire to have an aesthetically pleasing nose and the ability of the surgeon to deliver the desired results within surgical and anatomical constraints.

Commonest deformities of the nose that are treated by rhinoplasty are:

1. Saddle nose: depressed nasal dorsum requiring augmentation
2. Humped nose.
3. Crooked nose.
4. Tip deformities: Inadequate tip projection / definition (round tip), bifid tip, boxy tip, flared nostrils.
5. Cleft tip nose.
6. Postraumatic / surgical deformities

CONTRAINDICATIONS

1. Anatomic unsuitability.
2. Emotional inadequacy.
3. Medically unfit.
4. Relative contraindication is a young patient (prepubertal)

Anatomy

1. Bony vault-Nasal bones, frontal process of maxilla.
2. Cartilagenous vault - Upper lateral cartilages.
3. Tip: Lower lateral cartilages (alar cartilages), accessory cartilages, fibrofatty tissue.
4. Septum:

   Bony parts

   a. Perpendicular plate of ethmoid
   b. Vomer
   c. Crest of maxilla and palatine bones

   Cartilagenous part   :   quadrangular cartilages

   Membranous septum :   between caudal border of septum and medial crura of alar cartilage

   Sensory innervation (for local anaesthesia):
   - External nose   :   Anterior ethmoidal nerve, branches from nasociliary, infra orbital, infratrochlear and supratrochlear nerves.
   - Internal aspects: Branches of nasociliary nerve and sphenopalatine ganglion

PREOPERATIVE

Clinical examination

1. External :   The nose has to be viewed from the frontal, profile, oblique and worm's eye view (from below)
2. Internal :   The septum, vestibule, valve area, posterior choanae and the turbinate size have to be seen.

3. To determine what is unattractive above the nose eg: a hump, inadequate projection of dorsum, alar flare, round tip etc.

The operative plan is made after clinical examination, surface measurements and photographic analysis.

ANAESTHESIA

Most surgeons prefer hypotensive general anaesthesia. It can be done under local anaesthesia.

POSITION

Supine position with neck extension by a pillow under the shoulder and minimal head high tilt.

OPERATION

It is divided into five components:

Component I:

Exposure

a) **Open approach**: In this approach a bilateral rim incision is taken which is connected by a transcolumellar incision.

Advantages of an open approach:

a) It gives excellent exposure to the entire nasal framework.

b) It preserves the tip-septal angle relationship

c) It makes it easier to operate on the tip.

Indications of an open approach:

1. For revision rhinoplasty cases

2. When the surgeon is relatively inexperienced.

b) **Closed approach** : It entails the use of a rim incision, inter-cartilagenous and intracartilagenous transfixion incisions.

Rim incision	:	It is useful to approach the tip.
Intercartilagenous incision	:	It gives excellent exposure for the bony and cartilagenous dorsum
Intracartilagenous incision	:	It is useful when cephalic trim of the cartilage is indicated. Through the alar cartilage, the portion of the cartilage cephalad to the incision is removed.

Advantages of a closed approach:

• It avoids a transcolumellar scar

Disadvantages:

1. It gives poor exposure

2. It is difficult to approach the tip through this procedure

3. The transfixion incision disturbs the tip-septal angle relationship.

Component II:

In this step, **degloving of the skin** from the bony and cartilagenous septum is carried out. The entire skin of the dorsum has to be degloved as the loose skin evenly drapes over the changed framework.

Component III:

In this step, modification of the bony and cartilagenous dorsum is carried out by:

a) **Reduction / augmentation**

b) **Narrowing of the vault**

a) Reduction : In this step, removal of the cartilagenous hump is done with a knife / rasp. Removal of bony hump is done with an osteotome or a rasp. Removal by a push-rasp is safer.

b) Augmentation : Most Indian patients require an augmentation rather than a reduction.

Materials used for augmentation are:

i) Cartilage:

Septal / conchal.

Septal cartilage is in the same operative field. It is the best material to augment the dorsum as it is straight in shape and has least chances of resorption. Also the septum can be corrected in the same step.

ii) Bone

a) Iliac crest bone: It can be sculptured into a desired shape and large amounts can be harvested. There are chances of resorption, which may be uneven producing deformities.

b) Calvarial graft : It has the least chances of resorption. However its harvesting requires special instruments and sculpturing is a little difficult.

iii) Implants

- They can be of silastic or portex material
- They are available in different shapes and sizes
- It requires extreme aseptic precautions for insertion.
- It is ideally not to be inserted through an intranasal incision.
- It should not be used along with major nose work like osteotomies etc.
- There are chances of infection and extrusion.

  However implants are tolerated well by Indians than Caucasians.

c) Narrowing of the vault:

It is always necessary along with hump reduction to close the open-roof.

It is achieved by:

i) **Lateral osteotomy**:

It may be **external** (transcutaneous) with a 2mm. osteotome or **internal** along the edge of the pyriform aperture. The frontal process of the maxilla is broken along a line joining the ala to a point approximately 5mm. medial to the medial canthus

ii) **Medial osteotomy** and out fracture:

It is done on either side of the bony septum (perpendicular plate of ethmoid) with a 8-10 mm. osteotome to separate the nasal bones from septal attachment. At the end, the osteotome is swung laterally to break the superior attachment of the nasal bones with the frontal bone (out-fracture).

In-fracture : The loose nasal bones are compressed along the line of lateral osteotomy so as to achieve a medial shift and narrowing of the vault.

Component IV: Tip work.

A drooping tip can be corrected by:

a) Cephalic trim of alar cartilage

b) Hitching the alar cartilage to the septum

c) Excision of caudal septum

d) Invagination procedure-the septal angle is invaginated between the two medial crura and domes and sutured.

e) Umbrella type tip graft.

A boxy tip can be corrected by:

1. Scoring the domes

2. Dome transection

3. Tip graft.

An inadequately projecting tip can be corrected by:

1. Scoring or cross-hatching the domes
2. Umbrella graft or an onlay graft.

The flaring of the ala can be corrected by alar wedge resection.

Component V: Closure and splintage

Closure is achieved by 4-0 absorbable sutures.

Nasal packing is usually not required unless extensive septal work has been done.

The nasal dorsum is covered with an adhesive tape. The tip is splinted to the dorsum by a 'u' shaped adhesive tape. Splintage with Plaster of Paris is indicated in cases of onlay grafting and osteotomies. It is to be maintained for one week.

Ancillary procedures: These are procedures to improve the profile and harmony of facial features along with a rhinoplasty:

i) Forehead augmetation or reduction.
ii) Malar or chin implants
iii) Genioplasty.

10. ADENOIDECTOMY

It is an operation in which the nasopharyngeal lymphoid tissue-adenoids is removed surgically.
It is usually performed along with a tonsillectomy.

INDICATIONS

1. Persistent or recurrent enlargement of adenoids leading to
   - Severe nasal obstruction
   - Mouth breathing
   - Adenoid facies
   - Nasal discharge
   - Obstructive sleep apnoea
   - Failure to thrive
2. Secondary infection giving rise to
   - Otitis media
   - Bronchitis
   - Cervical adenitis

CONTRAINDICATIONS

1. Blood dyscrasias
   i)   Haemophilia
   ii) Purpura
   iii) Leukaemias
2. Submucous cleft palate. In these cases, velopharyngeal insufficiency can develop postoperatively as the adenoids help to close the velopharynx
3. Upper respiratory tract infections
4. Systemic disorders
   - Hypertension
   - Diabetes mellitus
   - Tuberculosis
   - Anaemia
5. Epidemic of polio. (rare nowadays)

   Adenoidectomy is performed only in children as the adenoid tissue undergoes atrophy by the age of puberty. It can be done in children under 5 yrs. of age where tonsillectomy is contraindicated

PREOPERATIVE

ANAESTHESIA

General anaesthesia with orotracheal intubation. It is always performed under general anaesthesia as it is performed in children.

POSITION

Supine position with less extension than that for tonsillectomy ie; Rose's position with less extension of neck. The reduction in extension is to prevent damage to atlanto-occipital joint during curettage.

PROCEDURE

Palpation of nasopharynx

Under general anaesthesia, after application of a mouth-gag an index finger is passed behind the soft palate to assess

- Width of nasopharynx
- Size of adenoids
- To feel any abnormal pulsations
- To push adenoids medially

Insertion of curette

The broadest adenoid curette has to be selected to fit in the postnasal space without encroaching on the eustachian tube orifices. After palpation of adenoids, the tongue is depressed and the adenoid curette, held like a pen is passed into the oropharynx just behind the soft palate. It is passed with the blade facing the footend. Once it reaches behind the uvula, it is rotated by 180^0, thus facing superiorly, without damaging the uvula and posterior pharyngeal wall.

> **Methods of Adenoidectomy :**
> Using adenoid curette
> Using adenotome
> Finger dissection (in the past)

Curettage of adenoids

Now the grip is changed to that of a dagger and the adenoid curette is brought in contact with the posterior edge of the bony nasal septum. It is ensured that the curette is in the midline and then the adenoids are shaved away with a sweeping downward movement of the wrist, maintaining a constant steady pressure. The curettage should not be too deep as it may injure submucosal vessels running horizontally at the junction of roof and posterior wall of nasopharynx. The whole adenoid mass is thus shaved off with the blade of an adenoid curette with cage. The cage prevents the adenoid tissue or its fragments from falling into lower respiratory tract. Alternatively, the central mass of the adenoid is removed with a curette without a cage and the adenoid is delivered out of the oropharynx with Luc's forceps. The remaining lateral masses are removed with a smaller curette.

Haemostasis

Following removal of the adenoids, an adenoid pack made of rolled up gauze is put in the postnasal space to achieve haemostasis. It is left in place for 4-5 minutes if only adenoidectomy is to be performed. (If adenoidectomy is combined with tonsillectomy, the pack is left in the postnasal space, till the whole procedure of tonsillectomy is completed and removed thereafter).

After the adenoid pack is removed, the nasopharynx is palpated for any adenoid tags. If tags are present, they are removed using a small sized adenoid curette or a Luc's forceps or a conchotome.

COMPLICATIONS

1. **Haemorrhage**
   a) **Primary haemorrhage** occurs at the time of surgery. It is due to :
      - Adenoid tags
      - Deep curettage leading to damage to pharyngeal mucosa

      Adenoid tags if present are removed followed by repacking for a while. Damage to mucosa may require repacking for a longer time or rarely a postnasal pack which is to be removed within 48 hrs. Intravenous antibiotics need to be given along with the packing.

      Also the soft palate can be retracted with retractors or with two simple rubber catheters passed through the nose and brought out through the oral cavity and any bleeding vessel is looked for. A bleeding vessel high in the nasopharynx is detected by flexing the patient's head so that the nasopharynx is no longer dependent. Bleeding points can be cauterized with a silver nitrate stick or with electrocautery.

   b) **Reactionary haemorrhage** occurs within 12 hours of surgery and may require a postnasal pack for control.

   c) **Secondary haemorrhage** occurs due to sepsis between 5-10 days. It requires intravenous antibiotics, styptics, sedation followed by postnasal packing if bleeding is not controlled. Blood transfusion is required in rare instances.

2. **Trauma** to surrounding structures

   a) Eustachian tube openings leading to fibrosis and secretory otitis media.

   b) Palate

   c) Uvula

   d) Tongue

   e) Teeth

3. **Incomplete removal** leading to persistence of symptoms.

4. **Otitis media** due to spread of infection to the middle ear via the eustachian tube

5. **Subluxation of atlanto-occipital joint** due to trauma, infection, decalcification of verterbra or laxity of anterior vertebral ligament.

6. **Hypernasality** due to velopharyngeal insufficiency, especially if performed in patients with a submucous cleft.

7. **Aspiration pneumonia** due to aspiration of blood and secretions into the respiratory tract.

8. **Torticollis** occurs due to damage to aponeurosis of vertebrae or prevertebral muscles

9. **Secondary atrophic pharyngitis** can occur if excessive pharyngeal mucosa is stripped off during adenoid curettage.

11. TONSILLECTOMY

DEFINITION

It is an operation performed for removal of palatine tonsils

INDICATIONS

I. Local

II. Focal

III. Systemic

IV. General

V. As an approach

I. Local

These are indications which are related to the pathology in the tonsil

- Hypertrophied tonsils causing obstruction to respiration or deglutition (most important indication)
- Chronic tonsillitis: recurrent attacks of acute tonsillitis (4-5 attacks / year)
- Following an attack of quinsy (Interval tonsillectomy performed 4-6 weeks later)
- Carriers of Diphtheria
- Tonsillolith
- Tonsillar cyst
- Foreign body embedded in tonsil
- Benign tumours of tonsil
- Excision biopsy in suspected malignancy of tonsil
- Part of treatment of sleep apnoea syndrome

> **ABSOLUTE INDICATIONS**
> - Hypertrophied tonsils obstructing respiration or deglutition
> - Sleep apnoea syndrome

II. Focal

When recurrent tonsillitis affects regional / surrounding structures, tonsillectomy is indicated

- Persistent non-specific jugulodigastric lymphadenitis or suppurative cervical lymphadenitis requiring drainage.
- Tuberculous cervical lymphadenitis where tonsils are the source of infection
- Aural infections (secretory / chronic suppurative otitis media) due to recurrent tonsillitis.

III. Systemic

Recurrent tonsillitis becomes a focus of sepsis for various systems of the body

1. Respiratory system	• Chronic bronchitis
	• Exacerbation of asthma
2. Cardiovascular system	• Rheumatic heart disease
	• Subacute bacterial endocarditis
3. Renal	• Acute glomerulonephritis
4. Cutaneous	• Urticaria
	• Erythema multiforme
5. Ophthalmic	• Phlyctenular conjunctivitis
	• Choroiditis
6. Bones / joints	• Rheumatoid arthritis

IV. General

- Dyspepsia
- Debility
- Failure to thrive/grow
- Secondary anaemia
- Febrile convulsions

V. Approach to

- Styloid process for Eagle's syndrome
- Glossopharyngeal nerve for glossopharyngeal neuralgia
- Distal end of branchial fistula tract in posterior faucial pillar

Indications For Unilateral Tonsillectomy :
- Excision biopsy in suspected malignancy or ulcer on tonsil
- Excision biopsy in lymphomas / tumours
- Tonsillolith
- Tonsillar cyst
- Tonsillar foreign body
- Styloidectomy
- Glossopharyngeal neurectomy

CONTRAINDICATIONS

Absolute

These are contraindications which impose a danger to life

1. Blood dyscrasias
   - Haemophilla
   - Purpura
   - Leukaemia

2. Pulsatile tonsils

   Aneurysm of Internal carotid artery

3. Abnormal / anomalous tortuous vessel in posterior pharyngeal wall (ascending pharyngeal artery)

Relative

These are contraindications in which the operation can be performed after cure of disease.

- Acute tonsillitis	- Risk of haemorrhage

- Upper respiratory tract infection
  - Coryza
  - Granular pharyngitis
	- It may flare up after the surgery

- Age below 5 yrs	- Tonsils may act as immunedefence organs - May lead to compensatory hypertrophy of other lymphoid tissue - Blood loss may not be well tolerated - Difficult surgery as operative space is less and risk of anaesthesia remains
- Diabetes - Hypertension - Asthma, allergy - Epidemic of poliomyelitis - Pregnancy - Menstruation - Oral contraceptive use	- Surgery can precipitate bulbar poliomyelitis

PROCEDURE

Preoperative

- Written informed valid consent
- Injection Atropine 0.6 mg intramuscularly half an hour prior to surgery

- Injection Tetanus toxoid 0.5 ml intramuscularly one day prior to surgery
- Systemic antibiotics if required

Anaesthesia

General anaesthesia with endotracheal intubation.

The endotracheal tube is either cuffed or a tight throat pack is kept surrounding the tube to prevent aspiration of blood and secretions into the lower respiratory tract. The tube can be passed transorally or transnasally. Transoral route is preferred if adenoidectomy is to be performed.

Local anaesthesia

It is used in adults. It is used along with intravenous sedation and local infiltration of peritonsillar tissue and pillars with 2% Xylocaine with 1:1,00,000 adrenaline.

Advantages of local anaesthesia :

- Risk of general anaesthesia is avoided
- Faster procedure
- Less haemorrhage

Position

Supine position with flexion of neck and extension of head.

DISSECTION METHOD TONSILLECTOMY

Mouth is kept open with a mouth gag (Doyen's / Boyle-Davis / Jenning's). Tongue is depressed with a tongue depressor. Under local anaesthesia, the patient is instructed to keep the mouth open.

Incision : An inverted 'J' shaped incision is taken submucosally along the edge of the anterior pillar after it is stretched by depressing the tongue. The incision is taken with a tonsillar knife (no: 12 blade on a Bard-Parker handle) from lateral border of tongue to the base of the uvula. The medial lip of the incision is held with Dennis-Brown tonsil holding forceps and the lateral lip is pushed laterally to expose the plane of dissection-the tonsillar capsule. Dissection of the tonsil is then carried out in the plane between the capsule and the fossa with the help of Mollison's tonsillar dissector and pieces of roller gauze. This blunt dissection separates the tonsil with its capsule from the loose areolar-tissue which binds it to its bed, and also achieves haemostasis. The tonsil is dissected free from its fossa except at the pedicle / lower pole which contains the insertion of the palatoglossus muscle in addition to blood vessels.

Snaring : Eve's tonsillar snare is passed around the pedicle and the tonsil is separated by crushing and cutting the pedicle. The tonsil is held with forceps while snaring so that it doesn't fall freely into the hypopharynx. The other tonsil is similarly removed.

Haemostasis : The tonsillar fossa is packed with roller gauze for a while to control oozing. After removal of gauze, the fossa is checked for any bleeding points. Haemostasis is achieved by contraction and retraction of blood vessels. Some bleeding points still remain, which are ligated by cross clamping. They are first held with straight tonsillar artery forceps followed by cross clamping with curved (Negus) artery forceps and then tied with silk or linen. The ligatures are not to be removed, they slough off by 7-10 days.

POST-OPERATIVE MANAGEMENT

1. Position
   - Left-lateral position
   - Knee and hip of upper leg flexed
   - Lower arm flexed at the elbow and shoulder and placed below the head of the patient.
   - This prevents the patient from aspiration in case of haemorrhage and also from rolling under the effect of anaesthesia

2. Monitoring of temperature, pulse and respiration every four hourly

3. Medical treatment

   a) Immediate :
      - Injectable antibiotics
      - Injectable analgesics
      - Hydrogen peroxide gargles on the day of the surgery to clear the fossa.

   b) Later :
      - Antibiotic syrup for one week
      - Antiinflammatory analgesic syrup
      - Condy's gargles (1:4000 potassium permanganate 3-4 times/day for 7-10 days)

4. Diet :
   - Nil by mouth for six hours
   - Cold liquid feeds orally after six hours eg: cold milk, ice cream.
   - It is followed by soft, cold, non-spicy diet for a week to ten days. eg:- bread and milk, mashed potatoes
   - Avoid lime juice (acidic), hot drinks (vasodilatation and bleeding)
   - Hard spicy foods are avoided for 10 days.
   - Each feed is followed by antibiotic gargles.

5. The patient is asked to lake semisolid feeds soon as it prevents stiffness of pharyngeal muscles. Chewing a chewing gum also helps for the same and alleviates pain.

6. Patient is asked to follow up after 1 week.

COMPLICATIONS

I. Intraoperative

Anaesthetic	Arrhythmias, Hypertension / Hypotension
Surgical	
Primary haemorrhage (Average blood loss in Tonsillectomy = 50 ml)	Arterial in nature Controlled by ligatures May be more if the operation is performed on inflamed tonsils.
Trauma	To anterior/posterior pillars Tongue Teeth Uvula Palate
Aspiration	**Aspiration of :** • Blood • Tonsillar tags • Adenoid tags **Diagnosis :** Cough and fever postoperatively **Prevention :** • Cuffed endotracheal tube/pack around the tube • Rose's position intra-operativelly (Head-low with extension at atlanto-occipital joint with sand bag under shoulders) • Post operative left lateral position

II. Postoperative

1. Reactionary haemorrhage

It occurs 6-24 hrs. after surgery

Causes :

- Clot in fossa preventing retraction of pharyngeal constrictors
- Slipping of ligature
- Dislodgement of clot by excessive coughing or straining
- Failure to ligate all bleeding vessels intra-operatively.
- Wearing off effect of local anaesthesia with adrenaline
- Rise in blood pressure as patient comes out of general anaesthesia
- Increase in venous pressure due to coughing

Clinical features

- Rattling noise during breathing.
- Swallowing movements postoperatively (child swallowing blood)
- Raised pulse, respiration
- Fall in blood pressure in severe bleeding
- Pale child in a state of shock and sweating over the forehead in severe bleeding
- Spitting out of blood by adults and older children.

Management

- Secure airway by postoperative tonsillar position.
- Assess blood loss
- Start Intravenous fluids
- TPR / B.P. monitoring
- Removal of clot from fossa :
  - Small clot comes out with hydrogen peroxide gargles
  - Larger clot requires a swab for removal
- Ligature of bleeding vessel
  - Under general anaesthesia/sedation
- Supportive therapy :
  - Vitamin C, K
  - Calcium
  - Styptics etc.

If the above methods fail :

- Pillar suturing : Approximation of anterior and posterior pillars by suturing with tightly packed gelfoam within.
- Ligation of external carotid artery.
- Blood transfusion.

2. Secondary haemorrhage

It occurs between 5-7 days.

Causes :
- Sepsis / infection in the fossa
- Sloughing off of the walls of the ligated vessels.

Clinical features

- Pain in oropharynx
- Rise in temperature
- Diffuse bleeding
- Tonsillar fossa covered with unhealthy granulations or slough.

Management

- Admission to hospital
- TPR / B.P. monitoring
- Hydrogen peroxide gargles
- Intravenous high generation antibiotics
- Intravenous fluids
- Packing the fossa with gauze.
- Cauterization with trichloroacetic acid (TCA)
- If bleeding is more and still continues, (> 1/10th of blood volume) fresh blood transfusion can be given. It replaces coagulation factors.
- Pillar suturing
- External carotid artery ligation.

3. **Oedema of uvula**
4. **Aspiration pneumonia**
5. **Change of voice** can occur due to
   - Damage to uvula
   - Damage to anterior pillars
   - Fibrosis of anterior pillars/soft palate
6. **Acute suppurative cervical lymphadenitis**
   - Due to spread of infection from septic tonsils
   - Can lead to septicaemial/pyaemia
7. **Reflex otalgia**
   - Irritation of glossopharyngeal nerve endings
8. **Otitis media**
9. **Dislocation of temporomandibular joint**
10. **Dislocation of atlanto occipital joint** can occur if a patient is shifted from operation table with a hyperextended joint and neck not supported.
11. **Subacute bacterial endocarditis**
12. **Exacerbation of granular pharyngitis**
13. **Recurrent / residual tonsillitis :** Infection of tonsillar tags.
14. **Quinsy** in residual tonsil/tonsillar tag.

12. THYROIDECTOMY

- Dr. Rajiv Joshi

INDICATIONS

I have seen a subtotal thyroidectomy (STT) being performed in a female patient aged 45 years with secondary thyrotoxicosis.

Before taking such a patient for surgery, I would like to confirm that the toxicity is reasonably controlled and she has got adequate medical treatment to prevent development of thyrotoxic crisis / 'storm' on the operation table.

PRE-OPERATIVE PREPARATION

Pre-operatively:

- Carbimazole   40 mg / day
- Diazepam   10 mg / day
- Propranolol   40 mg TDS
- Lugol's iodine   7 to 10 days prior to surgery

Response to therapy is judged by:

- Sleeping pulse rate.
- Daily weight gain.
- Good sleep pattern.

Fitness for anaesthesia is taken

Indirect laryngoscopy is done (IDL) to rule out recurrent laryngeal nerve paralysis.

Pre-operative:

- Shaving of neck in a male patient
- Inj. Atropine 0.6 mg intramuscular ½ hour prior to surgery.
- Inj. Ampicillin 1gm intravenous on operation table.
- Written consent.
- Blood grouping and cross-matching done.

Anaesthesia:

General anaesthesia with endotracheal intubation.

Position:

Supine position with neck extended with a pillow below each scapula, doughnut (ring) under the head and sand bags by the side of the neck as to maintain the thyroid cartilage, chin and suprasternal notch in the same straight line.

Anti-Trendelenburg position of table (head high to prevent venous congestion)

Parts painted and draped.

Incision:

Kocher's skin crease incision i.e. a curvilinear skin crease incision 2 cms above the suprasternal notch with the concavity facing upwards and extending from one sternomastoid to the other. Prior to taking the incision, it is marked with a thick twine (thread).

Saline and adrenaline is infiltrated along the line of the incision. The skin is incised with a knife (no. 23 blade mounted on a no. 34 Bard Parker handle). Alternatively a No. 15 blade mounted on a No. 3 Bard Parker handle can also be used (More cosmetic, thin scar).

Exposure:

The subcutaneous tissue and platysma are incised in one layer and flaps are raised. The upper flap is raised till the hyoid bone and lower flap till the suprasternal notch. The 2 flaps are retracted by using a pair of Joll's self-retaining thyroid retractors or retracted using skin stitches on either flap.

Anterior jugular vein coursing vertically is undermined using a mixter and ligated and divided. The deep fascia is incised vertically avoiding the veins and the 'strap muscles'.

If the lesion is small, retraction of the strap muscles laterally suffices. If it is big, the strap muscles are divided.

The strap muscles are divided as high as possible because:

● The nerve supply (ansa cervicalis) is from below.

● It prevents fromation of a hypertrophied scar which is a possibility when the skin incision and division of the muscle are in the same line.

The thyroid gland is exposed laterally upto the sternomastoids.

DEVASCULARISATION

First hug the middle, then kiss the superior and stay away from inferior.

● The middle thyroid veins are dissected, hooked up with a mixter, ligated and divided as close to the gland as possible to avoid tumour emboli to be released.

● Dissection is carried onto the superior pole. The superior thyroid artery and vein are hooked up, ligated and divided as close to the superior pole as possible - to avoid injury to nerve.

Dissection is now carried out downwards to inferior pole and inferior thyroid artery is ligated in continuity as far from the inferior pole as possible using 1-0 chromic catgut and a leash of inferior thyroid veins are ligated individually. Ligation in continuity serves 2 purposes:

● Recurrent laryngeal nerve division is prevented.

● Helps in maintaining blood supply to the parathyroid gland.

In a Subtotal thyroidectomy, do not search for recurrent laryngeal nerve, whereas in hemithyroidectomy the nerve is preferably identified.

The same procedure is carried out on the opposite side.

SUBTOTAL THYROIDECTOMY (STT)

Division of isthmus is carried out by applying clamps close to each lobe and the raw surface is ligated (using chromic catgut) to achieve haemostasis.

Clamps are applied all round the gland / multiple mosquitoes are thrust into the capsule of the gland from all sides and the diseased tissue is cut above the clamps.

Each of the bleeders are under run with chromic catgut and perfect haemostasis is achieved.

Alternatively the 2 edges or 2 poles of the lobes are approximated using 2-0 chromic catgut, continuous locking sutures.

In subtotal thyroidectomy for multinodular goitre, if diagnosis is in doubt, a frozen section is done if malignancy is suspected.

HEMITHYROIDECTOMY (HT)

In a hemithyroidectomy, the diseased lobe and isthmus are removed in which case the concerned lobe is devascularised as described earlier with the inferior thyroid artery divided.

The isthmus is separated from the trachea by blunt dissection using a peanut and the isthmus is hooked up with a mixter, clamped close to the opposite lobe and divided.

The raw surface on the side of the opposite lobe is ligated with a 2-0 chromic catgut. The whole diseased lobe and the isthmus are then dissected off the trachea taking care to protect the recurrent laryngeal nerve.

Closure:

- After achieving haemostasis, either a corrugated rubber drain or preferably a suction drain is left anterior to the trachea in the thyroid fossa and the drain is brought out through a separate stab incision by the side of the neck.
- Shoulder pads are now removed and the strap muscles are sutured with 2-0 chromic catgut using interrupted sutures.
- Deep fascia is sutured vertically with 2-0 chromic catgut interrupted sutures (to allow adequate drainage in case haemostasis is not achieved)
- Platysma is sutured with a 2-0 plain catgut - interrupted sutures.
- Skin is approximated with subcuticular stitches or 4-0 silk interrupted sutures or using skin clips e.g. Mitchell's Kifa, Cushing's etc.
- Thyroid dressing is given.
- During extubation, movements of the vocal cords are checked to rule out recurrent laryngeal nerve damage.

Post-operative orders:

- Nil by mouth for 8-10 hours.
- After that, oral fluids.
- Antibiotics / analgesics
- Tincture benzoin inhalations.
- Removal of drain usually by about 48 hours (once purpose is served).
- Suture removal by 5th day.
- Clips removal by 4th day.

COMPLICATIONS OF THYROIDECTOMY

Complications of anaesthesia

- Damage to vocal cords and oedema.
- Difficult intubation.

Complications of surgery

- **Intra-operative**
  - Primary haemorrhage.
  - Damage to trachea.
  - Damage to external laryngeal nerve.
  - Damage to recurrent laryngeal nerve
  - Tracheomalacia (collapse of trachea - respiratory distress)
  - Damage to carotid arteries, internal jugular vein.
  - Thyroid crisis / "storm".

- **Immediate post-operative**
  1. Breathlessness:
     Causes:
     - Tracheomalacia.
     - Vocal cord palsy.
     - Large haematoma compressing trachea
     - Tracheobronchial secretions.
     - Laryngismus stridulus.
     - Damage to pleura as in large / retrosternal goitre.

- Laryngeal oedema due to difficult intubation.
2. Reactionary haemorrhage
3. Hoarseness of voice - due to:
   - Vocal cord palsy (damage to recurrent laryngeal nerve)
   - Irritation of vocal cords due to intubation.
4. Wound complications:
   - Oedema of the flap.
   - Accumulation of serum.
   - Haematoma.
   - Infection (sepsis)
5. Thyroid crisis

- **Delayed post-operative**
  - Hypothyroidism
  - Hypoparathyroidism.
  - Recurrence of thyrotoxicosis.
  - Hypertrophied scar and keloid formation
  - Hoarseness of voice - due to fibrosis leading to entrapment of recurrent laryngeal nerve.

TREATMENT OF COMPLICATIONS OF THYROID SURGERY

- **Haematoma** - Compression on trachea causing respiratory problems.

  Rx: Open up sutures over the deep fascia and evacuate the haematoma.

  Prevention:
  - Good haemostasis.
  - Leave a drain
  - Interrupted sutures
  - Remove extension and check for haemostasis.

- **Recurrent laryngeal nerve damage:**

  Rx : Repaired by microsurgical technique and nerve graft using greater auricular nerve:
  - King's operation.
  - Woodword's operation.

- **Vocal cord palsy:**

  Hoarseness of voice.

  Rx:
  - Injection of Teflon paste into vocal cords.
  - Arytenoidectomy (excision of cartilage)

- **Parathyroid damage:**

  Diagnosis : Recognised by the fact that the gland turns bluish black on minimal trauma and sinks when put in a bowl of normal saline (D/D is Fat which will float)

  Treatment : In cases where all 4 parathyroids have been removed, as in total thyroidectomy one of them is reimplanted in the forearm after slicing it into multiple pieces (to facilitate revascularisation).

  Advantages: Of implanting the gland in forearm are:
  - Easy to implant
  - Easily recognisable, if pathological changes occur and if removal is necessary.

Reimplantation in sternomastoid muscle is not preferred as it lies in the field of irradiation.

- **Treatment of thyroid crisis:**
  - Patient is shifted to an air-conditioned, dark and silent room.
  - Nasal oxygen
  - Constant monitoring of vital parameters.
  - Tepid sponging.
  - Resotration of fluid and electrolyte balance.
  - Anti-thyroid drugs
  - Steroids.
  - Digoxin / β - blockers
  - Antihistaminics
  - Propranolol
  - Na iodide, Lugol's iodine

- **Treatment of tracheomalacia**
  - Low and permanent tracheostomy

13. TRACHEOSTOMY

DEFINITION

Tracheostomy is an operative procedure in which the anterior wall of trachea is connected to the exterior or sutured to the skin of the anterior neck.

History:

Antonio Brasovolo (1546)	–	1st reported successful Tracheostomy.
Heister (1718)	–	Coined the term Tracheostomy.
Caren	–	1st successful Paediatric Tracheostomy.

INDICATIONS

Signs of Laryngeal obstruction:
- Inspiratory stridor
- Prominence of sternocleidomastoid muscle
- Indrawing of suprasternal, epigastrium and intercostal spaces
- Cyanosis

INDICATIONS

I. Obstructive

II. Non-obstructive

I. Obstructive

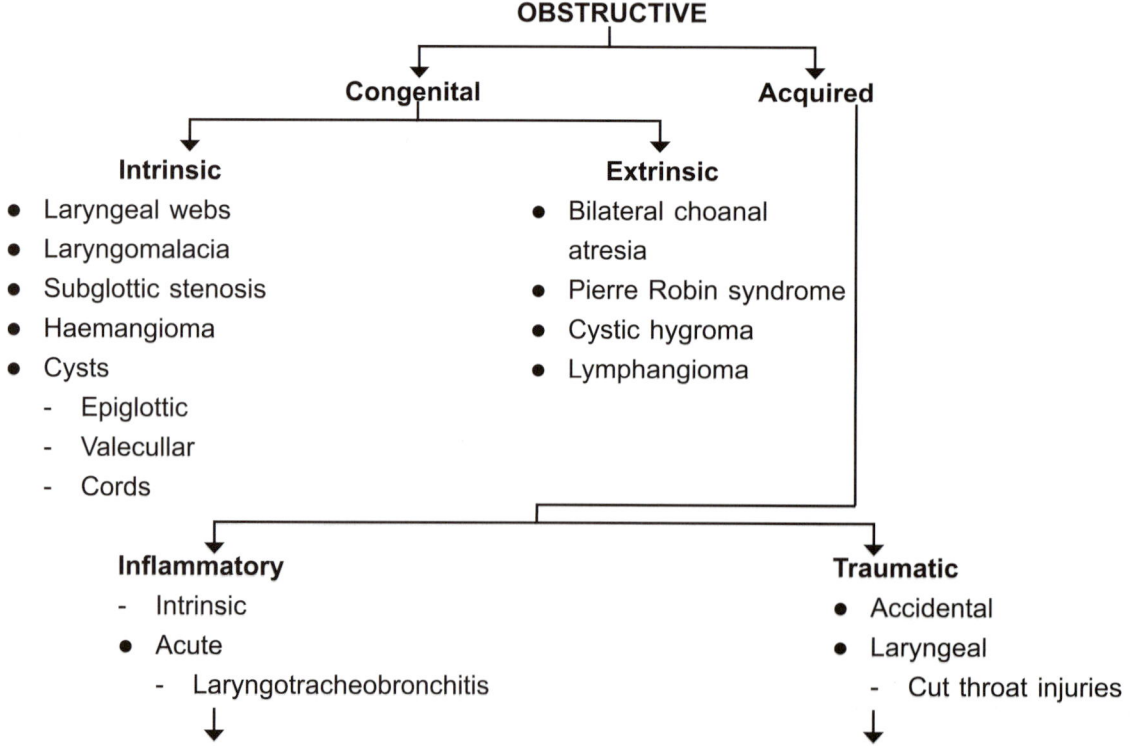

OBSTRUCTIVE

Congenital   Acquired

Intrinsic
- Laryngeal webs
- Laryngomalacia
- Subglottic stenosis
- Haemangioma
- Cysts
  - Epiglottic
  - Valecullar
  - Cords

Extrinsic
- Bilateral choanal atresia
- Pierre Robin syndrome
- Cystic hygroma
- Lymphangioma

Inflammatory
- Intrinsic
- Acute
  - Laryngotracheobronchitis

Traumatic
- Accidental
- Laryngeal
  - Cut throat injuries

342

- Epiglottitis
  - Diphtheric laryngitis in children
- Chronic
  - Tuberculosis
  - Syphilis
  - Scleroma
- Extrinsic
  - Ludwig's angina
  - Parapharyngeal abscess
  - Retropharyngeal abscess

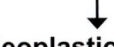

Neoplastic:

1. Benign:
   - Recurrent respiratory papillomatosis
   - Adenoma
2. Malignant:
   - Ca larynx
   - Ca thyroid
   - Ca oesophagus
   - Bronchogenic carcinoma
   - Mediastinal masses
   - Lymphomas
   - Cervical lymphadenopathy - secondary metastasis

- Strangulation
  - Corrosive poisoning
- Extralaryngeal
  - Faciomaxillary injuries
  - Haematoma base tongue

- Surgical
  - Thyroidectomy
  - Cardiac surgeries

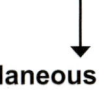

Miscellaneous

- Foreign body in air passages
- Angioneurotic oedema

---

5 Common indications:
- Head injury
- Tetanus
- Laryngeal trauma
- Ca larynx
- GBS (Guillain Barre syndrome)

II. Non-obstructive

1. Respiratory insufficiency:
   a. Central:
      i. Coma due to
         - Uraemia
         - Head injuries
         - Cerebrovascular accidents
         - Hepatic dysfunction
         - Diabetes ketoacidosis
      ii. Respiratory centre depression:
         - Fracture base skull
         - Barbiturate poisoning
         - Bulbar poliomyelitis
         - Injuries to spinal cord
   b. Peripheral / neuromuscular
      - Guillain Barre syndrome
      - Tetanus
   c. Pulmonary:
      - Pneumothorax
      - Pneumomediastinum

- Fracture sites
- Flail chest

2. Tracheobronchial toilet:
   - Bronchopneumonia
   - Bronchiectasis
3. IPPV
4. Post - surgical
   - Total laryngectomy
   - Total glossectomy
   - Mandibulectomy
   - Laryngofissure

CONTRAINDICATIONS

There are no contraindications for an emergency tracheostomy

The following contraindications are for elective tracheostomy:

1. Bleeding disorders
2. Diabetes mellitus
3. Hypertension
4. General debility

Types of tracheostomy:

According to

I. Purpose
   - Temporary
   - Permanent
II. Timing
   - Elective
   - Emergency
III. Level
   - High
   - Mid
   - Low

> **Indications of permanent tracheostomy:**
> - Carcinoma larynx
> - Carcinoma hypopharynx
> - Cancer thyroid
> - Bilateral abductor paralysis of vocal cord

Functions of tracheostomy

- Relieves upper airway obstruction
- Decreases dead space by > 1/3rd / almost 50%
- Can be used for:
  - Intermittent positive pressure ventilation
  - Anaesthesia
  - To deliver medications
  - Humidification
- Protects against aspiration
- Reduces air flow resistance
- Provides access for tracheobronchial toilet by aspirating secretions and permitting gas diffusion.

PROCEDURE

- **Pre-procedure orders:**
  - Written informed consent (except in emergency)
  - Injection Atropine 0.6 mg intramuscularly
  - Injection T. T. 0.5 cc intramuscularly
  - X-ray neck to note position of the trachea.

- **Anaesthesia:**
  - No anaesthesia is required in acute emergency.
  - General or local anaesthesia can be used.

    The patient may be already intubated

  Local Anaesthesia:
  - Infiltration of 2% Xylocaine with adrenaline 1:1,00,000 is done in a rhomboid shape bounded by submental region above, suprasternal notch below and sternomastoids laterally. It is also injected along the line of the incision.

> **Advantages of a pre-intubated patient:**
> - Procedure can be done without haste.
> - There are decrease chest movements during the procedure.
> - Decrease intrathoracic pressure leads to:
>   - Decrease bleeding-
>   - Less chance of damage to dome of pleura.

- **Position:**
  - Supine position.
  - Full extension of head and neck.
  - Pillow is kept below shoulders
  - Chin, Adam's apple and suprasternal notch should be in one line
  - No extension is given in a child.

- **Incision:** The incision on the skin of the neck can be:

INCISION	ADVANTAGES	DISADVANTAGES
1. **Horizontal:** • 5 cm incision • 2 cm below lower border of cricoid	• Better scar • Cosmesis	• Increase bleeding • Not in line with deeper tissues.
2. **Vertical:** • An incision midway between cricoid cartilage and suprasternal notch	• Faster procedure • Decrease bleeding • In line with deeper tissues	• Poor scar

- **Midline dissection:**
  - Deepening of incision is carried out through the
    - Skin
    - Subcutaneous tissue and
    - Superficial layer of deep fascia
  - Separation of strap muscles-Sternothyroid and Sternohyoid, is done in the midline
  - Incision and wide separation of pretracheal fascia is achieved.
  - After separating the pretracheal fascia, the trachea may be visible.

- **Identification of trachea:**
  The trachea is identified by the following features:
  - Midline structure ideally.
  - White cartilagenous rings.
  - Rings feel firm on palpation
  - Movement with respiration is present.

- Aspiration of air occurs with syringe and needle.
- Injection of Xylocaine causes-initial cough.

- **Incision on trachea:**
    - After identifying the trachea an incision is taken on it.
    - Achieve complete haemostasis before incising the trachea.
    - Inject 1ml of 4% Xylocaine into tracheal lumen to anaesthetise the mucosa
    - Types of tracheal incision.

> **Before tracheal incision:**
> - Achieve complete haemostasis.
> - Take skin stay sutures.
> - Confirmation of trachea.
> - Suction apparatus with tube should be ready.

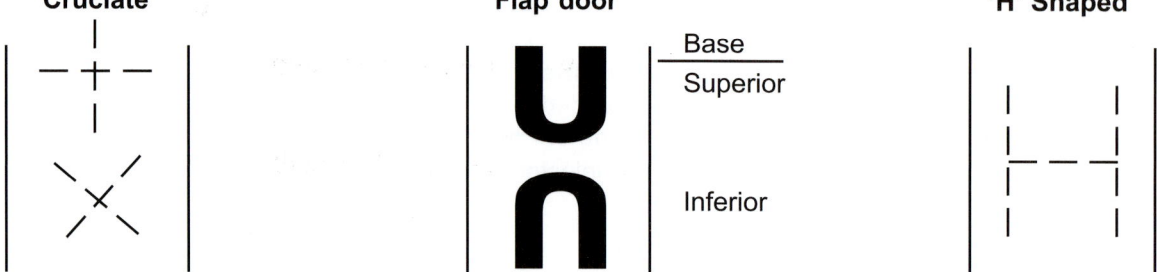

Cruciate   **Flap door**   **'H' Shaped**

Base / Superior / Inferior

- Incision should be between 2nd and 4th tracheal ring.
- 1st ring is avoided to prevent damage to cricoid cartilage and subsequent subglottic stenosis.

- **An ideal opening on the trachea is:**
    - Of optimal size
    - No ragged edges
    - Not round, or circumferential contraction with stenosis occurs

Different technique should be carried out for the following variations of trachea:

• Soft / malleable trachea	• Seen in children • Stay sutures on trachea are needed
• Hard / calcified trachea	• It is seen in elderly • Removal of some part of anterior tracheal wall may be required • Bone cutting instruments may be needed to open the trachea
• Carcinoma larynx patient	• High incision is taken

In case of an emergency tracheostomy:
- It is to be performed faster as anoxia causes death in 4-5 minutes
- Local anaesthetic solution is not injected into the lumen as the cough that occurs may worsen the distress.
- Also the anaesthetic should not infiltrate paratracheal gutters to cause more respiratory distress by paralysis of recurrent laryngeal nerves.

Tracheostomy tube insertion:
After making a tracheal incision, a tracheostomy tube is inserted.
- Previously selected tube

Size	Sex
7.5 mm - 8 mm $\longrightarrow$	Females
8.5 mm - 9 mm $\longrightarrow$	Males

- Cuff is checked for leak
- Tapes are tied to the tube flanges and a dilator is inserted in the tracheal opening
- The tracheostomy tube with the obturator within is inserted in the opening.
- On insertion, obturator is immediately removed.
- Confirm entry into trachea
- Secure / fix the tube
- Aspirate blood, mucus, secretions.

The following tests are used to confirm tracheostomy tube in the trachea:
- Air blast over the tube opening
- Auscultatory confirmation of air entry in both the lungs
- Cotton-wool test: moving of cotton wick due to air blast from the tube opening
- X-ray neck / chest to demonstrate the tube
- Catheter:
    - Passage of catheter through the tube opening into the lungs.
    - Air aspiration from the outer end of the catheter.

Fixation of the tracheostomy tube:
- Fixation is done after relief of neck extension.
- It is done with steritape and dressing gauze.
- Suturing of skin is carried out if required.
- Cuff is inflated with 3-5 ml of air.
- Cuff usually lodges between 4th and 7th tracheal ring.

Post-procedure orders:
- No sedation, no atropine and no drugs should be given which depress the respiratory centre.
- X-ray chest - PA view to check for position of the tube.
- Proper suction:
    - ½ hourly (Tracheostomy decreases efficiency of coughing)
    - Suction catheter diameter should be $\frac{1}{3}$rd of inner diameter of tracheostomy tube.
    - Catheter is to be inserted for approximately 15 cms, at peak of inspiration
    - Multiple eyed lubricated, catheter is preferred.
    - Suction is to be done after instillation of 5% $NaHCO_3$ / saline at the end of inspiration.
- Deflation of cuff should be done during expiration, for 5 minutes every hourly, followed by reinflation
- For metal tubes, inner tube has to be removed, cleaned and replaced every 4 hourly.
- Single moist gauze piece should be kept over the stoma or a humidification tent in which oxygen or compressed air is passed through sterlized water at the rate of 5-7 litres / min. should be used to humidify the inhaled air.
- Chest physiotherapy for lung ventilation and to prevent pulmonary infection.
- Expectorants, antibiotics and antiinflammatory drugs.
- To keep the following by the side of the patient:
    - Suction apparatus.
    - Tracheostomy tray.
    - Bell, note-pad and a slate.

Humidified air can be provided by:
- Moist gauze
- Steam tent
- Droplet infusion
- Commercial humidifier

Sequelae following tracheostomy:
- Loss of speech as air bypasses the larynx

- Loss of smell as air bypasses the nose
- Loss of laryngeal protective mechanism, therefore increased risk of foreign body aspiration.
- Swimming is not permitted.
- Overhead shower bath is avoidable.
- Inability to perform strenuous exercises as the subglottic pressure cannot be built up (difficult fixation of chest)

HOME CARE OF TRACHEOSTOMY TUBE:

- Cleaning the inner tube
- Boiling the inner tube
- Changing the tracheostomy tube
  - → First change is within three to five days of procedure
  - → Subsequent changes are every weekly
- Suctioning
- Fixing of tube
- Child is protected from water and sand
- Speech therapy for valved tube patients.

DECANNULATION:

Hospital Set-up:

Pre-procedure:

- There should not be any aspiration during eating
- Lateral X'ray-neck
- Xerogram / CT. scan / MRI
- Endoscopic examination
- To compare peak inspiratory air flow through mouth and through tracheostomy tube
- Granulations or fibrotic tissue from the tract should be removed

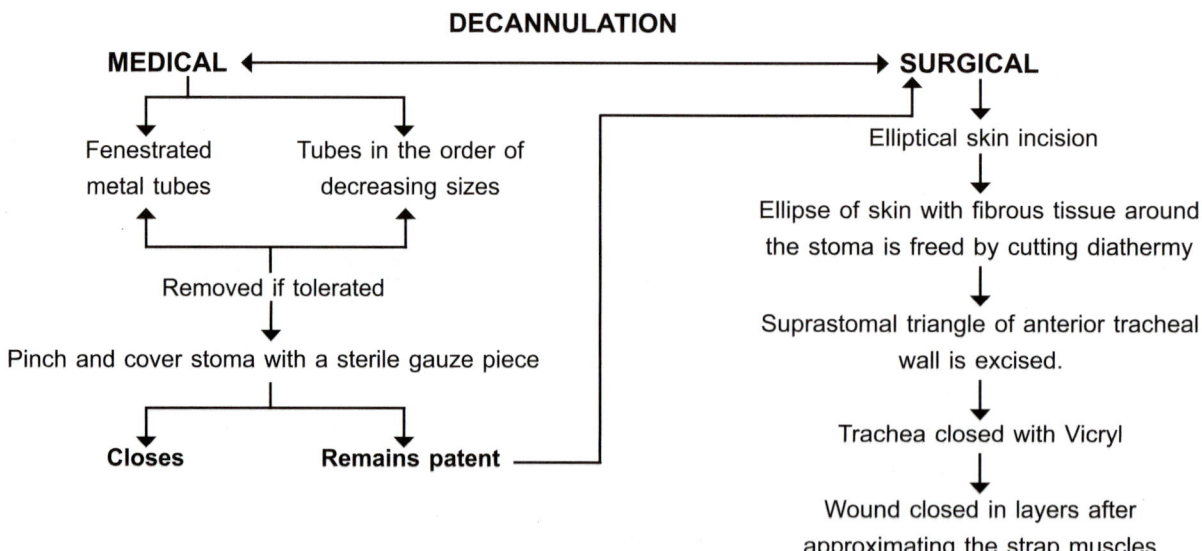

PAEDIATRIC TRACHEOSTOMY:

- The following important anatomical features are present in children:
  - Distance
    → Cricoid to suprasternal notch:
      - Neonates - 2.5 cm
      - 10 yr old - 6 cm
- Level
  → Cricoid cartilage:
    - Infant C3
    - Puberty C6
- Soft trachea
- Highly mobile neck
- Recurrent laryngeal nerves lie laterally
- Pretracheal pad of fat is present in the suprasternal notch
- On extension - mediastinal contents appear in the neck
- High pleural dome
- Large vessels are present in the midline
- Thymus may be present

PROCEDURE

- Suitably warmed infant
- Supine position
- Partial / no extension of the neck
- Prevent lolling of head by a head ring
- GA + Saline + Adrenaline (locally) (1: 2,00,000)
- Incision: vertical incision on skin and trachea is preferred
- Keep first tracheal ring intact
- Slit muscle from down to up
- Do not damage the post-tracheal wall.
- Pass tracheostomy tube:
  → Metal - with introducer
  → Portex - pinch with an artery forceps and insert
  → Rail-roading over a simple rubber catheter
- Stay sutures are essential

TRACHEOSTOMY TUBES

History:
- Intially the tubes were made up of bone, rubber and crude metal.
- The paediatric tubes were a smaller version of the adult tube.
- With further advancement the tubes were made of silver and the inner tube was added.
- Negus - added a valve to the tube for phonation
- Wilson - developed a silver paediatric tube with funnel shaped opening to be attached to a respirator.
- A window was also present on the outer tube to allow transglottic breathing prior to decannulation.
- Alder Hey tube - This was a modification of the previous tube with addition of a window and a valve to the inner tube.

- Polyvinylchloride and silicone rubber tubes.

> **Ideal tube:** An ideal tracheostomy tube should fulfill the following criteria:
> - All parts should be snugly fitting.
> - Inner tube should project slightly beyond the outer tube
> - Optimum air flow should be achieved
>   - Shorter shaft
>   - Greater radius of curvature
>   - Smooth inner surface
> - Non-toxic material with minimal tissue reactivity.
> - Comfortable / easy to change / easy to clean / easy to connect to a ventilator

PARTS OF A TRACHEOSTOMY TUBE

Metal

- Outer tube
- Inner tube
- Pilot / blunt ended obturator

Portex

- Tube
- Flanges

Materials used:

- German silver
- Polyvinyl chloride
- Rubber
- Silicon
- Latex

Tracheostomy tubes:

Metallic tubes

- Chevalier Jackson tube
  - German silver tube
  - Outer tube, inner tube, pilot, shield, luer lock
  - Inner tube is longer than the outer tube. It is removed when it gets blocked, keeping the outer tube patent
  - The obturator / pilot helps in an atraumatic entry and tracheal dilatation
  - Luer lock prevents dislodging of tube by coughing / pressure exerted during expiration
- Fuller tube
  - Outer biflanged tube
  - Bivalved

  Advantages:
  - Valve helps in phonation
  - Biflange acts as a tracheal dilator, easy introduction.

  Disadvantages:
  - Tube tip can cause irritation and is sharp
  - Broken flanges can act as a foreign body.
- Durham's tube
  - Ajustable flange
  - Made to fit any neck

- Colledge's tube
  - Used after laryngectomy
- Hollinger tracheostomy tube
  - Rotating lock, attached to shield at 75^0 as opposed to other tubes
  - Funnel shaped opening provides easy installation of aspiration catheters.
- Alder Hey's tube
  - Large radius of curvature
  - Silver tube
  - Inner tube has valve and window

Non-Metallic

- Portex
  - Portex stands for the name of the company
  - Blue radioopaque line
  - Cuff for
    - IPPV
    - Self-retaining
    - To prevent aspiration
  - High volume low pressure cuff
  - Sizes 3-10 (difference of 0.5)
  - Cuff starts 5.5 onwards
  - There is no inner tube. The whole tube is to be replaced or taken out and cleaned when blocked.
- Radcliffe tube
  - Rubber tube
  - Irritant to tissues
  - Used for irradiation

DOW Corning:

- Silastic tube

Kistner plastic tube:

- Extends only to the intraluminal surface of the tracheal fenestra
- Tube should fit snugly. The tracheostomy opening should be smaller than the diameter of the tube.
- Made of polyvinyl plastic
- One way valve - speech occurs without occluding the tube
- Non-irritant
- Used for patients for radiotherapy

Olympic tracheostomy tube:

- Same as above
- Adaptor is present for IPPV

Salpekar:

- Double cuffed tube
- Alternate cuff inflated by turns to prevent tracheal stenosis

DIFFERENCES BETWEEN METAL AND PORTEX TUBES:

METAL	PORTEX
• Consists of two tubes, hence less chances of getting blocked	• More chances of getting blocked

• No cuff present	• Cuff present
	  - Can give IPPV
	  - Prevents aspiration
	  - Less chances of accidental decannulation

• Cannot be used in patients who have to undergo:
  - MRI
  - Radiotherapy
	• Can be used for the same

• Some patients cannot tolerate this tube	• Can be used in patients who do not tolerate metallic tubes
• Usually used in long term tracheostomies	• Usually used in short term tracheostomies.

Advantages and Disadvantages of Tracheostomy:

ADVANTAGES	DISADVANTAGES
• It can be kept for a longer time	• It is a formal surgical procedure
• Patient can swallow	• It reduces cough efficiency
• It decreases dead space by 50%	• It takes more time than intubation
• It decreases respiratory resistance	• Greater bacterial colonization rate
• Tracheal stenosis is not very common	• Permanent scar occurs
• Tracheal toilet is easier	• Decannulation can be difficult
• No risk of main stem bronchus intubation	

MINITRACHEOSTOMY: (Mathews and Hopkinson)

Main indications:

- To remove chest secretions
- For treatment of respiratory failure

It consist of a vertical stab incision (coniotomy) made through the cricothyroid membrane under local anaesthesia, allowing insertion of a 4 mm. cannula attached to a high frequency jet ventillator. A minitracheostomy kit is also available.

PERCUTANEOUS TRACHEOSTOMY:

- Puncture trachea at the chosen level with a needle and cannula

    Pass guide wire by Seldinger's technique

    Gradually dilate stoma with increasing size dilators

    Pass the tracheostomy tube.

- Schachner (Rapitrae system)
    - Tracheotome passed over the guide wire
    - Dilate tract fully in one step
    - Opening dilated to pass the tracheostomy tube
    - Creation of false passage is a likely complication

CRICOTHYROIDOTOMY: (Laryngotomy)

(Mainly used as an emergency procedure)

Three Methods:

- Using an intravenous catheter
- Cricothyrotome or disposable Nu Trake's cricothyroidotomy device
- Formal surgical procedure

DECIDING THE SIZE OF TUBE:

Clinical assessment	For an intubated patient, No of portex tube is same as that of the endotracheal tube.
Portex tube number	formula Age < 8 yrs $\dfrac{Age}{3} + 3.5$ > 8 yrs $\dfrac{Age}{3} + 4.5$
Change of tube	Metal to Portex: $\dfrac{Metal\ no: - 2}{4}$ Portex to metal: Portex no: x π
	(Portex no: x 4) + 2 = Metal No

COMPLICATIONS

COMPLICATIONS	FEATURES	TREATMENT
ANAESTHESIA	• Anaphylaxis • Cardiac arrest • Hypotension	
SURGERY **I. Immediate complications** 1) Vasovagal attack		• Atropine prior to procedure. • Injecting 4% Xylocaine in tracheal lumen.
2) Haemorrhage: from a) Anterior jugular vein / Anterior communicating vein.		• Midline dissection
b) Thyroid isthmus / gland		• Retract Isthmus upwards. • Avoid its transaction. • Clamp, cut and ligate isthmus before proceeding.
c) Inferiod thyroid vein		• Avoid blind dissection in suprasternal notch.
d) Tracheal wall		• Suction with cauterisation. • Tight fitting tracheostomy tube.

e) Anomalous vessel
  - Thyroidia ima
  - Innominate artery
	May be high in children.	• Midline dissection

3) Damage to surrounding structures: 1. Apical pleura	Pneumothorax results (Post-op X'ray +) • Small	• Suture tear of pleura • Small pneumothorax will get absorbed
	• Large	• Oxygen • Antibiotics • Sedatives • Insertion of ICD
	• Tension	• Aspiration of upper anterior thorax with 14-16 gauge needle.
2. Oesophagus	Tracheo-oesophageal fistula. may result • Small	• Conservative management with nasogastric tube.
	• Large	• Surgical closure. Both Trachea and Oesophagus to be sutured separately with inter position of soft tissue.
3. Carotid artery 4. Recurrent laryngeal nerve	• Major bleeding • Hoarseness • Respiratory distress.	• Use of proper surgical technique. • Midline dissection
4) Failure to establish respiration	**Reasons:** 1. Vagal stimutation.	• Atropine to be given
	2. Central respiratory failure	• Administer Carbogen (90% O_2 +

COMPLICATIONS	FEATURES	TREATMENT
	Respiratory centre ⇓ Used to high CO_2 ⇓ Tracheostomy ⇓ ⇓ CO_2 + ⇑ O_2 ⇓ Drive for respiration gets lost	10% CO_2) • Partial obstruction of stoma: O_2 / CO_2 saturation change occurs gradually for the respiratory centre to adopt. • Mouth to tracheostomy tube breathing: Exhaled air has 4% CO_2.
	3. Blockage of tube	• Regular suction and change of tube.
	4. Creation of a false passage	• Reinsert the tube
5. Cardiac failure	**Reasons:** • Fast rise in pH	
	• Increase adrenaline	
	• Increase in K^+ levels	
6. Air embolism	• Large neck veins may be inadvertantly opened during surgery.	• Head-low position to be given • Conservative management.
7. Hypotension	• Due to sudden decrease in CO_2 levels.	• I. V. fluids • Vasopressors
II. Intermediate complications 　1. Displaced tube.	**Reasons:** • Improper placement • Excessive movement of patient • Excessive coughing • Chest physiotherapy • Loose fixation of tube. **Factors affecting dislodgement:** • Length of tube • Thickness of neck • Post-op emphysema, oedema, haematoma • Distance between skin and anterior tracheal wall	• Tying tube flanges to skin • Securing tapes with neck in flexion.
2. Blocked tube	**It leads to:** • Airway obstruction • Difficult catheter suction	• Regular suction • Tube change
3. Emphysema		
4. Tracheitis		
5. Pneumothorax		
6. Local infection of skin wound		• Change of dressing • Skin creams
7. Tracheo-arterial fistula		
III. Delayed complications 　1. Bleeding 　　a) Reactionary bleeding (after 48 hours)	**Causes:** • Loss of effect of adrenaline • Reestablishment of normal B. P. /	

COMPLICATIONS	FEATURES	TREATMENT
b) Secondary bleeding (5th 8th day)	rise in B. P. ● Repeated paroxysms of cough. ● Granuloma formation 　- Due to infection 　- Pressure necrosis of high innominate artery	● Antibiotics ● Coagulants
2. Delayed tracheo-oesophageal fistula (5th-7th day)	**Causes:** ● Tube pressure ● Overinflated cuff with RT in situ. **Symptoms:** ● Increase secretions ● Skin irritation ● Infection ● Poor phonation	● Endoscopic examination ● Right curvature tube ● Conservative management. ● Surgical closure
3. Surgical emphysema: ● Air leak into subcutaneous tissue which is prevented from escaping. ● Usually confined to the neck ● It may present on the 1st day and is self-limiting (by 7th day).	**Causes:** ● Pretracheal fascia not adequately opened. ● Uncuffed tube. ● Coughing (excessive) ● Tight sutures of skin causing ball-valve effect. ● Large tracheostomy opening with a small tube. ● Obstruction to egress of air. ● **Symptoms:** Discomfort, pyrexia.	● Use of cuffed tubes ● Release of skin and subcutaneous sutures ● Multiple incisions over affected area. ● Treatment of cough. ● Reassurance.
4. Profuse bronchorrhoea	**Cause:** ● Irritation due to tube ● Endotracheal aspiration of food	
5. Pneumothorax	Diagnosed if dyspnoea does not improve after the procedure.	
6. Pneumomediastinum	● Positive HAMMAN's sign. ● Respiratory rate increases. ● X-ray chest oblique lateral view: air in mediastinum	● Oxygen ● Antibiotics ● Sedatives
7. Tracheobronchial infection / Pneumonia	**Organisms:** ● Pseudomonas ● Proteus ● Aerobacter ● Fungi	● Appropriate antibiotics ● Aspiration of secretions
8. Crusting	● Dry weather ● Non-humidified air going to the patient	● Wet gauze over stoma ● Use of humidification tent
9. Atelectasis	● Partial atelectasis is due to aspiration of blood and secretions ● Total atelectasis is due to	● Conservative management. ● Readjust the tube

COMPLICATIONS	FEATURES	TREATMENT
	improper placement of tube into one bronchus leading to a collapse	• Shorter tube to be used
10. Aerophagia	• Seen in infants and elderly • Swallowing movements occur post tracheostomy. • Abdominal distension, vomiting, dyspnoea.	• Decannulation • Change tube to different size. • RT aspiration.

IV. Late complications
1. Laryngeal stenosis
	Causes:
	• High tracheostomy leading to perichondritis
	• Improper curve of tube
	• Chemical irritation by sterilizing agents / component of tube.
	• Damage to mucosa during procedure.
	• Movements of tracheostomy tube because of ventilation / deglutition.
	• Improper care.
	  - Non-deflated cuff
	  - Oversized / overinflated cuff.
	Ideal cuff pressure: 15-25 mm of H_2O
		• Prophytactic antibiotics, steroids.
		• Surgical management.

2. Tracheitis		
3. Tracheal stenosis.	**Causes:** • Tracheal resection • Tracheal infection • Repeated incisions • Scar contracture	• Tracheal dilatation • Initial ulcer can be allowed to heal secondarily or excised with primary closure.
4. Tracheomalacia	**Causes:** • Large part of tracheal wall excised. • Pressure necrosis	

5. Difficult decannulation	**Cause:**
	• Dependence of tube
	• Indication for tracheostomy is still present.
	• Granulations in trachea around the stoma.
	• Tracheal oedema.
	• Inability to tolerate upper airway resistance on decannulation
	  - Laryngo tracheal stenosis
	  - Tracheomalacia
		Endoscopy is done to assess the larynx / trachea.
		Rx:
		• Decannulation as early as possible.
		• Partial increasing blockage of tube.
		• Surgical closure.

6. Persistent tracheocutaneous fistula.	**Symptoms:** • Skin irritation	• It heals if present for less than 16 weeks

COMPLICATIONS	FEATURES	TREATMENT
- Seen after long-term tracheostomies	● Poor phonation	● Surgical closure with excision of old scar tissue.
7. Depressed scar / keloid formation.	● Poor cosmesis	

14. RADICAL NECK DISSECTION

- Dr. Shridhar Iyer

It is enbloc removal of all lymph bearing area between the clavicle and the mandible and horizontally from the midline to the trapezius posteriorly.

A specimen of radical neck dissection contains:

1. External jugular vein
2. Internal jugular vein
3. Sternocleidomastoid muscle
4. Omohyoid muscle.
5. Submandibular salivary gland
6. Tail of parotid gland
7. Accessory nerve
8. Sensory branches of cervical plexus.
9. The following lymph nodes are removed:
   - Lymph nodes of submandibular triangle
   - Deep cervical lymph nodes
   - Posterior triangle nodes
   - Supraclavicular nodes.

Lymph node groups not removed:

1. Superficial nodes of the preauricular, postauricular and occipital region
2. Nodes in the parotid gland
3. Retropharyngeal, lateral pharyngeal nodes
4. Prelaryngeal and paratracheal nodes.

TERMINOLOGY

1. **Conservation or functional neck dissection** : It is an alternative to radical neck dissection in which any of the following structures are preserved:
   a) Accessory nerve
   b) Cervical plexus branches
   c) Branches to trapezius, sternomastoid muscle
   d) Part of internal jugular vein.

2. **BOCCA'S operation** : It entails removal of lymph nodes and fascia as a single block with preservation of internal jugular vein, sternomastoid and accessory nerve.

3. **Suprahyoid neck dissection**

   It includes removal of nodes above the level of hyoid bone.

4. **Supraomohyoid neck dissection**

   It is an operation which involves dissection of anterior triangle of neck preserving the internal jugular vein, sternocleidomastoid muscle and accessory nerve.

5. **Elective neck dissection**

   It is carried out in patients with no palpable disease in the neck but a high incidence of subclinical disease (20-40%).

Occult metastases is commonly seen in the following carcinomas:

1. Nasopharynx
2. Supraglottis
3. Oral cavity (floor of mouth, tongue)
4. Pharynx

6. **Block dissection :**

   It is removal of primary tumour in continuity with an enlarged mass of nodes. This procedure leaves behind smaller involved nodes and is therefore not preferred.

Assessment of cervical lymph nodes:

1. **History and examination:**
   - Presence of swelling in the neck
   - Palpation of anterior and posterior triangles

   Retropharyngeal and parapharyngeal nodes are not amicable to palpation
   - The following structures can be mistaken for enlarged nodes:
     - Transverse process of atlas
     - Carotid bifurcation
     - Submandibular salivary gland.

2. **Radiology**
   a) C. T. Scan: The three criteria on C. T. scan to denote a node as metastatic are:
      i) Size of node: A likely node is suspected to be metastatic if its size is more than 1.5 cm in submandibular and jugulodigastric group and >1 cm in all other groups. C. T. scan is preferred over MRI for nodes less than 1.3 cm in size.
      ii) Peripheral enhancement
      iii) Central necrosis (low attenuation area)
   b) M. R. I.: Enlarged nodes and nodes with central necrosis are well shown by MRI. It differentiates nodes from surrounding tissues better than C. T. Scan.
   c) Ultrasound: Metastatic nodes show a heterogeneous appearance with a solid and cystic image.
   d) Radioisotopes: It demonstrates metastatic nodes (not until they are 2 cm in size) and not normal nodes.

Neck Dissection

History   :   The operation of systemic radical excision of regional lymphatics was described by Crile in 1906. This was popularised by Hayes Martin and has since become a standard procedure of head and neck surgery. Subsequently Bocca advocated that radicality should be directed against the tumour and not the neck and in 1967 Bocca and Pignataro popularised the conservative neck dissection. As more conservative dissection were described there was an increasing confusion on terminology, till Suen and Goepfert and recentty Robbins, Medina et al standardised the nomenclature.

Radial Neck Dissection

INDICATIONS

1. With resection of primary carcinoma in head and neck when clinically positive cervical node is present
2. Nodal involvement beyond 1st echelon group.
3. Clinically positive nodes when surgery is the only treatment planned
4. Regional metastasis after primary has been controlled by radiation and/or surgery
5. Clinically positive node after previous radiation.

CONTRAINDICATIONS

1. Uncontrollable primary site

2. Distant metastasis

3. Fixed nodes

4. Life expectancy <3 months.

Fixity to carotid artery, brachial plexus, prevertebral fascia and mandible are relative contraindications.

PRE-OPERATIVE

ANAESTHESIA

General anaesthesia is used. Tracheostomy is needed for a bilateral neck dissection.

Shaving from angle of mouth to the nipple.

POSITION : Supine

Neck extended and head turned to the opposite side.

Incisions for Radical Neck Dissection

INCISION	ADVANTAGE	DISADVANTAGE
Crile	-	• The 3 point junction of the in cision may lie on the carotids
MacFee	• Viability of skin flap is maintained • Preferred in already irradiated patients	Restricted access
Horizontal 'T' or half - H	• Good access • Protects carotid artery • Healing of horizontal incision is better • Conforms to main cutaneous blood vessels of neck	• Vertical limb may heal with scar contracture

• Other incisions
  - 'S' shaped incision
  - Modified Schobinger
  - Unilateral apron flap

Modified Schobinger incision

The first-limb (horizontal limb) begins at the chin and descends to the hyoid bone and passes 3cm below the angle of mandible to reach the mastoid. The vertical limb begins just posterior to the carotid pulsation (so that three point suture doesn't lie on the carotid) perpendicular to the horizontal limb and drops to the clavicle in a lazy 'S' to reach upto the midpoint of the clavicle.

If the patient has been irradiated, then a double horizontal incision is taken which protects against wound breakdown. The first horizontal incision is same as the horizontal limb. The second incision lies 2cm above the clavicle starting at the anterior border of trapezius and ending medially at the midline.

Limits of dissection

• Mandible (horizontal vamus)

• Clavicle

• Midline

• Anterior border of trapezius.

Contents :   -   Fat, fascia, lymph nodes
             -   Sternocleidomastoid
             -   Omohyoid
                 -   Cervical nerve roots, Cutaneus branches

- Accessory nerve
- I JV with the sheath
- Submandibular gland and tail of the parotid gland.

Flaps are raised in the subplatysmal plane. Skin is incised down to and through the platysma. In the posterior part of the neck, the platysma is very thin and the fibres of the sternomastoid are inserted directly on the skin, which may cause some bleeding. Care is taken not to make the flap very thin posteriorly and to retain some sternocleidomastoid muscle insertion on the flap.

The skin is held with skin hooks by the assistant and lifted upwards and dissection is done with adequate countertraction.

Flaps are raised upto the mandible superiorly, clavicle inferiorly, anterior border of trapezius posteriorly and midline anteriorly. Care is taken not to damage the spinal accessory nerve while raising the posterior flap which may happen if the flap is too thick.

Care is taken not to damage the lower branches of facial nerve (rima-mandibularis) while raising the superior flap. This may be achieved by:

1. Ligating and dividing the facial vessels on the submandibular gland and lifting them over the mandible, keeping the ligature long. (Hayes Martin technique).

    This manoeuvre may cause damage by pressure of the suture if the course of the nerve is lower than usual and will also cause compromise in removal of pre and post facial nodes.

2. Incising the deep fascia over the submandibular gland and elevating the flap with the deep fascia; so that the nerve remains protected.

The flaps are held apart by stay sutures

The External jugular and anterior jugular veins are ligated and divided superiorly and inferiorly. The lower end of the stenomastoid muscle is divided next, just above the clavicle using electrocautery. The lower end of divided muscle should not be transfixed as it may cause bunching up and necrosis. The carotid sheath is exposed and incised transversely. The internal jugular vein is identified and dissected. The vagus nerve is identified between the carotid and internal jugular vein, this step is important to prevent accidental ligation / transection of vagus. Three ligatures are used to transfix the internal jugular vein and division is between top and 2nd stitch.

On the left side, care must be taken to prevent damage to the thoracic duct. The sternomastoid and internal jugular vein are raised for a little distance. Middle thyroid vein may be ligated at this stage.

Supraclavicular Dissection

The fascia and fat just above the clavicle is sharply divided and traction is applied to it.

The omohyoid muscle now visible is divided with a cautery without clamping.

The fatpad and fascia is held with Allis or Babcocks forceps and, traction is applied to it and dissection is continued in a plane just above the prevertebral fascia. The supraclavicular nerves are divided. Care is taken to protect the transverse cervical artery and vein which run in this triangle (Especially if a trapezius myocutaneous or osteomyocutaneous flap is planned). The ascending branch of the transverse cervical runs alongside the phrenic nerve but above the prevertebral fascia and is divided and ligated and the specimen is freed from the supraclavicular fossa. Care is taken not to breach the prevertebral fascia as the phrenic nerve and brachial plexus run beneath it.

Sometimes if the ascending branch of transverse cervical is damaged and bleeds, blind plunging of hemostat to catch it may cause injury to phrenic nerve. The Phrenic nerve lies beneath the prevertebral fascia on the scalenus anterior muscle and runs from above down from a lateral to medial direction.

The Chassaignac's triangle (between the longus colli and scalenus anterior) is cleared where scalene nodes are present. Care is taken on left side to prevent damage to thoracic duct. At this point, the anaesthetist is asked to give positive pressure ventilation, and if a leak is detected, it is ligated with figure of 'S' stitch immediately. The supraclavicular dissection is done upto the anterior border of trapezius.

The operation now is continued in an upward direction towards the posterior triangle.

The Accessory nerve runs in the 'roof' of the posterior triangle and must be identified and dissected before dissecting in posterior triangle if it is to be protected (as in MND).

The nerve exits the sternomastoid muscle at the junction of the upper $\frac{1}{3}^{rd}$ and lower $\frac{2}{3}^{rd}$ and then has a sinuous course before reaching the lower anterior border of trapezius. The point of exit is known as Erbs point and in the operation it is identified 1 cm above the point where the greater auricular nerve winds around the sternomastoid muscle.

This dissection is carried upto the mastoid tip.

- The dissection continues clinging the fascia from anterior border of trapezius upto the mastoid tip where the sternomastoid and trapezius insert. The sternomastoid is divided from the mastoid tip. At this point, the tail of the parotid is also divided taking care to secure the retromandibular vein. Firm downward traction is applied to the sternomastoid and the digastric muscle (posterior belly is identified). Posterior belly of digastric is retracted upwards with a langenback retractor. Here the upper end of internal jugular vein along with the accessory are identified. The accessory nerve is divided and care is taken to identify and secure any tributaries of internal jugular vein.

- The internal jugular vein is ligated and divided between double ligatures.

    The specimen is next released from the posterior triangle by applying a series of tissue forceps and applying traction and releasing the cutaneous branches of cervical plexus.

- The internal jugular vein is dissected with the carotid sheath with manoeuvre of traction countertraction and is dissected off the carotid and vagus.

Identify and preserve the hypoglossal nerve as it traverses across the external carotid artery.

The occipital artery crosses the posterior part of the IJV and should be secured.

At this stage the specimen consisting of inferior belly of omohyoid / sternomastoid, IJV, fat, fascia and nodes from supraclavicular triangle and posterior triangle are lifted off and dissected free anteriorly (from strap muscles).

As the specimen is released, ansa cervicalis, superior thyroid vein and the facial venous trunk are identified and divided.

Anteriorly the omohyoid (superior belly) is released from its attachment to hyoid and the specimen is now pedicled to the submandibular region.

Dissection of submandibular triangle

The specimen is now attached superiorly only. The submental triangle is cleared (between anterior bellies of digastric muscle).

The fat, lymph nodes and fascia are now elevated upto the anterior end of the submandibular gland. The anterior end of submandibular gland is identified and dissected upto the posterior border of mylohyoid. The posterior border of mylohyoid is retracted to reveal the submandibular duct. Here the lingual nerve is seen to loop down and attach to submandibular ganglion. The lingual nerve is freed by detaching it from the ganglion and then dividing the submandibular duct, between ligatures as there may be a blood vessel along with it.

Bleeding from submental artery is encountered which is diathermised.

The facial artery and vein are ligated at the lower border of mandible and the specimen is pulled towards posterior flap.

The facial artery is again encountered as it enters the submandibular gland, winding above the superior border of digastric.

The facial artery is ligated and divided and the specimen is removed.

Haemostasis is achieved

A check is made for chyle leak and bleeding

Wound is closed in two layers (platysma and skin) after keeping suction drains.

Complications:
1. Bleeding:
   Sources:
   a) IJV-internal jugular vein lower end :

Treatment   :

Pack / Pressure

1. HEAD LOW (danger of air embolism)

2. Good suction, keep vascular clamps ready

3. Release and see if clamps can be applied

4. If not, repack

5. Excise medial end of clavicle and access the subclavian vein for vascular control.

b) IJV internal jugular vein upper end   :

1. Head low position

2. Pack, control the area by firm pressure with finger.

3. Retract the posterior belly of digastric well or divide it and then control the bleeding. If the vessel cannot be secured, pack jugular foramen with muscle and oversew. In some cases, removal of mastoid tip may help gaining exposure.

c) Damage to carotid arteries:

It occurs while dissecting off (adherent) tumour from the vessel wall.

Post operative bleeding is recognised as neck swelling.

Damage to common carotid artery and internal carotid artery is repaired after vascular clamps are applied and heparin is started.

2. Nerve injuries:

The marginal mandibular, vagus, phrenic, brachial plexus, facial, hypoglossal and lingual nerves are likely to be damaged.

Nerve repair must be performed if vagus, phrenic or brachial plexus is injured.

Nerves which are deliberately divided are:

1. Accessory nerve   :   Its division gives rise to shoulder syndrome which includes pain in the shoulder joint, limitation of abduction and drooping of affected shoulder.

2. Branches of cervical plexus:

   • Lesser occipital

   • Greater auricular nerve

   • Transverse cutaneous nerves of the neck

   • Supraclavicular branch

   • Nerve to trapezius

3. The descendens hypoglossi

3. Chylous fistula:

There is no disgrace in damaging or cutting a thoracic duct whilst operating on left side of the neck. Indeed it may be necessary while doing radical surgery low in the neck or mediastinum. It is disastrous to fail to recognise a leak.

Operating loop may be used to identify and secure it.

If injury is unrecognised, it doesn't usually manifest itself until the patient is subsequently fed, and at this time, the suction drain increases dramatically. Many small leaks (< 400 ml / day) will settle with conservative treatment.

1. Fat free diet (Medium chain triglycerides recommended)

2. Pressure over supraclavicular fossa.

If drainage is 500 ml / day for 2-3 days, reexploration should be done.

Chyle has specific gravity > 1.012

Fat content 1-3%

Protein content 3%

It produces intense inflammatory response, probably due to alkaline pH or inflammatory vasoactive substances produced by leukocytes.

4. Raised intra cranial tension :   It is not commonly seen as bilateral radical neck dissection is almost never done simultaneously.

Bilateral neck dissection where internal jugular vein is present on one side may sometimes lead to this complication if the vessel gets thrombosed.

As a staged procedure if, bilateral dissection is done then pre-operative tracheostomy is a must.

Treatment   :

- Head up position / Airway management (tracheostomy SOS)
- No constricting dressings
- Diuretics
- Steroids
- Mannitol
- Subarachnoid - peritoneal shunting

5. Seroma

6. Infection

Late Complications

1. Shoulder Syndrome ;

    It causes long standing pain and inability to perform certain manoeuvres involving abduction of shoulder. (Abduction beyond 45^0 becomes almost impossible) The best way to avoid this complication is to preserve the accessory nerve and branches from cervical plexus to trapezius (C3 & C4). If these cannot be preserved, then it is mandatory to start post-operative shoulder physiotherapy.

2. Carotid artery rupture :   It is due to necrosis of the arterial wall because of infection in and around the artery. It occurs in patient's treated with preoperative radiotherapy and those who develop postoperative fistula. It is rarely seen nowadays and there is no need to cover the carotid with muscle. If the adventitia of the carotid is dissected off due to adherent node then it may be prudent to cover it with levator scapulae flap. If it occurs, a warning bleed usually occurs prior to the rupture. The wound is reopened and the carotid artery ligated. Blood transfusion may be required and a cuffed portex tracheostomy tube is introduced to protect the airway. Carotid artery rupture is associated with a high mortality rate and risk of hemiplegia.

3. Wound infection

    The following factors affect healing of the wound:

    i)   Contamination of surgical field

    ii) Incontinuity removal of primary tumour and neck node specimen

    iii) Flap necrosis and wound breakdown

    iv) Postoperative fistula

    v)   Postoperative wound breakdown

15. COMPOSITE RESECTION/SEGMENTAL/ HEMIMANDIBULECTOMY/"COMMANDO OPERATION"

Composite resection, "En bloc" resection of various tissues with the lymphatics.

INDICATIONS

1. Primary tumours of oral cavity and tumours of oropharynx (eg. tonsil) which extend to involve the mandible.
2. Tumours with extensive soft tissue involvement around the mandible requiring the need to sacrifice an intervening segment of mandible to accomplish in confirmity resection.

INCISION

Standard trifurcate incision for neck dissection beginning at the mastoid tip and curving anteriorly, remaining approximately 2 finger breadths below the body of the mandible upto the midline of neck at level of hyoid bone. The incision then turns upwards dividing the skin and soft tissues of chin and lower lip in midline. The vertical limb begins perpendicular to the horizontal limb and posterior to the carotid bifurcation. The incision may be modified depending on individual merits of the case. eg: angle splitting incision is taken if the primary is too close to angle of the mouth

PROCEDURE

The steps of radical neck dissection/modified neck dissection/supraomohyoid dissection are first carried out.

As the operation proceeds cephalad to level I, no attempt is made to dissect the contents of the submandibular triangle, which remain attached, through the floor of the mouth and soft tissues medial to the mandible to the primary site.

The sternomastoid is divided at upper end and digastric muscle (posterior belly) is exposed.

The tail of the partoid gland is divided and the retromandibular vein is ligated and cut.

The upper end of the internal jugular vein is divided and the stump is doubly ligated.

The neck dissection specimen is now pedicled to the mandible at level I.

At this point the neck incision is extended upwards in the midline dividing the chin and the lower lip in its full thickness

A tongue stitch is taken and the throat is packed.

A mucosal incision is placed in the gingivobuccal sulcus remaining close to the attached gingiva.

The lower cheek flap is now elevated remaining right over the cortex of the mandible from lateral of the midline to the angle of the mandible, keeping as much musculature in the cheek flap as possible depending on the primary tumour. Using cautery, the masseter is detached from the mandible.

This manoeuvre provides exposure to the entire lateral cortex of the mandible from the mandibular notch to the symphysis menti.

All the muscular attachments over the coronoid process including the tendon of temporalis muscle are divided.

The mandible is divided above the entry of the inferior alveolar nerve, usually through the mandibular notch at its ascending ramus leaving the condyloid process but excising the coronoid process.

Care is taken that the power saw does not cut through the tissues medial to the mandible otherwise brisk haemorrhage will result from laceration of the pterygoid muscles.

The mandible is now divided at the appropriate place depending on the site, size, surface, extent of the tumour and the extent of soft tissue disease contiguous to the mandible. A straight cut is made through the mandible (usually just distal to the mental foramen)

The mandible, now divided at two places, permits its lateral retraction.

With gentle traction on the mandibular segment, mucosal incision is marked around the tumour medial to the mandible.

Using electrocautery, three dimensional resection of primary tumour with generous cuff of mucosa and soft tissue is done (1-1.5cm.)

The attachments of mylohyoid, digastric and medial pterygoid muscles are divided.

Once all the medial attachments are removed, the specimen is detached.

Frozen sections from appropriate areas are obtained.

Haemostasis is checked.

Appropriate reconstruction is planned and primary closure of mucosa (buccal mucosa with floor of mouth mucosa) using interrupted 3/0 vicryl sutures (mattress or single) is carried out if there is not much mucosal loss.

The closure continues upto the mucosal aspect of the lip.

The vermilion is now accurately approximated using 5/0 Ethilon. The lip musculature is also approximated.

Drains are placed in the neck.

The neck is now closed along with the chin in two layers after confirming haemostasis and absence of chyle leak on the left side.

Reconstruction:

Each patient's defect must be considered individually

The primary indication for bone reconstruction for lateral segmental defects is restoration of mastication.

a. Dentate mandible / patients wearing dentures / young patients: Bone reconstruction.

b. Edentulous patients not wearing dentures: Soft tissue replacement.

Soft tissue replacement is accomplished by:

1. Pectoralis major myocutaneous flap (most commonly used)
2. Pectoralis major flap with deltopectoral flap (if there is skin loss > 6 cm)
3. Bipedicled pectoralis major myocutaneous flap (if skin loss < 6 cm)
4. Trapezius myocutaneous flap

Bony reconstruction is by (Composite tissue transfer with microvascular anastomosis is 'State of the art')

1. Free fibula flap
2. Iliac crest free flap

Advantages of bony reconstruction:

1. Good restoration of function and cosmesis
2. Early radiotherapy is possible
3. Flap loss and failure are less as compared to other methods of bone reconstruction.

Disadvantages:

1. Complex procedure
2. Complications may delay radiotherapy

   While describing a case of mandibulectomy/composite resection

Mention:

1. Type of mandibulectomy
2. Site of lesion in oral cavity

   (e.g. This is a description of composite resection with a lateral segmental mandibulectomy for a case of T4 squamous carcinoma of buccal mucosa (alveolus/floor mouth/tongue)

Types of mandibulectomies:

1. Segmental
   - Lateral
   - Arch
2. Hemimandibulectomy
3. Arch saving hemimandibulectomy
4. Marginal mandibulectomy

Other methods of bone reconstruction:

- Pectoralis major osteomyocutaneous flap
- Trapezius osteomyocutaneous flap
- Latissimus dorsi flap
- Reconstruction plates
- Titanium trays
- Corticocancellous grafts
- Cadaver mandibular bone
- Osseointegrated implants.

All the above have significant rates of complications, hence not commonly used.

If bone reconstruction is contemplated, microvascular free composite tissue transfer is the best.

Middle $\frac{1}{3}^{rd}$ or anterior segment resection results in debilitating deformity if not reconstructed. Hence "Reconstruction of bone is mandatory".

COMPLICATIONS

1. Orocutaneous fistula
2. Flap necrosis
3. Mandibular deviation

   The medial pterygoid action causes displacement of the remaining mandibular segment medially. This mal-occlusion can be prevented by 'bite guide' fitted immediately especially after hemimandibulectomy
4. Stump tenderness/osteomyelitis
5. Complications of neck dissection

16. DIRECT LARYNGOSCOPY

This is a procedure in which the larynx is directly examined with a laryngoscope.

INDICATIONS

Diagnostic
1. When a lesion on indirect laryngoscopy needs further evaluation.
2. Diagnosis of
   - Congenital laryngeal web
   - Laryngomalacia
   - Vocal cord paralysis
   - Benign and malignant tumours
   - Chronic laryngitis
   - Laryngeal keratosis
   - Laryngeal foreign body
3. Overhanging epiglottis impeding view of endolarynx
4. To evelute the blind areas on indirect laryngoscopy
5. To examine larynx in children in whom indirect laryngoscopy may not be possible
6. As a part of panendoscopy
7. To take diagnostic biopsy.

Therapeutic
1. Removal of foreign bodies from larynx, hypopharynx
2. Removal of thickened secretions, crusts
3. Removal of vocal cord nodules, cysts, polyps, benign tumours etc.
4. For endotracheal intubation in general anaesthesia
5. Direct laryngoscopy with a detachable blade is used to pass a bronchoscope, particularly in children.
6. To inject Teflon paste in unilateral vocal cord paralysis.

CONTRAINDICATIONS

Absolute
Disease of the cervical spine. In caries spine, direct laryngoscopy can lead to spinal cord damage and quadriplegia.

Relative
1. Trismus or ankylosis of temporomandibular joint
2. Short, thick neck
3. Long incisor teeth
4. Systemic disorders
   - Diabetes
   - Hypertension
   - Cardiac abnormalities

PREOPERATIVE

ANAESTHESIA

Local or General anaesthesia

Local anaesthesia :   The oral cavity and oropharynx are sprayed with 4% Xylocaine spray. The larynx is sprayed with a laryngeal atomizer

A cotton wool soaked in 4% Xylocaine is placed in both pyriform fossa with a Krause's laryngeal forceps for five minutes. This is to anaesthetise the internal laryngeal nerve running under the mucosa of the pyriform fossa. The subglottis is anaesthetized by instilling Xylocaine through the glottis while the patient holds his tongue and says 'EEE'

General anaesthesia :   This is preferred as it allows detailed examination and adequate relaxation and control over the airway. A smaller size endotracheal tube is preferred.

POSITION

(BOYCE'S position)

Supine position with flexion of neck and extension of atlanto-occipital joint. This particular position brings the larynx in direct axis with the oral cavity and facilitates introduction of the scope.

PROCEDURE

The laryngoscope is held in the right hand and passed from the right side of the mouth. The upper lip and teeth are protected with a thick layer of gauze to prevent injury during the scopy. The endoscope is introduced from the right angle of mouth to the lateral side of tongue till the posterior part of tongue is reached. It is then shifted to the midline and the base of the tongue is elevated. This brings the epiglottis into view. The tip of the laryngoscope is passed behind the epiglottis and the epiglottis is lifted by lifting the handle of the laryngoscope upwards. This brings the posterior part of the larynx into view. By proper manipulation of the scope, keeping in mind to avoid pressure on the lip and teeth, the whole of the larynx especially the blind areas are visualized for any pathology.

The following structures are visualized on direct laryngoscopy.

- Valeculla
- Base tongue
- Lingual surface of epiglottis
- Aryepiglottic fold
- Pyriform sinus
- Post cricoid region

- Interarytenoid region
- True vocal cords
- False vocal cords
- Anterior commissure
- Posterior commissure

> **Blind areas of larynx :**
>
> (Difficult to visualize areas of larynx)
>
> - Laryngeal surface of epiglottis below its tubercle
> - Ventricle of larynx
> - Anterior commissure
> - Subglottis

The laryngoscope is then gently withdrawn. A microlaryngoscope abuts against the true vocal cords while a direct laryngoscope is only introduced upto the epiglottis to visualize the supraglottis and glottis. A straight blade laryngoscope is only used to examine the larynx and to pass a rigid bronchoscope. The anterior commissure laryngoscope is used to visualize the anterior part of glottis, anterior commissure, subglottis and to fix the vocal cords for therapeutic purposes.

COMPLICATIONS

1. Trauma to lips, teeth, gum, tongue, palate etc
2. Damage to cervical spine or spinal cord
3. Laryngospasm or stridor may be precipitated.
4. Anaesthetic complication like hypertension, cardiac and respiratory arrest.

Direct Laryngoscopy in children

It is indicated in children having stridor with feeding difficulties. It differs from adult laryngoscopy in that the tip of the laryngoscope is not placed behind the epiglottis, but anterior to the epiglottis in the valeculla. This manoeuvre brings the laryngeal inlet in line with the optical axis of the laryngoscope and allows a good view of the larynx. Also in this way, the tip of the laryngoscope does not press on the aryepiglottic fold which would restrict cord movements in a case of cord paralysis.

Stridor is common in infancy and childhood because of certain anatomical differences between adult and infantile larynx.

LARYNX	INFANT	ADULT
1. Position	1. Higher in the neck, therefore the air current enters more straight into the larynx.	1. Lower in the neck The pharynx, larynx and trachea meet at an acute angle.
2. Laryngeal aperture	2. Smaller and narrow especially in the subglottic region.	2. Large and wide
3. Antero-posterior diameter of glottis	3. The lumen of the larynx and trachea is smaller in proportion to the body as a whole. Glottis 7 mm Subglottis 6 mm (4 mm is stenosis)	3. The larynx and trachea are proportionate to the body.
4. Epiglottis	4. - Folded - Funnel shaped - Infantile	4. - Leaf-liked - Not curled
5. Cartilages	5. Softer and more pliable	5. Tough
6. Neuromuscular apparatus	6. Hyperexcitable Hypersensitive	6. Normal response Normal response
7. Mucosa	7. Loose and less fibrous	7. Less loose

INDIRECT LARYNGOSCOPY	DIRECT LARYNGOSCOPY
1. Mirror image of larynx	1. Direct visualization
2. Inverted image obtained	2. True image is seen
3. Two-dimensional image	3. Three-dimensional visualization
4. Inadequate visualization of anterior commissure, ventricle and subglottic region	4. Good visualization of entire larynx with its blind areas.
5. Overhanging epiglottis may hamper view	5. Epiglottis is lifted up with the tip of the scope
6. Out patient's procedure	6. Operative procedure
7. No anaesthesia is usually required	7. General anaesthesia is preferable.

Types of Laryngoscopes

TYPE	USE
Mackintosh laryngoscope	Endotracheal intubation
Jackson's direct laryngoscope (with a sliding blade)	Most commonly used for direct laryngoscopy. It has distal illumination.
Negus laryngoscope	Direct laryngoscopy. It has a wide proximal end and proximal illumination
Anterior commissure laryngoscope	It has a bevelled end and is used to view the anterior commissure and for vocal cord operations.

17. BRONCHOSCOPY

INDICATIONS

Diagnostic

- Patients with respiratory disease of long duration.
  - Diagnosis of:
    - Unexplained chronic cough, sputum production.
    - Stridor.
    - Wheeze.
    - Haemoptysis.
  - Suspected foreign body
  - Paralysis of a vocal cord.
  - A mass in neck (thought to be metastatic carcinoma.)
  - Suspicion of tracheal, bronchial or pulmonary disease.
  - Sputum cytology suggestive of a malignant tumour.
  - Oesophageal and thyroid diseases involving the tracheobronchial tree.

> **Specific Indications for Bronchoscopy:**
> - Atelectasis
> - Emphysema
> - Parenchymal densities
> - Foreign body
> - Mediastinal masses
> - Pleural effusion

Therapeutic

- For aspiration of tracheobronchial secretions in atelectasis and bronchiectasis
- Removal of benign endobronchial neoplasms - such as papillomas, lipomas etc.
- Removal of foreign bodies and broncholiths.
- Drainage of lung abscess.
- Dilatation of bronchial stenosis.
- Lung lavage in asthma and cystic fibrosis
- Biopsy of a suspected tumour

CONTRAINDICATIONS

Absolute

- Aortic aneurysm.
- Bleeding tendencies.
- Recent massive haemoptysis of any cause.

Relative

- Acute respiratory infections
- Cervical spine ankylosis
- Trismus.

PREOPERATIVE

ANAESTHESIA

General anaesthesia is preferred. Ventilation is maintained by oxygen-venturi system.

POSITION

Supine position with head extended and the cervical spine flexed at the atlanto-occipital joint. The surgeons left hand steadies and controls the upper jaw. The upper teeth are protected with a double-layered gauze from pressure of the scope.

OPERATION

Insertion of bronchoscope with the aid of the laryngoscope: The direct laryngoscope is first passed lifting the epiglottis. The assistant holds the bronchoscope at its midpoint like a pencil and places the distal tip of the bronchoscope in the laryngoscope. The operator takes hold of the handle and advances the bronchoscope through the laryngoscope, supraglottis, the vocal cords and then into the trachea. Once the bronchoscope is in the trachea, the handle of the laryngoscope is rotated to the left, its slide is removed and then the laryngoscope is removed.

Insertion of only bronchoscope: In this method, the bronchoscope is inserted like an oesophagoscope. It is introduced through the right side of the mouth, following the tongue to the epiglottis. The epiglottis is elevated and using the left thumb as a fulcrum for the scope, it is advanced towards the glottis. Before entering the glottis the tip is rotated by 90^0 to the right. This makes the tip vertical and enables the scope to pass through the vertical axis of the glottis and to visualise the left vocal cord. It should be remembered that while withdrawing the bronchoscope, the opposite is followed ie; the tip of the scope is rotated to left by 90^0. So that the right vocal cord and its undersurface can be visualised. With gentle twisting movements, the bronchoscope is further advanced down the larynx into the trachea.

Inspection of trachea and carina: The scope is gently advanced visualising the tracheal walls till the sharp outline of the carina is seen.

The carina is evaluated for its position, sharpness, and mobility on respiration and cardiac contraction. Enlarged lymph nodes and masses may displace the carina. As a general rule, the right bronchus and its subdivisions are examined first. As the right bronchus is entered, the head and neck are turned to the left to allow a more direct passage of the scope. The handle of the bronchoscope is rotated to the right so that the tip of the bevel will enter the right bronchus. After bronchoscope has entered the right bronchus, the handle is rotated to the left so that the orifice of the upper lobe bronchus may be inspected. It ideally requires a lateral viewing telescope for adequate inspection.

All subsequent lobar bronchi are examined and as the bronchoscope is withdrawn, the head and neck are shifted back to the midline and then to the right as the left bronchus is entered. Entry into the left bronchus requires more caution as it is longer and curved at an oblique angle to the carina.

BRONCHO - PULMONARY SEGMENTS

RIGHT LUNG			LEFT LUNG			
Lobes	**Segments**		**Lobes**		**Segments**	
Upper	Apical	B1	**Upper**	Superior division	Apical Posterior	B1-2
	Posterior	B2			Anterior	B3
	Anterior	B3		Inferior division (Lingula)	Superior	B4
Middle	Lateral	B4			Inferior	B5
	Medial	B5			Apical	B6
Lower	Apical (Superior)	B6	**Lower**		Medial basal	B7
	Medial basal	B7			Anterior basal	B8
	Anterior basal	B8			Lateral basal	B9
	Lateral basal	B9			Posterior basal	B10
	Posterior basal	B10				

The bronchoscope is withdrawn to just below the carina. Bronchial washings are usually taken from each bronchial tree separately. Normal saline, 5 to 10 ml is injected through the bronchoscope and aspirated. The specimen may be sent for bacterial culture and sensitivity, acid fast smear and culture, fungus culture and cytologic examination. A large sample of biopsy can be taken. Biopsy is carried out at the end of the procedure, so that the bleeding that follows does not hamper visualization. It is required to fix the scope to the teeth before any therapeutic indication is carried out since the scope may move with respiratory movements.

COMPLICATIONS

- Trauma to surrounding structures.
- Arytenoid dislocation
- Laryngeal oedema
- Haemorrhage
- Bronchospasm
- Aspiration

Foreign Bodies of the Tracheobronchial Tree:

They are mainly seen in children. Common foreign bodies are seeds, nails, pins, beans, smooth objects like peanuts, peas and plastic toys. Foreign body in the tracheobronchial tree produces severe spasmodic cough which lasts for approximately half an hour and then subsides. Foreign bodies most frequently lodge into the right bronchus.

> **Foreign bodies are more common in the right bronchus because:**
> - Carina is slightly to the left
> - Right bronchus is larger in diameter than the left.
> - Right bronchus is a more direct extension of the trachea then the left.
> - Action of trachealis muscle.
> - Greater volume of air enters the right bronchus.

As the cough abates, auscultation of the chest may show signs of bronchial obstruction.

> **Types of bronchial obstruction**
> - Bypass valve.
> - Expiratory check / one way valve
> - Inspiratory check / stop valve

A foreign body in the bronchus may produce a bypass valve, an expiratory check or one way valve, or an inspiratory check or stop valve type of obstruction. The most common is the one-way valve, in which the air may enter the bronchus distal to the foreign body during inspiration but may not escape from the lung on expiration. This type of valve obstruction produces emphysema distal to the foreign body.

Signs of obstructive emphysema:

1. Respiratory system examination
    - increased resonance
    - decreased breath sounds
2. X'ray picture
    - emphysema obvious on expiratory film
    - increased radiolucency of lung is present distal to the foreign body
    - mediastinal shift to opposite side.
    - separation of ribs from eachother

Signs of stop-valve kind of obstruction:

1. Atelectasis of lung distal to the foreign body (absorption of air in the lung)
2. Shift of mediastinum to opposite side
3. Compensatory emphysema of the opposite lung for adequate ventilation
4. Respiratory distress, cyanosis and cardiorespiratory failure can occur.
5. Absent breath sounds on the affected side.

The stop valve kind of obstruction completely occludes the bronchus.

Smaller tracheal foreign bodies may move in the trachea during respiration. Radiography is not usually helpful with tracheal foreign bodies.

Vegetable foreign bodies produce severe inflammatory reactions which are particularly severe with peanuts and nuts which produce arachidonic bronchitis. After a latent period of 24 hours, the patient develops cough with purulent sputum and fever. Beans and peas are hygroscopic and swell as water is absorbed. Metallic and plastic foreign bodies that cause partial obstruction of a bronchus may be tolerated for long periods. General anaesthesia is used in most paediatric and adult patients for foreign body removal. Antibiotic therapy is required in patients with long standing foreign bodies.

The size of the ventilating bronchoscope should be appropriate to the patient. It should be small enough in diameter to reach the level of the foreign body and yet provide large working lumen as possible. An over sized bronchoscope can lead to subglottic oedema post-operatively.

Causes of subglottic oedema:
- Over sized bronchoscope
- Prolonged bronchoscopy
- Extensive manipulation during scopy.
- Trauma during extraction of foreign body.

Once the foreign body is seen, it is important not to displace the foreign body. Surrounding secretions should be gently suctioned away and the foreign body should be inspected for the best position of the bronchoscope for forceps application. Sharp or pointed foreign bodies may require disengagement from the mucous membrane before withdrawal. The distal tip of the bronchoscope should be as close as possible to the foreign body. There should be an adequate space around the foreign body needed for application of the particular forceps for that foreign body. **(Forcep space)**

Bronchial foreign bodies are removed by placing the distal end of the forceps beyond the centre of the foreign body so that it is not propelled distally as the forceps is closed. Care must be taken to avoid crushing fragile foreign bodies such as peanuts. Foreign bodies are usually withdrawn through the bronchoscope but if the foreign body is too large, it must be removed as a trailing foreign body. This is done by gently withdrawing the foreign body to the bevel of the bronchoscope, fixing it there and then the forceps, bronchoscope and foreign body are removed as one unit. The foreign body has to be manoeuvred at the level of the glottis for its passage through the narrow space. If there is subglottic swelling or expansion of foreign body, then a tracheostomy has to be performed and the foreign body removed by introducing the scope through the tracheostoma.

Principles of removal:
- Selection of an adequate size bronchoscope.
- Achieving best exposure of foreign body.
- Bronchoscope positioned close to foreign body without touching it and keeping adequate forcep space.
- The distal end of the forcep used should pass beyond the centre of the foreign body
- Small foreign bodies are removed through the scope while larger once are removed by trailing mechanism.

Chances of endobronchial oedema increase if the procedure takes more than half an hour.. After foreign body removal a check scopy is done to inspect the tracheobronchial tree for a second foreign body.

- Smooth foreign body in a peripheral bronchus can be removed by passing a Fogarty balloon catheter distal to the foreign body, gently inflating it and withdrawing it.
- Hollow foreign bodies can be removed by placing one blade of an alligator forceps inside and one outside.
- Pointed foreign bodies, such as nails, hooks and pins are almost always situated with the point directed superiorly. The point must be enclosed in the blades of the forceps to prevent perforation of the bronchus. If the point is already embedded in the mucous membrane, the foreign body must be pushed distally with the forceps to disengage the point. Klerf Arrowsmith safety pin closing forceps are used to close open safety pins and to remove them.

Methods of removal of an open safety pin:
- Disengagement from mucous membrane and closure of pin with closing forceps and then removal through the scope.
- If the tip is facing upwards and not closing, the pin can be rotated so that the tip faces downwards and then removed through the scope. (Retroversion)
- Gastroversion can be attempted in which the safety pin is pushed into the stomach, rotated to face the tip down, closed and then removed.

18. MICROLARYNGOSCOPY

It is a surgical procedure in which the endolarynx, especially the vocal cords are examined with the aid of an operating microscope.

Pre requisite

Indirect laryngoscopy is needed before microlaryngoscopy.

INDICATIONS

Diagnostic

To come to a diagnosis in a case of

1. Hoarseness of voice
2. Suspicion of laryngeal carcinoma
3. Biopsy from pathological lesions

Therapeutic

1. Removal of vocal cord nodules, polyps, granulomas.
2. Cauterisation of vocal cord ulcers
3. Stripping of vocal cords in Reinke's oedema.
4. Teflon injection in vocal cord palsy.

CONTRAINDICATIONS

1. General debility making general anaesthesia risky - myocardial infarction, embolism, arrhythmias, hypertension.
2. Patients in whom hyperextension of the cervical spine is difficult
   - Cervical spine disease/surgery
   - Tuberculosis
3. Small glottis

ANAESTHESIA

- A high level of co-operation between the surgeon and the anaesthesiologist is required
- General anaesthesia with a small sized endotracheal tube is preferred.

POSITION

- Supine position with no head rest and no sand bags under the shoulder.
- Protection of the teeth with rubber tubings or gauze pieces is required.

INTRODUCTION OF THE LARYNGOSCOPE

- The neck is placed in maximal flexion and the laryngoscope (largest possible size) is introduced from the corner of the mouth.
- The anaesthetic tube is followed passing the uvula, lifting the epiglottis and finally positioning the scope a few millimeters cranial to the anterior commissure of the vocal cords.
- The scope is then fixed in place with the chest holder.
- Both the vocal cords are visualised along their entire length.
- If the anterior commissure is difficult to visualize, larynx is pushed slightly posteriorly with externally applied manual pressure

EXAMINATION UNDER MICROSCOPE

- The initial light source is removed.
- Zeiss surgical microscope with a 400mm objective lens attached is placed in front of the laryngoscope
- Working distance between the laryngoscope and the microscope is approximately 20 cm and the eyepiece is adjusted.
- After proper suctioning, the following areas are examined.
  - Vocal cords
  - False cords
  - Ventricle
  - Subglottis
  - Arytenoid area

Documentation of the laryngeal findings is done.

POST OPERATIVE CARE

- Voice rest and speech therapy, if required

SECTION - IV
SURGICAL PATHOLOGY

– Dr. N. K. Behl

1. STAINING

For routine haematoxylin and eosin staining, tissue sections need to be processed as per the following steps:

1. Fixation - by formalin
2. Dehydration - by ascending grades of ethyl alcohol
3. Clearing - by xylene
4. Embedding - by paraffin.

This processing can be manual (hand processing) or automated (autotechnicon)

After tissue embedding in paraffin, blocks of paraffin are prepared and sections are cut (4-6 μ thick) on microtome. These sections are then stained.

Fixation

- **Purpose of fixation:**
  a) To study cell morphology as in living state (i.e. to prevent autolysis)
  b) To kill bacteria and other infectious organisms.
  c) To render tissue resistant to further steps of processing and staining.
- Amount of fixative used is 10 times the volume of the tissue
- Time required is 24 hours
- Mechanism of fixation is that it causes coagulation of proteins in the cell.

Types of fixatives

FIXATIVE	USED FOR	REMARKS (ADVANTAGE / DISADVANTAGE)
1. 10% Formalin	Routine processing Most commonly used.	Advantages 1. Cheap 2. Easily available 3. Rapidly penetrates tissue 4. No overhardening occurs even if tissue is kept for a long time 5. Permits wide range of staining. Disadvantages. 1. Irritant to conjunctiva, skin, mucosa 2. Allergic reactions can occur 3. Formalin pigment artefact may be created in the tissue
2. Bouin's fluid 3. Zenker's fluid	For liver and testicular biopsy For muscle biopsy and CNS studies	Disadvantages 1. Overhardening of tissue occurs if kept for a long time 2. Tissue is stained yellow due to the colour of fixative. So prolonged washing is required to remove the colour.
4. Alcohol	To preserve glycogen (which is water soluble)	Disadvantages 1. Over harden's tissue 2. Dissolves fat
5. Glutaraldehyde 6. Osmium tetraoxide	For electron microscopy	

Staining

Methods of staining:

1. Vital staining - applied in living tissue.
2. Routine staining - eg. Haematoxylin and Eosin. It differentiates between nucleus and cytoplasm

   Nucleus: stains blue (haematoxylin).

   Cytoplasm: stains pink (eosin).
3. Special staining - For specific structure identification and microorganisms

Special methods:

1. Immunological -   Immunohistochemistry.
   -    Immunofluorescence
   -    Immunoelectron microscopy
2. Flowcytometry
3. Molecular biology techniques

2. MICROBIOLOGY

The specimens sent for microbiology study (eg.: pus swab) should be sent in a sterile container to be processed without delay

Laboratory diagnosis of disease is:

1. Direct   :   isolation of organism by smear, culture and biochemical reaction (identification of organism)
2. Indirect   :   blood counts, serological and biochemical tests.
- Purpose of smear -
    1. Organism identification - cocci / bacill and gram +ve / gram -ve will help in selecting culture media.
    2. Presence of pus cells - indicates inflammation.

STAINS

1. Gram Stain

Smear is air dried and fixed by passing 3-4 times through the flame

⇓

Stain with Gentian violet or methyl violet for 1 to 1½ min (principal stain)

⇓

Wash with Gram's Iodine (1 min) (It is a mordant ie. fixes dye over smear)

⇓

Wash and add decolourising agent (spirit, alcohol, acetone) till blue colour comes out (15-25 sec.)

⇓

Lastly counterstain with safranin. (40 sec.)

⇓

Then wash, dry and see under oil lens.

Gram +ve: due to Mg - ribonucleate protein complex in cell wall, appears blue

Gram -ve: appears pink

2. AFB stain (Ziehl Neelsen stain)

Smears fixed by passing in flame and covered with carbol fuschin. It is kept warm for 8 min. Basic Fuschin is a dye, (warm dye penetrates better). Carbol acts as a mordant.

⇓

Wash and decolourise with 20% H_2SO_4 or 3% HCl for 2 min.

⇓

Counterstain with methylene blue or malachite green for about 1 min. Dry, see under oil lens

⇓

AFB look red.

3. CYTOLOGY

- Purpose - Rapid diagnosis of malignancy and other conditions eg. tuberculosis, Hashimoto's thyroiditis etc.
- Examination of cells which are obtained by
  1. Exfoliative cytology
  2. FNAC
  3. Imprint or crush smear from tissue pieces
  4. Brush cytology (through fibreoptic endoscopes)
- FNAC (Fine Needle aspiration cytology)
  - It is a most commonly used technique. It is an out-patient procedure.
  - Disposable syringe and needle (usually 23 no.) of variable length as per the need is taken. Negative pressure should be applied only after entering the lesion to be aspirated. The negative pressure should be released while removing needle out of the lesion.
  - USG or CT guided FNAC can be done especially for deep seated organs.
  - The material obtained in the needle is expressed on a glass slide, smears are prepared and rapid fixation in ether-alcohol is done for PAP staining while other remaining air dried smears are used for Giemsa staining. H and E staining can be done instead of PAP staining.
  - Complications (rare) :
    Local haematoma, very rarely dissemination of malignancy via needle tract may occur
  - Advantages :
    Rapid, easy, inexpensive and reliable if done by an experienced person.
  - Disadvantages :
    - Interpretation of smears needs experience
    - Inherent limitations in cases where diagnosis depends mainly on tissue architecture eg. in follicular carcinoma of thyroid where diagnosis of malignancy depends on capsular and vascular invasion and not on cytomorphology.
  - It is commonly used for diagnosis of enlargement or swelling of :
    Thyroid, lymph nodes, breast and salivary glands.

4. FROZEN SECTION

Indications

1. Rapid tissue processing and staining

   (Routine paraffin embedding and processing of tissue takes about 1 day)

   So it is useful for intraoperative diagnosis of tumours
2. For demonstration of
   a) fat (in routine processing, it is dissolved by alcohol)
   b) antigen - antibody reactions

Technique

1. Freezing microtome - rarely in use now since sections are thick.
2. Cryostat - Microtome enclosed in refrigerated chamber (20^0C) and can be operated to give thin sections
   - Tissue is hardened by rapid freezing with CO_2 gas and embedded in ice.

Disadvantages

(As compared to routine haematoxylin and eosin staining)

1. Morphology is less preserved
2. Sections are thicker
3. Bone and fatty tissue create problems in technique
4. Serial sections are difficult to obtain.

5. SPECIMENS

1. NASAL POLYP

Gross features

Appearance: Baloon like mucosal protrusion

Types of nasal polyps

1. Antrochoanal-unilateral, arising from maxillary antrum
2. Ethmoidal-bilateral, grape like masses from the ethmoid sinuses.

    Site: Nasal cavity, sometimes in paranasal sinuses

    Size: Variable. Usually 1-3 cm

    Number : Single or multiple, may be bilateral (in both nostrils)

    Shape   : Oval to elongated.

    Irregular in antro-choanal polyp.

External surface: Smooth or finely bosselated, whitish pale grey in colour with a shiny translucent appearance. Surface may be ulcerated

Cut surface: May show haemorrhage, necrosis, mucoid discharge and tiny cysts may be seen.

Consistency: Soft, tends to become firm with increase in fibro-collagenous tissue.

Modalities of treatment
- Steroids
- Polypectomy
- Caldwell Luc operation
- Ethmoidectomy
- FESS

Difference between Antrochoanal and Ethmoidal polyp.

FEATURES	ANTROCHOANAL	ETHMOIDAL
Age	Young adults and children	Elderly
Origin	Maxillary antrum	Ethmoid cells
Number	Single	Multiple
Shape	Trifoliate	Bunch of grapes.
Side	Unilateral	Bilateral
Size	Can grow very large	Small size
Vascularity	Avascular	Relatively vascular
Recurrence	Uncommon	Common
Extension	Backward	Forward
	Towards choanae	Towards anterior nares
Etiology	Infection	Allergy
Treatment	FESS/Caldwell-Luc operation/Polypectomy	Polypectomy / External Ethmoidectomy / FESS.
Prevention of recurrence	Caldwell-Luc / FESS	FESS / Antihistaminics / Topical / oral steroids

2. NASOPHARYNGEAL ANGIOFIBROMA

It is almost exclusively seen in males between 10 and 25 years age because this neoplasm is androgen - dependent.

- Origin from distinctive erectile - like fibrovascular stroma located in the postero-lateral wall of the roof of nose. Characteristic location is useful in case of a diagnostic problem.

- Gross: Polypoidal mass which bleeds severely on manipulation. It can extend into antrum, protrude below free edge of the soft palate and even into the orbit and cranial cavity.

  CT scan / MRI is required to see extension of mass.

- Microscopy:

  Blood vessels from capillary to venous size with surrounding characteristic fibrous tissue stroma which have "erectile tissue" appearance. (ie. loose, oedematous tissue with stellate fibroblasts, mast cells and collagenised tissue.)

  D/D from capillary haemangioma is necessary.

  Fate: May regress partially after puberty; but treatment is indicated. Surgery and radiotherapy are available. Recurrence may develop, usually within first year of treatment. Chemotherapy is added for a more aggressive tumour. Rarely sarcomatous transformation occurs.

3. NASOPHARYNGEAL CARCINOMA

- Incidence - leading cause of death in south east Asia and northern Africa.

  Age: Bimodal peak-at 15 to 25 years and at 60-70 years

- Etiopathogenesis - Combined action of genetic predisposition, environmental factors and Epstein Barr virus (EBV) infection

- Gross features - Tumour may be very difficult to detect. Random blind biopsies from nasopharyngeal area should be taken in suspected cases.

- Microscopy - types:

  1. Epidermoid or Squamous cell carcinoma (keratinization +)

     - older age group, less association with EBV, poor prognosis

  2. Non keratinising and undifferentiated (sometimes spindle cells)

     - More frequent than epidermoid carcinoma

     - Microscopically lymphocyte rich inflammatory infiltrate is common, hence also called lymphoepithelioma

  Growth pattern:

  Carcinoma cells can be in well formed aggregates or diffuse fashion. The diffuse pattern can be mistaken for lymphoma.

  3. Adenoid squamous carcinoma ⎤
  4. Papillary adenocarcinoma ⎦ — rare

  It has a strong tendency to metastasize to regional lymphnodes and commonest clinical presentation is cervical lymphadenopathy.

  Radiation therapy cures over half of the patients and survival is better in young individuals.

  In children, the most common types of nasopharyngeal malignancies are:

  1. Embryonal rhabdomyosarcoma

  2. Lymphoepithelioma

  3. Malignant lymphoma.

4. CARCINOMA OF MAXILLARY SINUS

- Incidence:
  - Malignant tumours of nasal cavities and paranasal sinuses represent only 3% of the all upper aerodigestive tumours (amongst these, tumours occur more frequently in maxillary sinus followed by nose and ethmoid sinus.)
- Types of malignant tumours
  - A. Primary tumours:
    - i. Epithelial
      - a) From the mucosa
        - Squamous cell carcinoma
        - Melanoma
      - b) From the mucous glands
        - Adenoid cystic carcinoma
        - Adeno carcinoma
      - c) From odontogenic epithelium - Ameloblastic carcinoma
    - ii. Non-epithelial
      - a) From bone - osteosarcoma
      - b) From cartilage - chondrosarcoma
      - c) From connective tissue - fibrosarcoma
  - B. Metastatic tumours -
    - More common in mandible than maxilla
    - Primary tumours in adults
      - Carcinoma from breast, lung, large bowel, prostate, kidney, thyroid, testis
    - Primary tumours in children
      - Adrenal neuroblastoma, embryonal rhabdomyosarcoma
      - Wilm's tumour.

Squamous cell carcinoma of maxillary sinus

Incidence:

- 80% of all malignancies of maxillary sinus.
- More frequent in men over 40 years of age
- Usually previous long history of chronic sinusitis

Presentation

- Unilateral nasal obstruction
- Persistent rhinorrhoea and epistaxis usually for more than 4 weeks.
- Tumours grow undetected until whole sinus is filled.

Diagnosis

- Anterior and posterior rhinoscopy can be useful in visualising tumour mass
- Radiology will be useful to determine extent of lesion and bone erosion.
- FNAC by sinus puncture and aspiration of contents
- Biopsy obtained by endoscopic guidance or surgical exploration.
- C. T. Scan
- Orthopantomogram

Gross: Irregular cauliflower like whitish grey necrotic tumour mass. There may be areas of haemorrhage and necrosis

Microscopic examination - Squamous cell carcinoma.

Classification

1. Ohngren's Classification
2. Moffets Classification
3. Ledermann's Classification
4. TNM Classification
5. Broder's Classification

Staging: Staging system can be considered as follows.

Ohngren's imaginary line from medial canthus of eye to angle of mandible divides maxilla in

a) Anteroinferior portion (Infrastructure)
b) Posterosuperior portion (Supra structure)

Treatment:

- Total / extended maxillectomy
- Radiotherapy and chemotherapy as adjuvant treatment.

Prognosis:

- Five year survival rate is around 30%
- Tumours of infrastructure are away from the eye and base of skull and may be resected more easily, hence carry better prognosis.

5. CARCINOMA OF ORAL CAVITY

- Leukoplakia
  - It is a clinical term for a white patch or plaque which is at least 5 mm in diameter, cannot be removed by rubbing and cannot be classified as any other diagnosable disease
  - Epidermoid carcinoma has been reported to develop in 1% to 6% of leukoplakia cases followed up for 10 years.

    It is usually seen in lesions with dysplastic epithelium.
- Squamous cell carcinoma
  - Predisposing factors
    - For lip carcinoma - sunlight, fair complexion
    - For oropharyngeal carcinoma - tobacco, alcohol, syphilis, oral sepsis, candidiasis
  - Incidence - Usually in males over the age of 50 years

    Common sites are -
    1. Floor of the mouth (especially at exit of Wharton's duct)
    2. Anterior pillar of soft palate and retromolar area
    3. Ventrolateral aspect of tongue
  - Apart from typical microscopic appearance, cells may have acantholysis with pseudoglandular appearance. Definite stromal invasion is the criteria for malignancy.
    - Role of frozen section is for evaluation of surgical margins.
    - After radiotherapy, abnormal appearing mucosa if seen, should not be biopsied till 6-8 weeks because interpretation of biopsy may be difficult and misleading.

- F. N. A. C. has main role in detecting lymph node metastases.
- Two morphological patterns which may create diagnostic difficulty in lymph node assessment include
  a) Cystic degeneration in metastatic deposits
  b) Extensive foreign body giant cell reaction around clumps of keratin without viable tumour cells.

Prognosis:

- Depends on stage, location and grade.
- Overall 5 year survival rate is:
  - CA of lower lip - 90%
  - CA of anterior tongue - 60%
  - CA of posterior tongue, floor, tonsil, gingiva - 40%
  - CA of soft palate - 20% to 30%

Other microscopic types

1. Verrucous carcinoma
2. Adenosquamous carcinoma
3. Basiloid carcinoma
4. Spindle cell carcinoma
5. Small cell carcinoma

- Spread and Metastases
  1. Direct Spread:
     a) Carcinoma lip - adjacent skin, orbicularis muscle, buccal mucosa, adjacent mandible and mental nerve.
     b) Tumours of floor of mouth - Sublingual gland, oris gingiva and mandible
     c) Tumours of tongue - Often on lateral and undersurface and remain localised for a long time. They eventually invade the floor of mouth
     d) Tumours of buccal mucosa - Infiltrates in underlying muscle and skin
     e) Tumours of gingiva - Quick spread to periosteum and oral mucosa
     f) Tumours of hard palate - Infiltrate in underlying bone but extension to maxillary antrum is very rare.
  2. Lymphatic spread:

     Important points -
     a) The more anterior is the tumour, the lower is the position of cervical lymph nodes involved.

GROUP OF LYMPH NODES SHOWING METASTASES	PRIMARY SITE OF CANCER
1. Upper cervical lymph nodes	1. Posterior tongue and oropharynx
2. Middle cervical lymph nodes	2. Anterior tongue
3. Lower cervical lymph nodes	3. Lip, gingivae, floor of mouth, hard palate.

     b) Cervical lymphnode enlargement due to metastases can be the initial clinical presentation (due to occult primary carcinoma)
     c) Cervical lymphnode metastases can undergo cystic degeneration and may be misdiagnosed as branchial cyst with malignant transformation.
     d) F. N. A. C. is a useful screening procedure.
     e) Mediastinal lymphnodes may be involved
  3. Haematogenous spread:

     Rarely seen - to lung, liver, bone.

Treatment:

- Surgery and radiotherapy in combination
- Radical neck dissection may be curative in early stages.

6. CARCINOMA OF LARYNX

Laryngeal carcinoma (invasive)

Incidence

- Men - 2.2% of all cancers
- Women - 0.4% of all cancers
- 96% are males, usually in 5th decade or beyond

Predisposing factors

1. Smoking. Risk increases with heavy alcohol consumption.
2. Chronic laryngitis
   - Types: According to location - % of total cases
     1. Glottic (60% to 65%)
        - From true vocal cords,
        - Tends to remain localised due to surrounding cartilage and paucity of lymphatic vessels. Prophylactic lymph node dissection is not indicated
     2. Supraglottic (30% to 35%)
        - From false cords, ventricles, epiglottis
        - Tends to spread to preepiglottic space but the oropharynx is protected by the thick hypoepiglottic ligament.
        - Average incidence of lymph node metastases is 40%
3. Transglottic (less than 5%)
   - Cancer spreading beyond laryngeal ventricle
   - Highest incidence of lymph node involvement (52%)
     So lymph node dissection should be done with total laryngectomy.
4. Infraglottic (Subglottic) (less than 5%)
   - Cancer involving true cords with subglottic extension of more than 1cm. or tumours confined to subglottic area only
   - Tends to involve cricoid cartilage, thyroid gland and trachea.
   - Management needs radical surgery with resection of trachea and clearance of paratracheal lymph nodes
- Tumours of pyriform fossa or post-cricoid areas are considered of pharyngeal origin.

Pathology

Gross - Usually 1-4 cm pink, grey ulcerated mass
      - Polypoid appearance in verrucous carcinomas

Microscopy (types)

1. Squamous cell carcinoma (90%)
   - Well differentiated
   - Moderately differentiated
   - Poorly differentiated

2. Verrucous carcinoma
   - Diagnosis based on deeper biopsy to demonstrate invasion.
3. Small cell (oat cell carcinoma) - (less than 0.5%)
   - In 6th - 7th decade and heavy smokers
   - Cells exhibit neuro-endocrine differentiation
   - Metastases common.
   - Prognosis is bad
4. Basiloid squamous carcinoma
   - In heavy smokers
   - Squamous cell carcinoma associated with small cells resembling basal cells.
   - Extremely aggressive behaviour.
5. Adenocarcinoma - very rare
6. Sarcomatoid carcinoma (spindle cell carcinoma)
   - Polypoid, usually supraglottic
   - High predilection for upper aerodigestive tract.
   - Cells are pleomorphic - sarcoma - like but immunohistochemistry indicates epithelial origin.

Prognosis

It depends on the following factors:

1. Clinical stage and site

   5 year survival
   - Glottic - 80%
   - Supraglottic - 64%   Stage IV <5%
   - Transglottic - 50%
   - Subglottic - 40%
2. Microscopic grade - poor prognosis in high grade tumours
3. DNA aneuploidy - worse prognosis
4. Host reaction - Langerhan cells in stroma carries a better prognosis

7. CARCINOMA OF OESOPHAGUS

It is usually an epidermoid carcinoma (squamous cell)

It is seen in men over 50 yrs. of age

It is common in China and other oriental countries

It is associated with:

a) Achalasia cardia

b) Stricture / web

c) Oesophagitis

d) Local irradiation

- Gross

  Site in oesophagus

  a) Upper $\frac{1}{3}^{rd}$ -   Rarest

  b) Middle $\frac{1}{3}^{rd}$ -   Commonest

  c) Lower $\frac{1}{3}^{rd}$ -   Follows middle $\frac{1}{3}^{rd}$

Tumour is usually circumferential, often ulcerated with sharply demarcated margins. On cut section greyish white tumour is seen invading the deeper wall. Due to rich lymphatic supply, lymphnode metastases are frequent. Metastases to liver, lung and adrenal glands are common.

Microscopy

- It is usually moderately differentiated squamous cell carcinoma.
- In situ carcinoma and superficial spreading variants have been described.
- Brush cytology should be used along with biopsy to improve diagnostic yield.

Treatment

- Surgery for lower $\frac{1}{3}^{rd}$
- Radiotherapy for upper $\frac{1}{3}^{rd}$ and middle $\frac{1}{3}^{rd}$.
- Prognosis is poor.
- 5 year survival after surgery is 4%

Other microscopic types:

1. Spindle cell carcinoma
2. Verrucous carcinoma
3. Adeno carcinoma
4. Adeno squamous carcinoma
5. Basiloid carcinoma
6. Small cell carcinoma.

Other tumours and tumour like lesions:

- Commonest benign tumour of oesophagus is leiomyoma
- Malignant melanoma - predilection for lower $\frac{1}{3}^{rd}$
- Inflammatory pseudotumour
- Amyloidosis

8. THYROGLOSSAL CYST

- It is a congenital abnormality - arising due to cystic change in a part of the persistent thyroglossal duct. The duct runs from foramen caecum of tongue to the thyroid isthmus. It usually passes through the hyoid bone.
- Common in children but can present later in life.
- Cystic change develops due to secretion of the lining cells.

  The cyst may be connected to foramen caecum or to skin or appears as a sinus. It may get infected.
- Microscopy -

  Cyst is lined by pseudostratified ciliated or squamous epithelium. Mucous glands and thyroid follicles are commonly seen in the adjacent stroma.
- Management -

  Surgical excision.

  It is important to include excision of middle third of the hyoid bone to minimize recurrence.

  When sinus is formed, entire tract should be excised.
- Thyroid tissue located within the cyst can undergo malignant change - (usually papillary carcinoma).

Causes of enlargement of thyroid

1. a) Development abnormality - Thyroglossal cyst
   b) Congenital - Dyshormonogenetic goitre

2. Autoimmune   -   Graves' disease
                 -    Hashimoto's thyroiditis
3. Inflammatory -   Infectious etiology
                 -    Granulomatous thyroiditis
                 -    Riedel's thyroiditis
4. Neoplastic enlargement
5. Iodine deficiency - Physiological / colloid / simple goitre.
6. Thyroid stimulators / autonomous behaviour - Multinodular goitre.

9. APPEARANCE IN THYROID LESIONS

1. **Simple goitre:**
    a) First stage (Due to compensatory hyperplasia of follicular cells)
       Size: Moderate, weight upto 150 gm.
       Shape: Maintained, enlargement is symmetrical, diffuse
       External and cut surface: Near normal brownish homogenous appearance.
       Consistency: Soft (Honey-comb appearance)
    b) Second stage (Due to involution of the stimulated follicular cells)
       Size: Moderate
       Shape: Maintained with symmetrical enlargement (diffuse)
       External surface: Near normal
       Cut surface: Brownish glossy and translucent due to excessive colloid (Hence also termed as colloid
                        goitre)
       Consistency: Soft
       In both these stages, enlargement of glands is diffuse, hence it is also termed as diffuse non-toxic goitre.
    c) Third stage (Due to recurrent episodes of hyperplasia and involution of follicular cells)
       It is also termed as Multi-Nodular Goitre
       Size: Massive, weight upto 2kg
       Shape: Irregular - asymmetrical enlargement
       External surface: Multiple bosselated areas corresponding to nodules of variable sizes
       Cut surface: Irregular nodules with variable amount of brownish gelatinous colloid.
       Consistency: Variable (Due to regressive changes)
       Regressive changes (in older lesions):   Areas of haemorrhage (reddish brown), fibrosis (whitish, firm
                                                 irregular), calcification (chalky white, gritty) cystic change(con-
                                                 taining colloid or haemorrhages)
       Extension: can compress adjacent trachea, oesophagus or may extend behind sternum or clavicles
                   (termed as intrathoracic or plunging goitre)
       Differential Diagnosis: (on gross examination)
       One nodule may be dominant (adenomatous goitre) so clinically or on gross examination may be misdi-
       agnosed as a neoplasm.
2. **Hashimoto's thyroiditis:**
    Size: Moderate
    Shape: Maintained usually, enlargement is symmetrical, diffuse, rarely irregular - resembling solitary thyroid
              nodule
    External surface: Pale brown

Cut surface: Lobular accentuation, pale grey-tan, finely nodular, whitish streaks due to fibrosis may be seen.

Consistency: Firm

Variant: Fibrosing variant - reveals small atrophic gland with extensive fibrosis. However gland is well demarcated from surrounding structures. (Differential diagnosis-Riedel's disease - where fibrosis is more extensive with extrathyroidal involvement.)

3. **Graves' disease:**

Size: Moderate, weight upto 150gm

Shape: Maintained, enlargement is symmetrical, diffuse

External surface: Smooth, brownish red appearance. Sometimes prominent vessels are seen.

Cut surface: Soft, meaty appearance resembling muscle. (due to its rich blood supply)

Consistency: Soft

4. **Toxic nodular goitre:**

It is a solitary thyroid nodule with hyper function (excessive secretion of thyroid hormone)

Size: Variable.

Shape: Distorted if nodule is large or if the nodule is part of a multinodular goitre.

External surface: Smooth or bosselated, brownish.

Cut surface: Brownish, rarely nodule may be capsulated (termed as follicular adenoma)

Consistency: Soft.

5. **Carcinoma of thyroid**

A) Papillary Carcinoma

B) Follicular Carcinoma

C) Medullary Carcinoma

D) Anaplastic Carcinoma

E) Metastases to thyroid.

A. **Papillary carcinoma**

Gross types :   i) Small (occult - clinically not palapable)

ii) Intrathyroidal (clinically palpable)

iii) Extrathyroidal(massive)

i) Small papillary carcinoma:

Size: Less than 1 cm. Thyroid is normal in size.

Shape: Maintained

External and cut surface:

● Near normal, except for the lesion

● Sometimes it may be associated with multinodular goitre or Hashimoto's thyroiditis

● Sometimes it is seen as an incidental finding in autopsies or in thyroidectomy done for other causes.

Appearance of lesion: Sclerotic white to a tan nodule.

Consistency: Firm

Presentation: May remain occult with cervical lymphnode metastases at presentation.

ii) Intrathyroidal papillary carcinoma

● Size: Lesion more than 1.5 cms, mild enlargement can occur.

● Shape: Usually maintained

● External surface and cut surface:

- Occasionally papillae, solid areas or haemorrhages are seen.

- Multicentric tumours are known.
- Fibrosis and calcification is common but necrosis is rare.
- Consistency: Variable, usually firm, if no cystic change has occured.
  Variations: Gross variants are -
  a) Encapsulated
  b) Invasive
  c) Diffuse
  d) Cystic

iii) Extrathyroidal papillary carcinoma.

Size - Moderate, nodule usually more than 5cm.

Shape - Irregular

External surface - Infiltration by tumour is often seen.

Cut surface - Nodule with infiltration is seen in surrounding structures

Consistency - Usually firm.

B. Follicular carcinoma

Types: i) Minimally invasive
         ii) Widely invasive

i) Minimally invasive follicular carcinoma

Size: Moderate, solitary nodule variable in size

Shape: Usually maintained, but may be enlarged at site corresponding to nodule (so may be irregular)

External surface: Capsule of thyroid appears intact.

Cut surface: Solitary, well circumscribed and encapsulated tan to pink nodule.

Central part is homogenous and regressive changes are not common.

Consistency: Soft.

- Gross appearance of follicular adenoma is similar. However, sometimes, follicular carcinomas may show thickening of capsule (response to tumour infiltration.)

ii) Widely invasive follicular carcinoma

Size: Moderate to massive

Shape: Often irregular

External surface: Gross infiltration of tumour is seen beyond thyroid capsule and in cervical veins.

Cut surface: Solid irregular mass with infiltration.

Consistency: Soft to firm.

Widely invasive follicular carcinomas are often non-curable by surgery and only tumour debulking is done.

C. Medullary carcinoma

Size: Mild to moderate, enlargement depends on the tumour size

Shape: May be distorted depending on the tumour.

Appearance of the tumour -----

- Site in thyroid: lateral upper ⅔rd of gland (highest 'C' cells)

External and cut surface   -   Solitary, whitish grey circumscribed nodule
                                -   Multicentricity known, especially in familial cases.
                                -   Regressive changes like calcification, haemorrhage or necrosis are rare.

Consistency: - Usually firm.

D. Anaplastic carcinoma

Size: Moderate to massive thyroid.

Shape: Usually distorted, irregular

External surface: Infilterated by tumour beyond thyroid capsule, extending in extrathyroidal tissue.

Cut surface: Tumour seen as whitish tan, fleshy irregular mass with haemorrhage and necrosis

Consistency: Soft to firm.

Anaplastic carcinomas are often non-curable by surgery and only tumour debulking is done.

10. LYMPHADENOPATHY

Causes of lymphadenopathy:

1. Infective -

   a) Bacterial

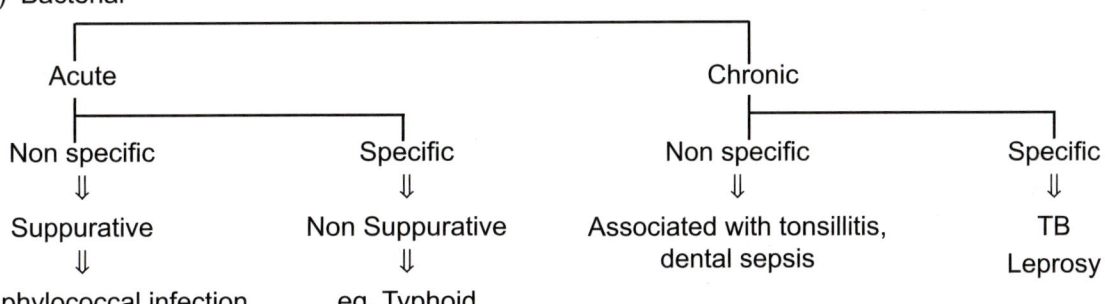

      b) Viral eg. Infectious mononucleosis

      c) Fungal eg. Histoplasmosis

      d) Parasitic eg. Toxoplasmosis, filariasis

2. Neoplastic -
   a) Primary - lymphoma
   b) Secondary - carcinoma
3. Reactive -
   Follicular hyperplasia, rheumatoid arthritis
4. Unknown etiology
   - Sarcoidosis
5. Iatrogenic
6. Immunological
   Immuno blastic lymphadenopathy
7. Associated with connective tissue disorders
   - SLE
   - Rheumatoid arthritis
   - Polyarteritis nodosa

11. TUBERCULOUS LYMPHADENITIS

- Sites -
    1. Upper deep cervical. (Tonsillar infection)
    2. Bronchial or hilar (Lung)
    3. Mesenteric (Intestine)
    4. Rarely inguinal / axillary
- Gross:

    The appearance depends on the stages of development which are:

    1. Hyperplasia
    2. Periadenitis
    3. Caseation
    4. Fibrosis and calcification
        - Enlarged, discrete but get matted with periadenitis. Firm (hyperplasia and fibrosis), soft (caseation) or hard (calcification) in consistency

            Skin is attached over the swelling and a sinus may form.
- Histopathology

    Loss of normal architecture and caseous necrosis with epitheloid cell granuloma, Langhan giant cells, lymphocytes, macrophages.

Primary Tuberculosis:
- Primary complex consists of three components:
- Focal lesion + draining lymphatics + regional lymph nodes

Secondary Tuberculosis:
- Reactivation or reinfection
- Hypersensitivity - manifests as caseous necrosis

12. LYMPHOMA

Lymphoma is a neoplastic proliferation or accumulation of cells native to lymphoid tissue ie. lymphocytes, histiocytes and stem cells.

Types :
1. Nodal - in lymph node
2. Extranodal - other sites containing lymphoid tissue. eg. gastrointestinal tract, brain, thymus, etc.
    Spread
    1. To other lymph nodes
    2. To viscera - (usually spleen, liver, bone marrow)
    3. Spill over into blood stream - leukaemia like blood picture.

Gross
- Enlarged lymphnodes, usually cervical. Sometimes mesenteric and axillary, rarely inguinal
- Size depends on stage and varies from few mm to several cms.
- Shape is round to oval. Enlargement of group of lymphnodes may occur but glands are discrete and fleshy without matting or caseous necrosis as in tuberculosis. Lymphnodes may be adherent due to periadenitis
- Cut surface - homogenous fish flesh appearance, foci of necrosis may be seen. Consistency is soft to firm.

Microscopy

Histological types:

1. Hodgkin's disease
2. Non Hodgkin's lymphoma

- Hodgkin's disease

  Diagnosis is based on histological features

  - Reed sternberg cell

    Large cells (15-45 μ), usually binucleate (mirror image appearance) with thick nuclear membrane and large eosinophilic inclusion like nucleolus. Variants of R-S cells have been described. (- lacunar, polypoid, pleomorphic)

  - In the background of R-S cell, the lymphnode usually shows loss of normal architecture with polymorphic cellular infiltrate (ie. lymphocytes, plasma cells, eosinophils, neutrophils)

  - Histrological types:

    1. Lymphocytic predominance
    2. Mixed cellularity
    3. Lymphocytic depletion
    4. Nodular sclerosis

  - Clinical features

    - Presents as lymphnode enlargement. (Primary extranodal Hodgkin's disease is very rare)
    - Can present with constitutional symptoms like fever etc.

- Non Hodgkin's lymphoma

  - Lymphomas other than Hodgkin's disease

    So this is a heterogenous group which includes nodal and extranodal lymphomas.

  - Classification is based on

    1. Cell type - T cell, B cell etc.
    2. Degree of differentiation
    3. Type of cellular infiltrate
    4. Pattern of growth
       - nodular or diffuse.

Staging of Lymphoma

Stage

1. Single group of lymphnodes involved
2. Two or more lymphnode groups on same side of diaphragm are involved
3. Disseminated lesions

Each stage has subgroups -

A. Without Symptoms
B. With Symptoms. (Fever, night sweats, loss of weight)

SECTION - V
RADIOLOGY

– Late Dr. Suren Kothari
– Dr. Jigna Rathod

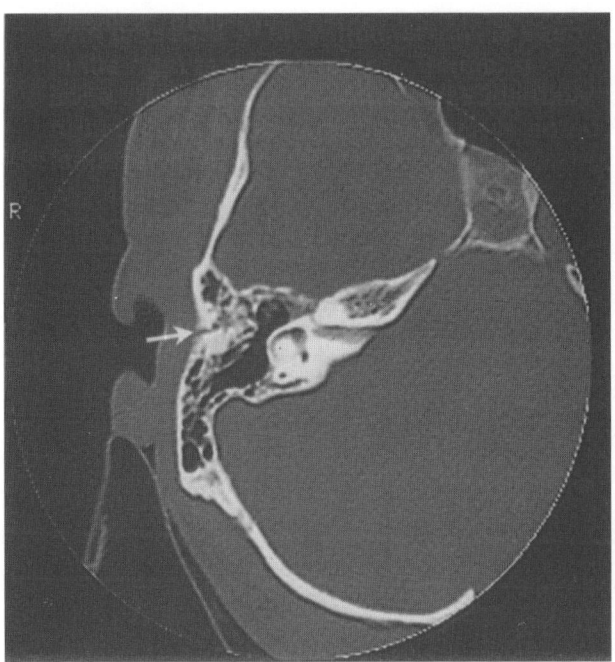

1. Axial high resolution CT scan showing longitudinal fracture through the right mastoid (arrow)

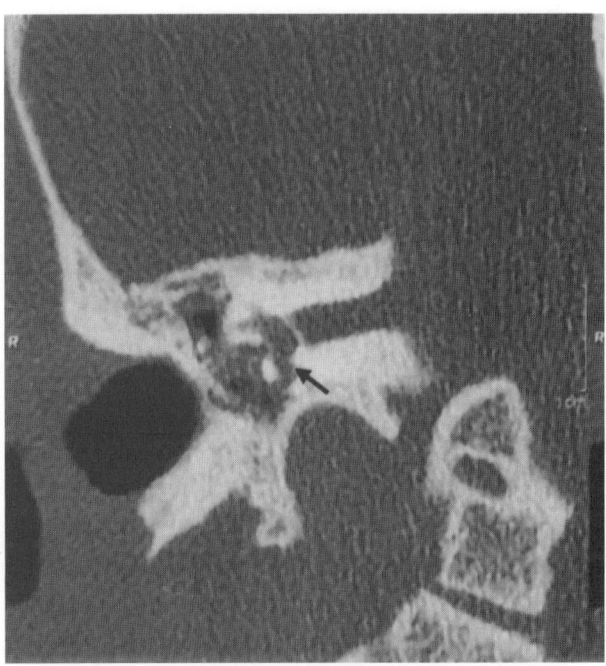

2. HRCT of temporal bone showing chronic sclerosing otitis media. Note soft tissue in middle ear and destruction of the bone.

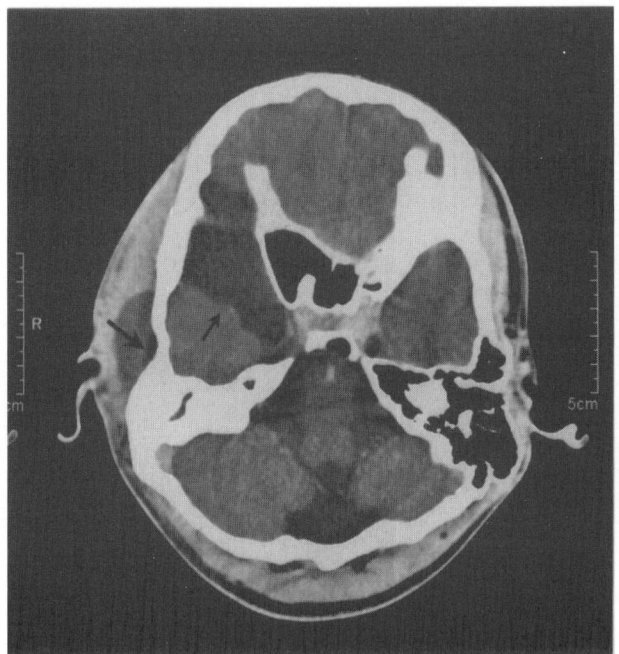

3. Axial CT scan of brain showing abscess in right temporal region. A well defined, peripherally enhancing low density lesion with presence of air within (arrow) is seen in the right temporal region. Temporal bone shows acute mastoiditis. Incidentally right temporal lobe arachnoid cyst is noted (small arrow).

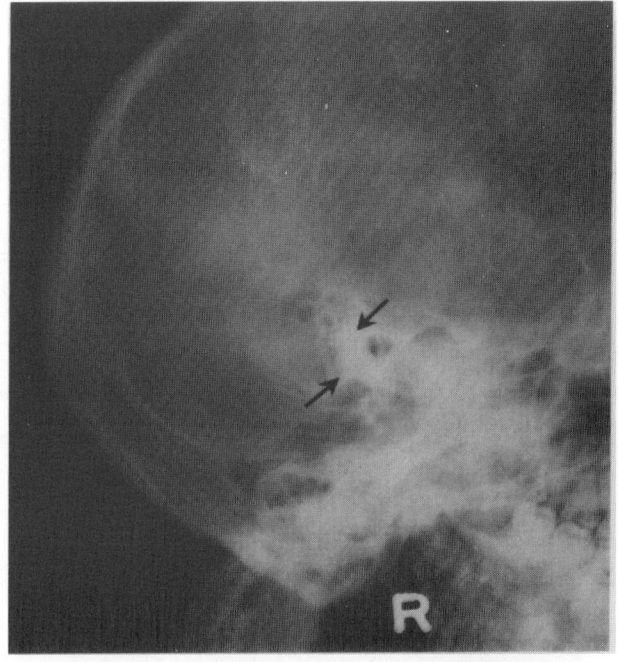

4. X-ray mastoid - sclerosing mastoiditis. Sclerosis of mastoid air cells is seen.

403

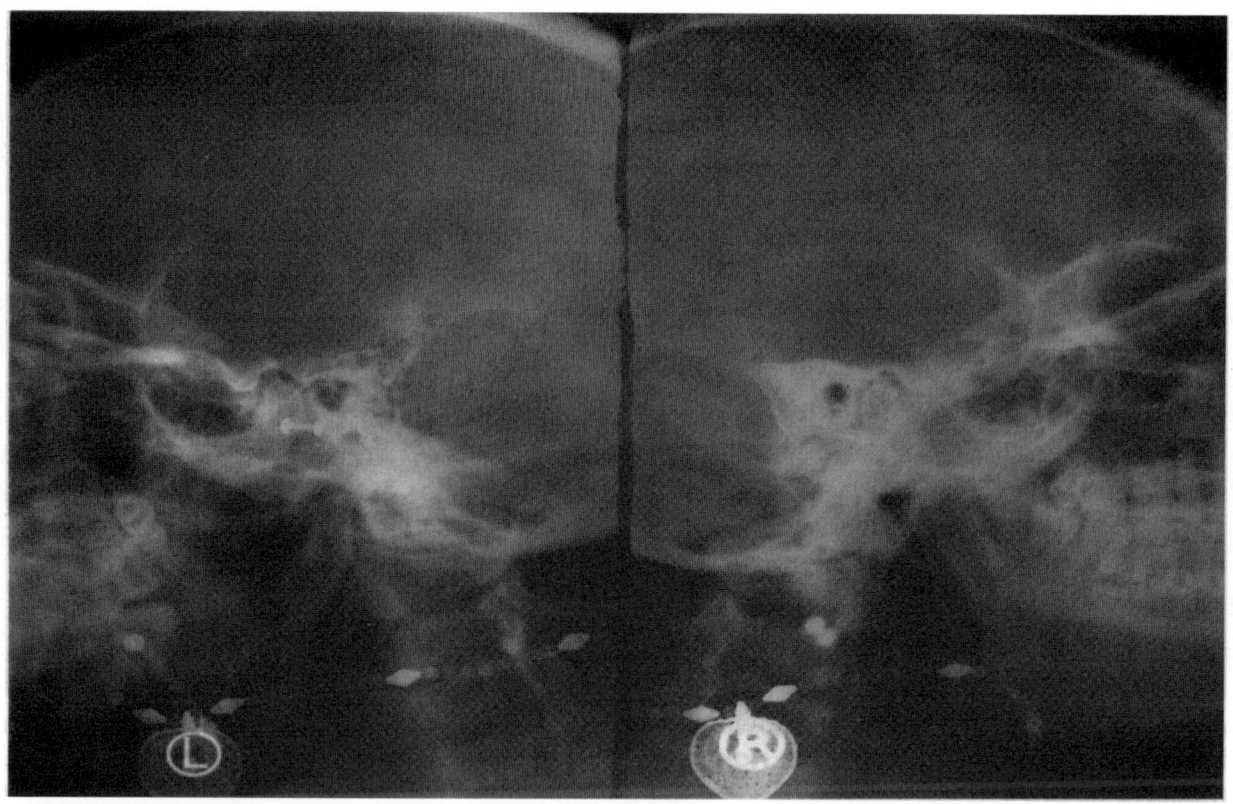

5. X-ray mastoid Schuller's view - sclerosing mastoiditis on right side. Note normal mastoid on the left side.

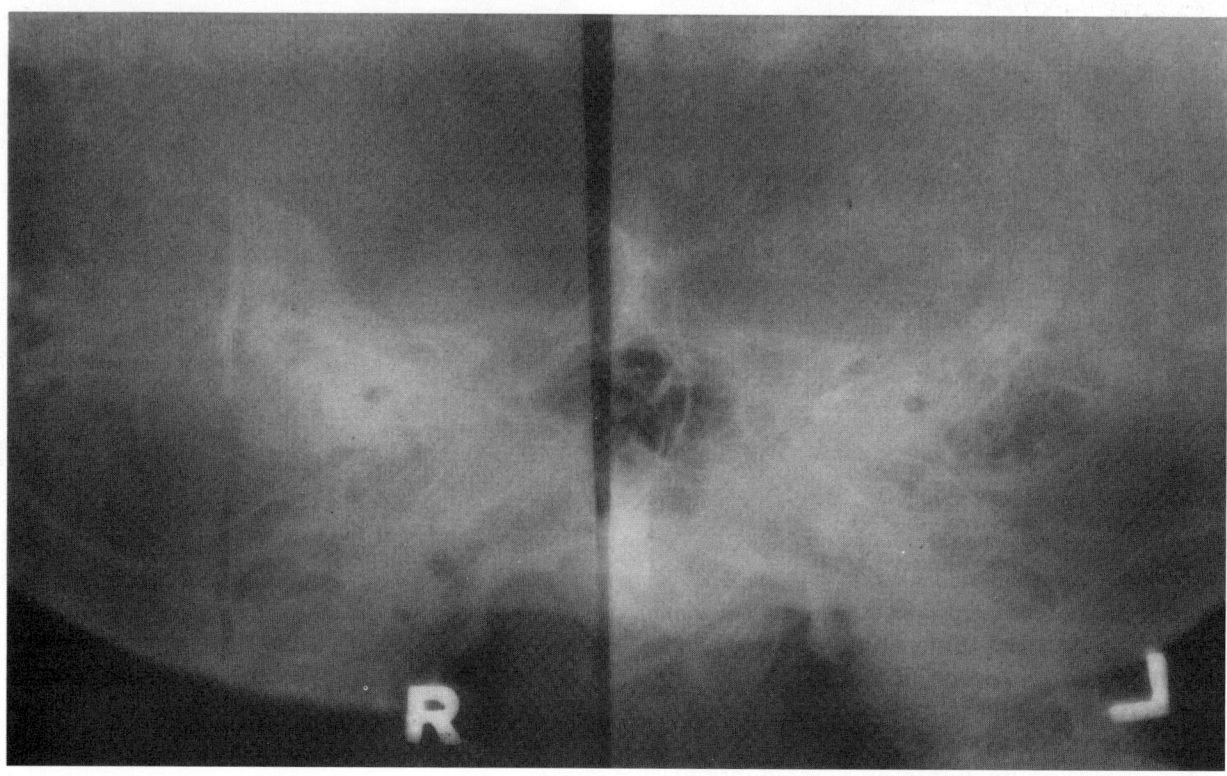

6. X-ray mastoid Schuller's view - sclerosing mastoiditis on right side. Note normal mastoid on the left side.

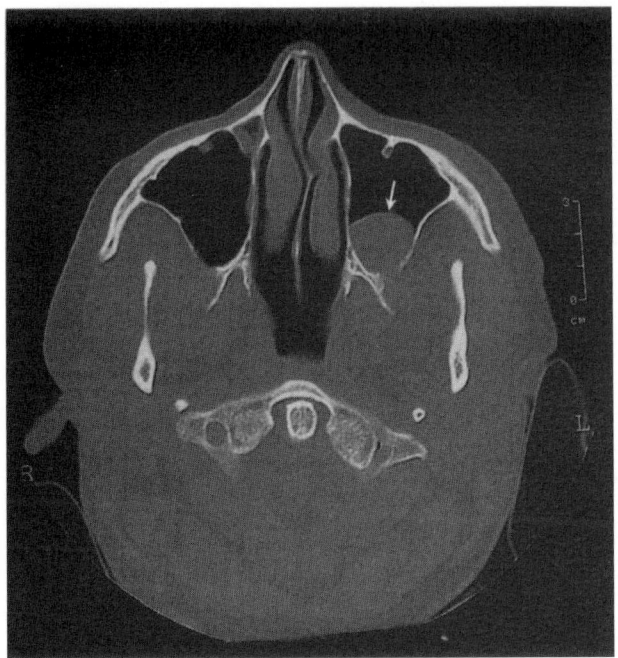

7. CT scan showing a polyp. The left maxillary antrum shows a homogenous low density lesion with convex margins (arrow).

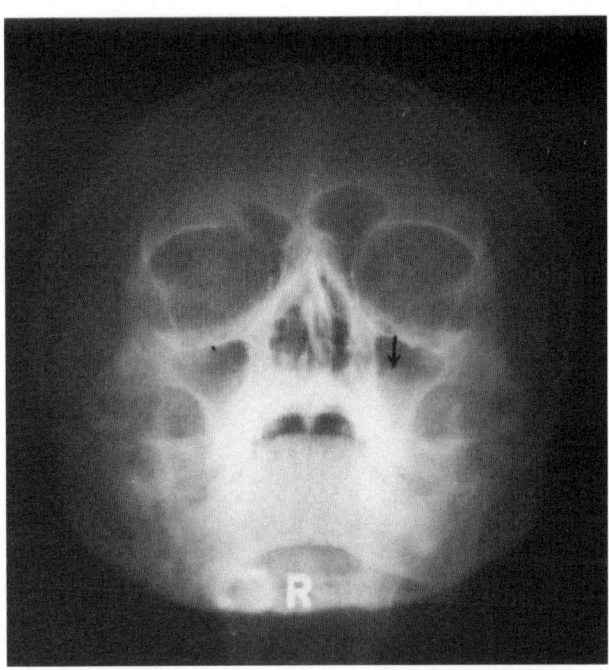

8. X-ray PNS - Water's view - polyp. A well-defined soft tissue opacity is seen in the left maxillary sinus with convex margins (arrow).

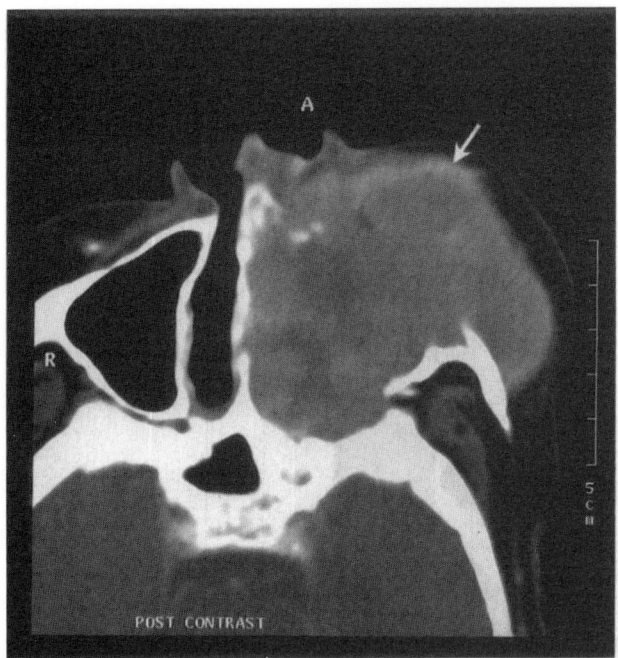

9. CT left maxillary carcinoma - contrast enhanced CT Scan shows a fairly large, ill-defined, heterogeneously enhancing soft tissue lesion involving left maxillary sinus with none erosion. Extra-antral soft tissue mass is seen anteriorly (arrow)

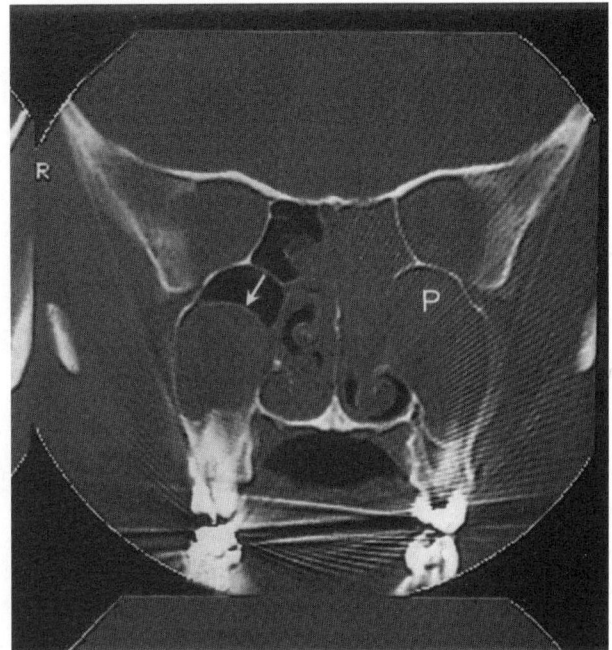

10. CT Scan showing antrochoanal polyp (P) on left side. The left maxillary sinus is completely filled with low density, homogenous mass expanding the bone, going through posterior choana into the nasopharynx. Polyps are noted in the right maxillary antra (small arrow) and in the left ethmoid sinus.

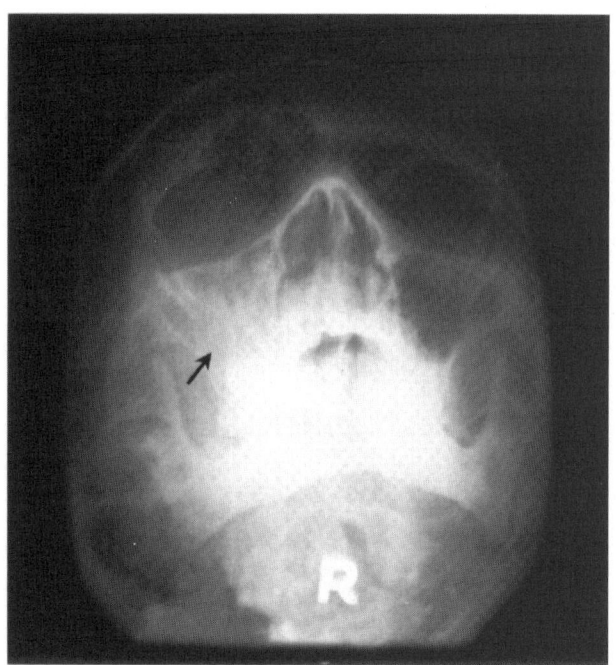

11. X-ray PNS - Water's view - Malignant neoplasm involving right maxillary sinus. Note haziness in right maxillary sinus with destruction of lateral wall of sinus (arrow).

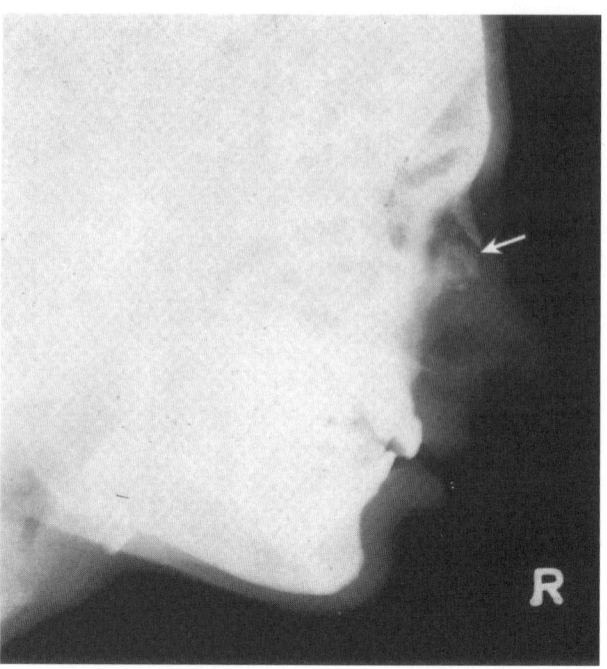

12. X-ray nasal bone - complex fracture involving nasal bone.

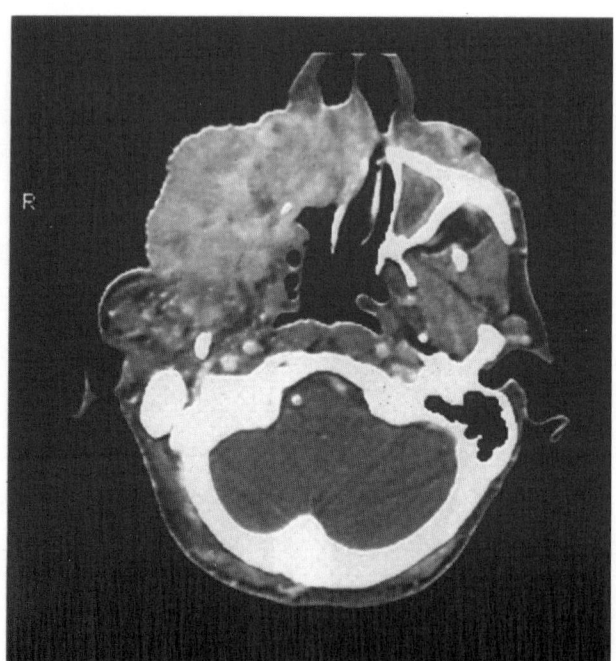

13. CT scan axial view of maxilla - Malignant neoplasm of right maxilla. Large ill-defined, lobulated, heterogeneously enhancing mass is seen involving the right maxillary sinus, overlying soft tissue and the nasal cavity.

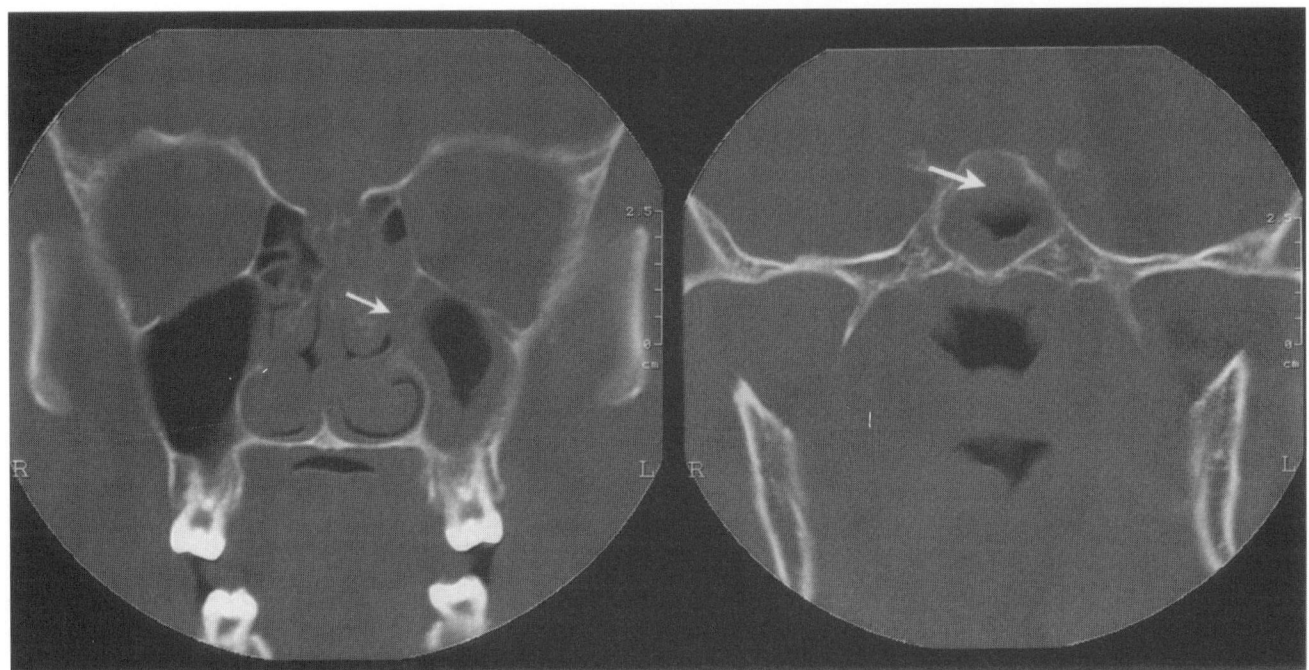

14. CT Scan of PNS - Sinusitis; mucosal thickening is noted in left maxillary sinus with blockage of osteomeatal complex (arrow). CT Scan of same patient through the sphenoid sinus reveals mucosal thickening in the sphenoid sinus (arrow).

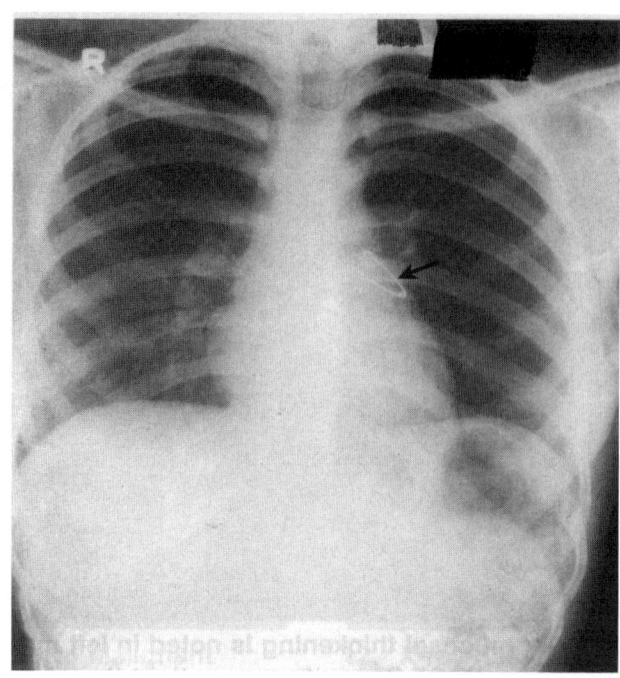

15. X-ray chest AP view shows foreign body - safety pin in left main bronchus (arrow)

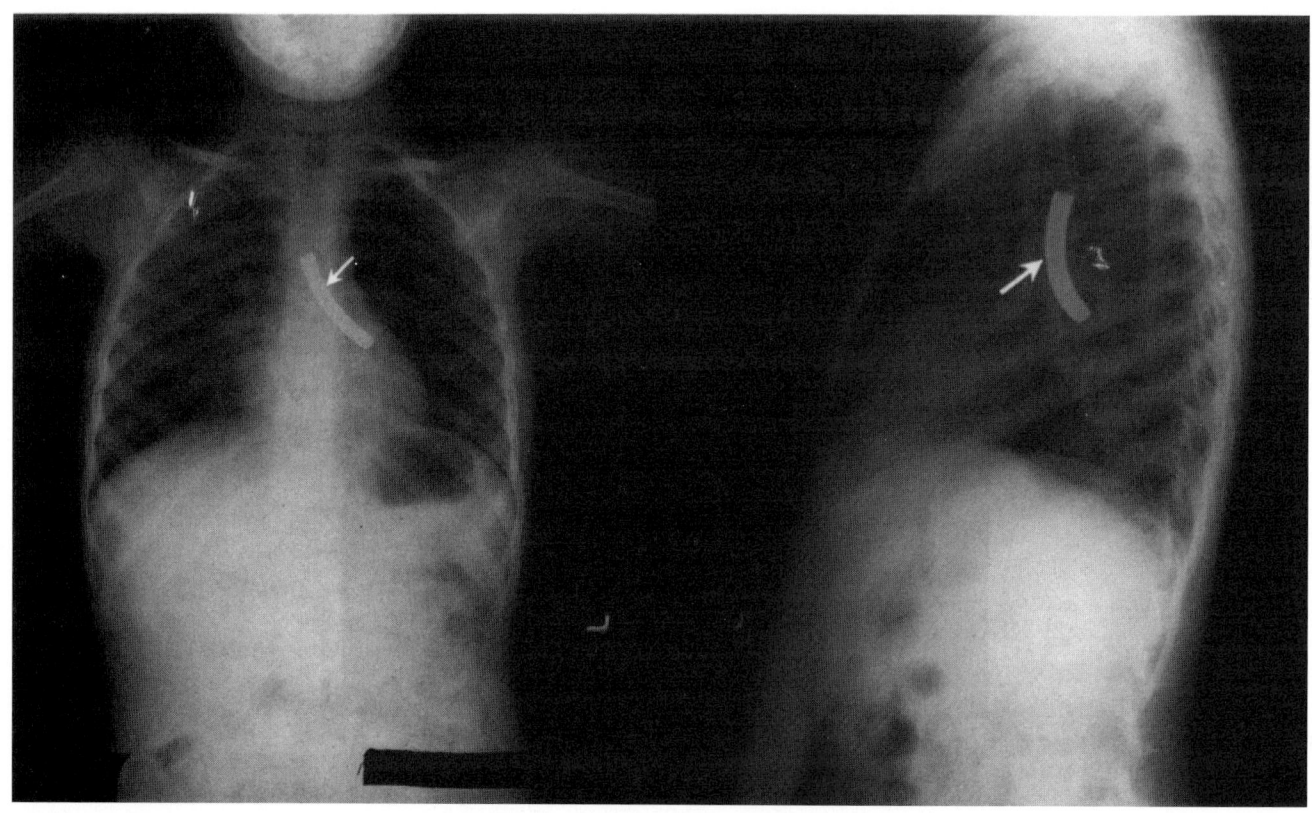

16. X-ray chest anteroposterior and left lateral view showing fracture tracheostomy tube as a foreign body in the left main bronchus.

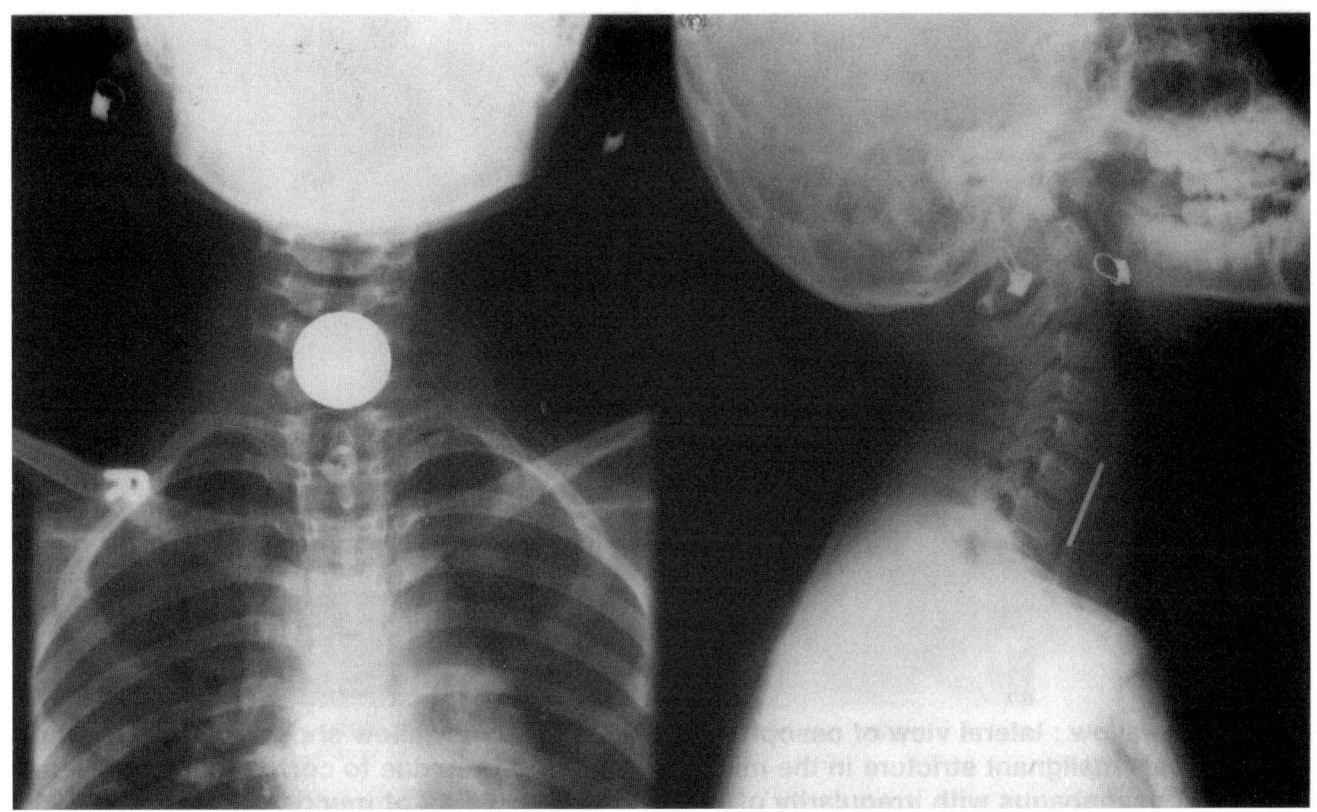

17. X-ray AP and Lateral views of neck showing presence of foreign body - coin in cervical oesophagus.

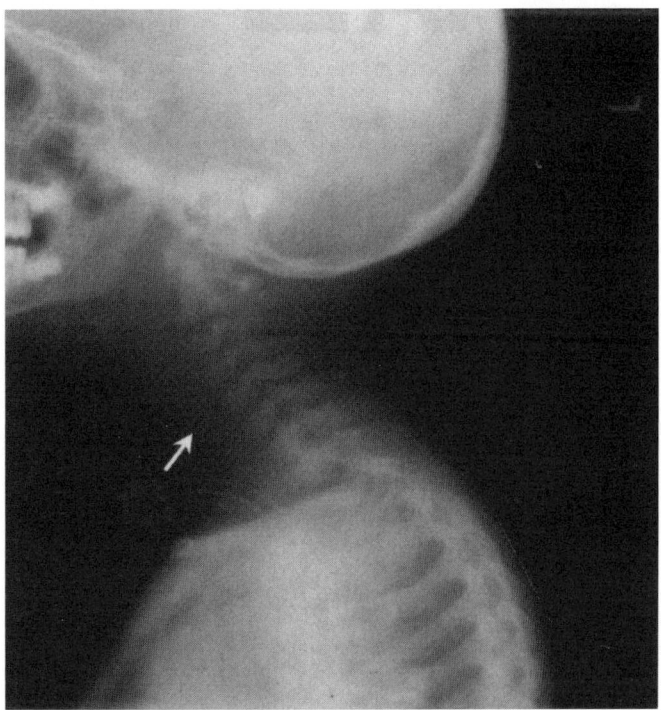

18. X-ray neck lateral view - Retropharyngeal abscess. A large soft tissue swelling in retropharyngeal and prevertebral region (arrow) with air is seen within the soft tissue. Tracheostomy tube is seen in situ.

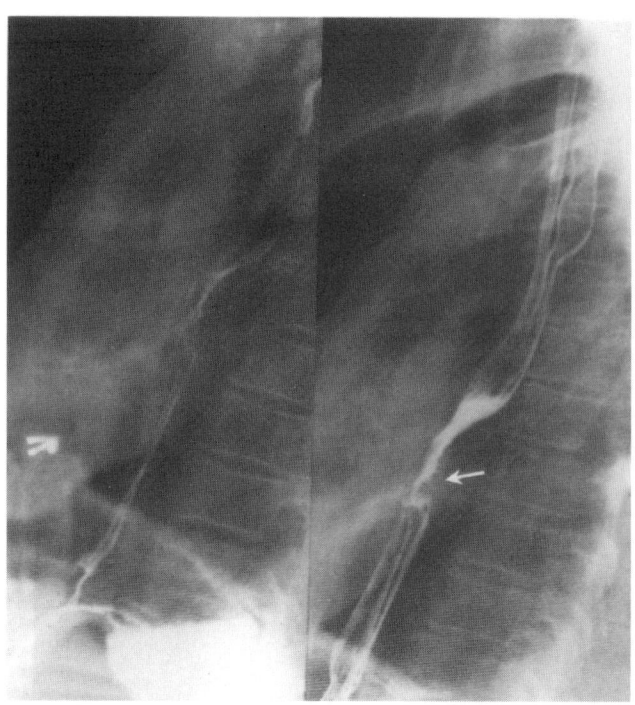

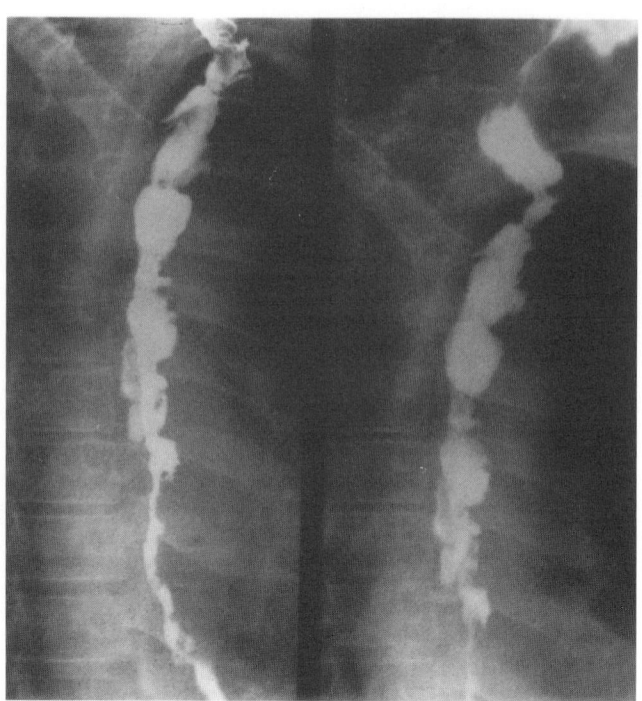

19. Barium swallow: Lateral view of oesophagus reveals malignant stricture in the mid thoracic oesophagus with irregularity of mucosa.

20. Barium swallow shows multiple irregular strictures due to corrosive burns. Note irregularity of mucosa.

EAR

NORMAL ANATOMY

Temporal bone is made up of five bony parts: squamous, mastoid, petrous, tympanic and styloid portions.

External ear: The lateral one-third of the EAC is cartilagenous. The vestibule is seen as a rounded lucent area in the bony labyrinth situated lateral and posterior to the fundus of internal auditory canal. The medial two thirds of the canal is osseous and lies within the tympanic bone. External auditory canal is covered by skin and periosteum.

Mastoid: There are three important landmarks of the mastoid - the mastoid antrum, the aditus ad antrum and the Koerner's septum. The aditus ad antrum connects epitympanum (attic) of middle ear cavity to the mastoid antrum. The Koerner's septum is a part of petrosquamosal suture. It runs posterolaterally through the mastoid air cells and serves as a partial barrier to extension of infection from lateral mastoid air cells to medial mastoid air cells, and it is also one of the important surgical landmarks.

Middle ear cavity: The middle ear is divided into the epitympanum (or attic), mesotympanum (tympanic cavity proper) and the hypotympanum. The epitympanum on coronal HRCT is the tympanic cavity above the line drawn between the inferior tip of the scutum and the tympanic portion of facial nerve canal. Into the epitympanum, projects the malleus head and the body and short process of the incus. On the axial CT, the head of the malleus and body of the incus form classical "ice-cream cone" sign, where the cone is formed by the body of the incus and ice-cream is formed by the head of malleus. Prussak's space is an important area, which can be assessed on coronal plane - this is the area between the incus and the lateral side wall of the epitympanum. This is the most commonest site for pars flaccida cholesteatoma. Within the mesotympanum, lies the rest of the ossicles (i.e. the manubrium of the malleus, long process of incus and stapes) and two muscles of the middle ear (i.e. tensor tympani and stapedius).

Inner ear: MR shows fluid spaces of the membranous labyrinth whereas CT shows bony labyrinth better. Bony labyrinth houses cochlea, vestibule, semicircular canals, and vestibular and cochlear acqueducts. Cochlea is situated anteroinferior to the vestibule and resembles a snail shell with a two and three quarter turns.

X'RAY MASTOID / SCHULLER'S VIEW

X'ray Mastoid

Schuller's view - The two sides are taken separately. The patient is lying in the lateral position and the side to be examined lies in contact with the X-ray plate. The central ray is directed at an angulation of 30^0 to prevent overlap of the other mastoid bone. This angulation of the X-ray beam makes it different from the lateral-skull view.

Structures seen are - External canal and tympanic cavity, temporo-mandibular joint, mastoid air cells, dural plate, sinus plate, dense bone of labyrinth. Schuller's view can document the extent of neoplastic and inflammatory lesions in the region of the tympanic cavity and the mastoid. Bone destruction due to cholesteatoma, mastoiditis, and middle ear effusions can be seen.

Types of mastoid:

1. Pneumatic - Air cells are seen not only covering the mastoid but also beyond the limit of the dural plate and the sinus plate.

2. Moderate pneumatisation - The air cells are seen filling up the mastoid cavity, however do not cross the confines of the dural and sinus plate.

3. Sclerotic - Absence of air cells is notable. The whole mastoid appears to be small in size with marked opacity. This is a common feature in chronic otitis media but however, sometimes also seen in normal patients.

4. Mastoid with radiolucent cavity - Here a single radiolucent shadow is seen in an otherwise sclerotic mastoid. Eventhough it indicates a disease, it may also be seen in normal patients.

Causes of a radiolucent cavity within the mastoid are:

- Cholesteatoma
- Operated mastoidectomy
- Large antral cell
- Large peri-antral cell
- Malignancy
- Eosinophilic granuloma
- Tuberculosis
- Multiple myeloma
- Skull metastasis from kidney, bronchus, breasts etc.
- Chronic mastoiditis with granulations

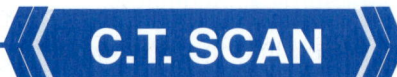

High resolution CT scan (HRCT) in axial and coronal planes is the primary imaging modality. CT Scan is poor in evaluating the otic labyrinth and internal auditory canal as it has poor soft tissue definition. HRCT gives good bony definition and is used to evaluate the air spaces and bony structures. In most cases intravenous contrast isn't needed. In case of CNS examination and vascular pathology contrast enhanced CT scans are required.

MRI

MRI has become the primary investigation of choice for the evaluation of the non osseous components of the temporal bone region including the major blood vessels, fluid spaces (cerebrospinal fluid, endolymph, perilymph) nerves, skin, fat and important structures surrounding the temporal bone.

T_1 and T_2 weighted images should be obtained using spinoecho (SE) sequences. Intravenous administration of contrast agent like gadolinium (Gd)-DTPA is needed in some cases e.g. when differentiating a haemangioma from a glomus tumour in dynamic turbo-FLASH T_1 weighted sequences.

Images in coronal, sagittal, and axial planes can be obtained and there is no radiation involved. Bony resolution is poor in MRI.

INFLAMMATORY DISEASE OF THE TEMPORAL BONE

MASTOIDITIS

Acute mastoiditis:

In this condition the middle ear appears more opaque than normal, and the ossicles may appear blurred. The mastoid antral outlines may also get blurred, and the air cells may get somewhat opaque. In addition to these changes, radiological evidence of the complications of acute mastoiditis may be seen. Imaging is performed in acute mastoiditis only if there is a clinical suspicion of coalescent mastoiditis.

This is diagnosed on CT by identification of thinning or the erosion of the mastoid septae.

The external mastoid cortex is looked at for any defect that can result in a subperiosteal abscess. If this defect occurs at the mastoid tip, the infection may extend inferiorly to the soft tissue of the neck and result in a Bezold's abscess. The inflammation can extend internally to the dura over the sigmoid sinus. The lateral sinus thrombosis can be due to direct extension or due to retrograde thrombophlebitis.

Spread of the debris into the labyrinth is usually via the round or the oval window. This is visible on the enhanced T_1 weighted images as a faint enhancement of the membranous labyrinth. Petrous apex infection occurs in individuals with a pneumatized petrous apex. The patients usually present with Gradenigo's syndrome. On CT this appears as erosive changes with abnormal enhancement of the adjacent meninges.

Granulation tissue in chronic otomastoiditis is probably the most common cause of middle ear debris and is diagnosed on CT by lack of bone erosion. The granulation tissue shows intense enhancement on MR unlike a cholesteatoma.

The CT appearance of tympanic cavity with cholesterol granuloma is similar to that of a granulation tissue. MR is diagnostic as this displays a bright signal on all spin echo pulse sequences. A quiet cholesteatoma is a concentrically enlarging collection of exfoliated keratin. This arises within the Prussak's space located between the neck of the malleus and the lateral attic wall. Cholesteatoma may result in an erosion of the tegmen tympani and the ossicular chain. It may also result in a labyrinthine fistula which usually occur at the level of the lateral semicircular canal.

Chronic mastoiditis:

It occurs as a sequel of acute mastoiditis, when the infection is not fully resolved, or if the infection is chronic by itself. Destruction of the cell walls takes place, with a concomitant reactive bony sclerosis, which may be extremely dense in character. Total obliteration of the air cells may result. In addition, the radiological signs of any of the complications of the condition may be seen.

Complications:

Labrynthitis may be tympanogenic, meningogenic, haematogenic or post traumatic. There is contrast enhancement of the membranous labyrinth on gadolinium enhanced T1W image. Once labrynthitis becomes a chronic process, membranous labyrinth is replaced with fibrous tissue and becomes ossified.

Otitis externa is usually a benign, self limited process, however it may become a life threatening condition in the elderly, diabetic or immunocompromised patients (malignant external otitis), Both CT and MRI give excellent delineation of soft tissue invasion in the subtemporal region and the status of the stylomastoid foramen. CT is needed for osseous erosion, involvement of the middle ear, mastoid and infratemporal facial nerve canal.

1. Abscess formation: Due to localised destruction of the cell walls, a large lucency is seen. This abscess may be surrounded by an area of sclerosis.

2. Cholesteatoma formation: The commonest site of appearance of the cholesteatoma is the 'attic', i.e. the epi-tympanic recess. It is usually a fairly well defined lucency in a typical site, with little or no surrounding sclerosis. There is invariably sclerosis of the mastoid process.

CHOLESTEATOMA

Cholesteatoma is an abnormal accumulation of the keratin producing squamous epithelium in the middle ear, epitympanum, petrous apex and or mastoid. The pathologically accurate term is keratomas. Cholesteatoma is a sac lined by keratinizing stratified squamous epithelium which is trapped and grows within the middle ear and other pneumatized areas of petrous bones.

TYPES OF CHOLESTEATOMA

1. Congenital cholesteatoma (epidermoids)
2. Acquired cholesteatoma: account for 98% of all the lesions and are further subdivided into
   a) Primary acquired - with no history of otitis media.
   b) Secondary acquired - with a past history of otitis media.

Congenital Cholesteatoma (also called Epidermoid or Primary Cholesteatoma):

These account for 2% of all cholesteatomas. They are similar to their intracranial counterparts. They are seen at five characteristic sites in the temporal bone - petrous apex, middle ear, mastoid, middle ear cavity and external auditory canal.

In the middle ear, there is a propensity for the formation of a congenital cholesteatoma near the junction of the eustachian tube and the anterior tympanic ring. Generally these cholesteatomas are seen anteriorly within the epitympanum or mesotympanum and in the vicinity of the incudostapedial articulation. High resolution CT scanning is advocated in the preoperative evaluation of these lesions as -

- Retrotympanic location of the pathology makes an exact determination of the lesion difficult only on the basis of clinical examination.
- CT is sensitive for the evaluation of spread of the lesion to the mastoid, epitympanum, middle ear and for evaluation of the ossicles.

Acquired cholesteatoma:

Primary acquired cholesteatomas usually arise from the pars flaccida. Secondary cholesteatomas usually arise from the pars tensa of the tympanic membrane. Pars flaccida type is more common in adults. Pars flaccida (attic) cholesteatoma begins in the Prussak's space. It displaces the ossicular chain medially. Commonly it expands in the posterosuperior direction initially via the superior incudal space to the attic and then further posteriorly through the aditus to the antrum and the mastoid. Pars tensa cholesteatoma are generally due to posterosuperior retraction of the ear drum. These lesions begin in the posterior tympanicum and often involves posterior recesses including the facial recess and sinus tympani.

CT Features of Cholesteatoma:

CT had three advantages over pluridirectional tomography. These advantages are, better demonstration of the soft tissue details, better spatial resolution and reduced radiation dose to the patients.

The features of cholesteatoma are:

a) Erosion and destruction of the scutum (lateral attic wall).

b) Widening of the aditus to antrum when the lesion extends into the antrum.

c) Displacement and or destruction of the ossicles.

d) Erosion into the facial canal.

e) Dehiscence of the tegmen tympani.

f) Destruction of the mastoid (automastoidectomy)

g) Formation of fistula between middle ear and the posterior and lateral semicircular canal and vestibule.

h) Erosion and sagging of the external canal roof.

i) Dehiscence of the sigmoid plate with or without venous sinus thrombosis.

j) In cases of petrous apex cholesteatomas, enlarged or dilated facial nerve canal which acts as a conduit connecting middle ear and petrous apex can be seen.

k) External ear cholesteatomas are seen as soft tissue lesions lateral to the tympanic membrane.

l) Since most of these lesions are associated with chronic mastoiditis, evidence of the same in form of opacification of the mastoid air cells, sclerosis of the mastoid air cells etc is seen.

BRAIN ABSCESS

Brain abscess may develop from temporal bone inflammatory processes by several mechanisms. Petrositis of the apical air cells can extend into the epidural and skull base spaces. In these instances CT Scanning will show the bony destruction with dural enhancement adjacent to the temporal bone. This is seen in Gradenigo's syndrome. Cholesteatomas can erode through the tegmen tympani or tegmen antri into the middle cranial fossa, or though the mastoid into the posterior cranial fossa. CT or MRI studies with contrast enhancement will show elevation and enhancement of the dura with extension of pus into the epidural space. Classic ring-enhancing lesions can also be seen. Otological brain abscess can be temporal or cerebellar, depending on the location of the abscess in the brain. Patients with recurrent cholesteatomas after radical mastoidectomies may develop intracranial spread of the infection. This occurs when the bony barriers have been surgically removed.

TEMPORAL BONE TUMOURS

Paragangliomas or glomus tumours are the most commonest tumours. These tumours are classified according to the location: Glomus tympanicum - only the middle ear is involved, and Glomus jugulare - only the jugular foramen is involved, and Glomus jugulotympanicum - both the middle ear and jugular foramen is involved.

On CT Scan, glomus tympanicum is seen as an intense enhancing globular soft tissue mass abutting the cochlear promontory in the middle ear cavity. Glomus jugulotympanicum is seen as an intensely enhancing mass extending from the jugular foramen into the middle ear cavity. The jugular spine and the bony floor of the middle ear are eroded. MRI may be sometimes used to complement CT findings, particularly to look for soft tissue extension at the base of the skull or intracranial extension. On MR a glomus tumor is seen as a soft tissue mass with multiple flow voids due to small vessels within the tumor. These small hypointese 'flow voids' often give rise to appearance called as "salt and pepper" appearance.

Miscellaneous temporal bone tumours like haemangioma, meningioma, adenomatous tumour and vascular metastases can also present with a vascular tympanic membrane. Rhabdomyosarcoma - It is the most common malignant paediatric middle ear tumour. About 7% lesions occur in middle ear region. These are highly malignant mesenchymal tumours seen in children below 5 years of age. CT scan shows an enhancing soft tissue tumour mass with destruction of the surrounding bone.

TRAUMA

In the setting of temporal bone trauma, CT and MRI are complimentary. MRI is recommended for patients in whom an intracranial abnormality is suspected. CT is recommended for those patients with post traumatic hearing loss, vertigo, CSF leak or seventh nerve palsy where bony detail is to be demonstrated. Temporal bone fractures are classified as longitudinal, transverse or mixed.

Temporal bone fractures are described as per their orientation to the long axis of the petrous bone and are accordingly considered as longitudinal or transverse. Number of fractures have both a longitudinal and transverse component and are best classified as mixed. The longitudinal fracture line, directed parallel to the long axis of petrous bone, usually results from a blow to the temporo-parietal region. The tympanic membrane is usually ruptured and an associated haemotympanum leads to secondary conductive hearing loss. Ossicles too are commonly involved.

The transverse fracture line, directed perpendicular to the long axis of the petrous pyramid, begins near the jugular foramen or foramen magnum and extends to the middle cranial fossa. The most common site of injury in transversely oriented fracture of temporal bone is within the labyrinth. Damage to the facial nerve occurs both in the horizontal as well as in the longitudinal component of the temporal bone fracture and may present as intraneural haematoma, impingement by fracture fragments or a complete resection.

Persistent vertigo may indicate a perilymph fistula. The presence of a pneumolabyrinth is highly suggestive in the absence of a demonstrable fracture. Vascular complications such as ICA occlusion, jugular vein and sigmoid sinus laceration should not be overlooked.

In patients with sensorineural hearing loss following trauma, MRI can help by demonstrating intralabyrinthine haemorrhage. Enhancement of labyrinth may indicate post traumatic labyrinthitis. When the hearing loss is conductive, CT can establish a diagnosis. Ossicular chain can be disrupted at multiple sites. The incus is vulnerable to fracture.

References

1. John R. Haaga, C. F. Lanzieri et al: CT and MRI of the Whole Body, third edition Part III.
2. K. C. Clark. Positioning in Radiography, ninth edition.
3. S. Howard Lee, Krishna C. V. G. Rao. Cranial MRI and CT, third edition. 477-504.
4. R. G. Grainger, D. J. Allison. Diagnostic Radiology.
5. Chakeres DW. A systematic method for evaluation of the temporal bone by CT. Radiology 1983; 146:97-106.
6. Borgan M. CT and MR imaging of the normal anatomy of the temporal bone. Semin Ultasound CT MR 1989; 10:178-194.

NOSE

VIEWS FOR PARANASAL SINUSES

1. OCCIPITO-MENTAL VIEW (WATER'S VIEW) :

This X-ray is ideally taken in the standing or sitting position. The patient's chin and the tip of his nose should gently touch the film. The film is taken with the patient's mouth kept open. In this view, the maxillary antra are seen free of any overlap of the petrous bones, and if the mouth is kept open, then the sphenoid sinus and nasopharynx may be seen. The frontal sinuses are also seen on this view, but a foreshortened view is obtained. The floor of the orbit is also demonstrated.

2. OCCIPITO-FRONTAL VIEW (CALDWELL'S VIEW) :

This view is also taken in the erect position. The patient is positioned with his forehead and the tip of his nose touching the film and the film is taken in the postero-anterior projection with the X-ray beam making angle of 20 with the orbito-meatal line. In this projection, the frontal sinuses, ethmoid sinuses and nasal septum are well demonstrated. Maxillary antra are not well demonstrated as they are overlapped by the petrous temporal bones.

A Caldwell's view can be grouped under the following headings :

a. Normal - There is individual variation in the size and the shape and asymmetry is seen in the paired sinuses also. Normally the frontal sinus shows a radiolucent shadow and individual cells are made out, giving it a scalloping (clove like) appearance.

b. Chronic frontal sinusitis - Increased opacity of the frontal sinuses is seen with absence of the normal scalloping (crenated outline of the sinuses). Such an appearance is also seen in a mucocele or pyocele, which results as a complication of chronic frontal sinusitis.

c. Osteoma - This lesion shows a marked opacity (denser than bone) in the frontal sinus. Patient is usually asymptomatic and the finding is incidental.

d. Pneumatization - Hypopneumatization of the frontal sinuses is common in severe erythroblastic anaemia, whether sickle cell or Cooley's type. Hyperpneumatization is a feature of acromegaly and Sturge-weber disease.

3. LATERAL VIEW

This view is of limited value, due to superimposition of bilateral structures. The sphenoid sinus is well visualized.

⟪ FUNCTIONAL ENDOSCOPIC SINUS SURGERY AND MUCOCILIARY DRAINAGE ⟫

Functional Endoscopic Sinus Surgery (FESS) is now the standard care for the treatment of uncomplicated inflammatory disease of the paranasal sinuses. Experienced otolaryngologists use it for treating complicated sinonasal conditions like mucocele, allergic fungal infections and localized benign neoplasms.

The health of the sinus cavity depends on the normal mucociliary clearance mechanism that propels the mucus and debris towards the drainage outlet. Maintenance of this mucociliary clearance depends upon adequate spacing between mucosal surfaces allowing room for both the sole phase of mucus in which the cilia beat and the superficial gel phase of mucus that transports the mucus and debris. Any disease process of the sinuses alters this mechanism causing loss of the adequate spacing resulting in jamming of the ciliary movement and inadequate drainage of the mucus. FESS treats sinusitis by reestablishing the normal mucociliary clearance. This concept of FESS as a functional surgery is to restore the normal ventilation through the narrow convolute drainage pathways, allowing peripheral mucociliary clearance to resume. The sinus mucosa then can heal by normal mechanisms. As FESS is a functional procedure it is important to recognize the functional areas of the paranasal sinuses like the frontal recess, osteomeatal unit (OMU) and the sphenoethmoid recess (SER). The extent of sino-nasal inflammatory disease, important anatomic landmarks and their variations can be easily depicted on CT scans, thereby providing a reliable 'road-map' to endoscopic surgery, aimed more at functional restoration and preservation. Advancement in the CT scan techniques like faster scan, higher spatial resolution, helical volume acquisitions etc enables the radiologists to provide invaluable information about frontal recess, OMU and SER.

Imaging Techniques :

Plain radiographs though widely available and inexpensive do not provide sufficient details for planning surgery. MRI with its excellent soft tissue contrast shows mucosa and secretions very well. However MR is limited in evaluation of the cortical bone and does not depict thin osseous structures. On the other hand CT scan shows excellent bone detail in the sinonasal region and is very good for soft tissue evaluation as well. CT thus remains the best technique to evaluate the presence, type and extent of the disease before planning any surgery.

Common indications of CT scan in evaluation of inflammatory paranasal sinus disease are :

1. Chronic and recurrent sinusitis.
2. Sino-nasal polyposis.
3. Evaluation of complications of acute sinusitis like periorbital cellulitis, mucocele, and in the assessment of intraocular and intracranial extent of the disease.
4. Headache with sinogenic cause.

INFLAMMATORY DISEASE OF THE PARANASAL SINUSES

1. **Acute Sinusitis** - Acute infection of the paranasal sinuses causes mucosal swelling and accumulation of fluid within the sinus. Maxillary antra are affected most frequently, followed by the frontal sinuses. In X-rays, the findings are-loss of lucency due to mucosal thickening or fluid content, opacification of the air passages with soft tissue and the presence of fluid. (useful diagnostic feature in a sinus). A fluid level is seen sometimes which has a concavity pointing upwards. The final confirmation of fluid level is done by repeating the plate in lying down position, resulting in obliteration of the fluid level. In allergic sinusitis the mucosa tends to show scalloped appearance and polypi may be seen occasionally.

    There are five major patterns of occlusion of the mucosal drainage channels. Three commonest are infundibular, osteomeatal unit, and sphenoethmoidal recess patterns. Additional patterns are sinonasal polyposis pattern (also called allergic sinusitis or hyperplastic rhinosinusitis) and unclassifiable pattern. On CT Scan there is smooth and nodular mucosal thickening produced due to submucosal oedema and mucosal inflammation.

2. **Chronic maxillary sinusitis -** Haziness (radio-opacity) of the sinus is seen. The mucosa may show persistent thickening in chronic sinusitis. Occasionally associated is some sclerosis and thickening of bony walls of the sinus, which may proceed to a marked reduction in the sinus volume. Chronic sinusitis is most often seen in the maxillary antra and then the frontal sinuses.

    On CT scan, osteitic thickening, due to long standing mucosal inflammation and reactive bony proliferation of the sinus walls is seen. Retention cysts are frequently seen in patients with sinusitis. These smooth rounded and sharply marginated cysts are usually found in the floor of the maxillary antrum, broad based along the inferior cortical margin. Retention cysts are difficult to distinguish from polyps, unless the polyp is clearly pedunculated. The retention cyst can fill a sinus cavity but it never causes bony expansion.

    Periosteal new bone formation, followed by sclerosis involving the posterolateral antral wall is seen following Caldwell-Luc antrostomy and should not be interpreted as indicative of infection. A persistent antral fluid level following dental extraction, particularly of a canine tooth, suggests the presence of an oro-antral fistula.

3. **Polyp -** Opacity is seen, as compared to the rest of the maxillary sinus. Here, there is a convexity which points upwards and a repeat plate shows no shift in opacity. Polyps are smoothly rounded or pedunculated soft tissue masses in the nose and sinus cavities, of relatively low density on the CT scan. They may obstruct the sinonasal drainage channels if located within the OMU, frontal recess and the sphenoethmoidal recess.

Polyps exert a pressure effect on the adjacent bony structures with resultant enlargement of the involved bony cavity. The process is gradual and causes expansion and distortion with relative preservation of the interspinous septations, a finding usually seen in the ethmoid sinuses. Antrochoanal polyps, (4-6% of the polypoidal disease) have distinct radiological appearances. It fills the maxillary antrum, then expands into the middle meatus eventually growing through the choana into the nasopharynx. They are usually of low density associated with smooth bony expansion of the maxillary sinus wall. MRI can help in differentiating polyp from a tumour.

4. **Granulomatous sinusitis -** Granulomatous diseases affecting the paranasal sinuses have both infectious and noninfectious causes. Infectious causes are actinomycosis, tuberculosis, syphilis, rhinoscleroma, and leprosy. Noninfectious causes are Wegener's granulomatosis, and sarcoidosis as well as foreign body reaction from beryllium, chromium salts and cocaine. All the granulomatous diseases are potentially dangerous and erode both the cartilage and the bone. On CT, they all have similar appearance starting with non specific soft tissue nodules along the nasal septum with marked mucosal thickening through out the nasal cavity. Perforations of the nasal septum then occurs, the hallmark of this group of disorders.

5. **Fungal sinusitis -** It is a diverse group of disorders that are categorised into four distinct clinical entities based on the host immunological status : invasive fungal sinusitis, chronic indolent sinusitis and mycetoma in the immunocompromised host, and allergic fungal sinusits in the immunological hypercompetent or atopic host. Invasive fungal sinusitis owing to mucormycosis and aspergillosis is an acutely fulminant disease characterised by marked erosion and bony destruction. It is commonly seen in diabetic patients. Chronic indolent sinusitis is a slowly growing disease and slowly progresses eventually destroying the bone. Mycetoma is associated with repeated facial trauma. It causes partial or complete opacification of the sinus cavity and may be associated with thickened mucosa. Mycetomas can be hyperdense on CT, scan and contain flocculent calcifications in about 25% of the cases. Allergic fungal sinusitis typically occurs in young adults with nasal polyposis. On CT the involved sinus contains peripheral rim of low attenuation, oedematous mucosa and complete opacification of the central cavity by homogenous high density material that is diagnostic of the disease.

6. **Mucocele -** A mucocele is an obstructive complication of chronic sinus inflammation, polyposis, trauma, surgery or tumour. The frontal sinus is most commonly affected followed by the ethmoid, maxillary and sphenoid sinuses. Radiologically smooth rounded enlargement of a completely opacified sinus cavity of an air cell is seen indicating the slow nature of the expansile process. The bony walls are thinned out. Mucopyocele is an infected mucocele and it causes rapid bony dehiscence. On CT, mucoceles are of low density and do not enhance following contrast administration thus differentiating them from polyps.

7. **Malignancy -** Opacity of the sinus is seen. Destruction of the walls of the maxillary sinus is diagnostic of malignancy. The distance between the antero-lateral wall of the maxilla to the coronoid process of the mandible is measured. Increased distance on one side suggests involvement of infratemporal fossa by a tumour (**Handousa's sign**). Squamous cell carcinoma accounts for 80-90% of the malignant tumors of the nose and paranasal sinuses. It arises most often from the lateral wall of the nasal cavity, or from the maxillary antrum. Most patients are Men in their sixth decade. CT scan shows a mass, bone destruction, extension of the tumour into the adjacent sinuses and surrounding compartments. Intracranial spread, in particular in the pterygopalatine fossa and intraorbital spread can be assessed. Metastatic lymphnodes may be recognized.

Other malignant tumours are adenocarcinoma, adenoid cystic carcinoma, olfactory neuroblastoma, plasmacytoma, lymphoma and chondrosarcoma.

Adenocarcinoma has predilection for the upper nasal cavity and the adjacent ethmoid cells. Adenoid cystic carcinoma commonly arises in the lower part of the nasal cavity and the maxillary antrum. Hard palate is commonly involved.

FRACTURE NASAL BONES

The patient sits erect with the head in the lateral position and the X-rays are directed to the root of the nose. Any disruption seen in the nasal bone architecture would indicate a fracture of the nasal bones.

Reduction of this fracture is done only as an elective procedure, i.e. for cosmetic reasons. Before doing so, the complications caused by fractured nasal bones are ruled out. They are CSF rhinorrhoea, epistaxis, septal haematoma, proptosis and oedema.

NORMAL ANATOMIC VARIATIONS ON CT SCAN

The variations in the anatomy of the paranasal sinuses are important because some of these variants can narrow the drainage channels predisposing to chronic recurrent sinusitis. Certain normal variants increase operative risk.

MIDDLE TURBINATE VARIATIONS

1. Concha bullosa - The middle nasal turbinate is usually a thin bony structure which may show varying amount of pneumatization. Balloon like or significant pneumatization of the middle turbinate is called as concha bullosa. When large, it may constrict the middle meatus or encroach upon the infundibulum. Concha bullosa may be bilateral and may occasionally contain polyps, mucocele and pyocele. True concha bullosa in normal population has a reported prevalence of 4 to 15% and in patients with chronic sinusitis it is as high as 33%.

2. Paradoxically curved middle turbinate - Middle nasal turbinate has a convexity which is directed medially towards the septum. When it is paradoxically curved towards the lateral sinus wall it is presumed that it may predispose to recurrent sinusitis due to narrowing of middle meatus. It is required to know that paradoxical curvature of the middle meatus is important in its anterior portion and not in the posterior portion.

NASAL SEPTUM VARIATION

Nasal septum variation is the second most common variation and is seen in upto 20% of the population. The deviation is usually at the junction of the nasal cartilage and the vomer. The deviated nasal septum or bony spur causes decrease in the area of the osteomeatal unit predisposing to obstruction. Synechiae formation between the turbinates and the lateral wall or with the uncinate process can lead to failure of FESS and recurrent sinusitis.

ETHMOID VARIATION

Haller cells are extensions of the middle ethmoid air cells placed laterally along the floor of the orbit. These can result in narrowing of the infundibulum predisposing to maxillary sinusitis.

These are more common in women. Sometimes large ethmoid bulla may contribute to sinus disease by obstructing middle meatus or infundibulum.

UNCINATE PROCESS VARIATION

Abnormal deviations of the uncinate process may narrow the drainage channels. Occasionally uncinate process is pneumatised which may narrow the maxillary infundibulum.

DANGEROUS NORMAL VARIANTS

Onodi cells are posterior ethmoid air cells that extend posteriorly and sometimes superior to sphenoid sinus, lying medially to the optic nerve. Onodi cells are in close relationship to the optic nerve and share a common wall with the sphenoid sinus, the sphenoethmoidal plate. In case of posterior ethmoidectomy the optic nerve may be at risk in these cases. Another dangerous variant is extensive pneumatization of the sphenoid sinus with aeration of the anterior clinoid process. The optic nerve lies just medial to the anterior clinoid process and nerve can be damaged if dissection extends posteriorly. Complete dehiscence of the optic nerve may be seen in 3-12% of the patients.

The integrity of the lamina papyracea is important when the uncinate process is located laterally or abuts the lamina. Resection of the uncinate process may be difficult and injury to the lamina may occur. Occasionally the nasolacrimal duct is located anterior to the maxillary sinus ostium and may be injured during anteriorly directed surgical enlargement of the ostium. Pre-operative CT should be carefully looked at for a low lying fovea ethmoidalis. Cribriform plate, roof of posterior ethmoid air cells and superior and lateral walls of the sphenoid sinus should be looked at carefully as these can predispose to CSF leak post operatively. Bulging of the carotid artery into the sphenoid sinus has to be noted. Rarely the carotid artery may traverse through the sphenoid sinus and injury to this artery during surgery can be fatal.

LARYNX, PHARYNX

TRACHEO-BRONCHIAL FOREIGN BODIES

These foreign bodies may lead to a life threatening situation due to obstruction caused in the respiratory passages. Coins form majority of the tracheal foreign bodies. Here antero-posterior view shows a vertical opaque slit and lateral neck plate shows the complete coin. This is because of the 'C' shaped cartilages of the trachea, resulting in the antero-posterior diameter greater than the transverse diameter.

Bronchial foreign bodies are divided into 3 types according to the air-flow pattern:

a. Bypass of air - Foreign bodies like buttons, rings or beads which have an opening within itself allow passage of air to either side. X-ray picture shows no abnormal findings other than the foreign body.

b. One sided airway obstruction - Metallic and other non-organic foreign bodies lead to an unilateral obstruction to the airway. On inspiration the bronchial diameter increases and this leads to the passage of air distal to the foreign body. On expiration as the bronchial diameter decreases, it leads to entrapment of air distal to the foreign body. These changes in airway pattern lead obstructive emphysema and therefore the X-ray findings and breathlessness.

c. Total airway obstruction - Vegetable foreign bodies like peas or groundnuts, swell up in the bronchus due to their hygroscopic nature. This causes impaction of the foreign body onto the bronchial wall. Air cannot pass distal to the foreign body, nor can escape out. This leads to collapse of the lung segment distal to the foreign body and compensatory emphysema of the remaining lung. Changes occur accordingly which are seen on the X-ray. The classical feature is a mediastinal shift-which being the change in position of the mediastinum with each phase of respiration on account of the collapse caused by the foreign body.

Lateral Skull (Nasopharynx)

Normally the nasopharynx is seen as a radiolucent shadow because it is occupied by air.

- Shift of the air shadow posteriorly occurs with an antrochoanal polyp, as it arises from anteriorly. The air shadow is reduced to a small outlining shadow around the polyp (**Crescent sign**).

- Shift of the radiolucent shadow anteriorly is seen with adenoids (children) and nasopharyngeal carcinoma (elderly), both of them arising posteriorly.

OESOPHAGEAL FOREIGN BODIES

The commonest foreign bodies lodged in the oesophagus are coins, marbles or traumatic foreign bodies like dentures, pins and meat bone.

a. Coin - They lodge in the oesophagus occupying a classical position that is in the transverse plane. This is due to the fact, that the transverse diameter is much greater than the longitudinal diameter. Therefore, on an antero-posterior view of the neck-chest, the whole coin can be seen showing a totally radio-opaque shadow. A lateral plate is also taken to confirm the exact position of the foregin body and also to rule out a second foreign body if overlapping the first. On a lateral plate a vertical slit like structure is seen.

b. Marble - These also give a radio-opaque shadow which is less dense as compared to a coin. The other feature being that on both antero-posterior and lateral X-ray film, a circular shaped foreign body is seen. The use of may forceps result in pushing the foreign body more distally. A folley's catheter is passed distal to the foreign body and the balloon is inflated. Gradually the catheter is removed and the foreign body is taken out.

c. Traumatic foreign bodies - Sharp foreign bodies can cause a complete vertical tear in the oesophageal wall during its removal. Traumatic foreign bodies are either pins or dentures.

OESOPHAGEAL STRICTURES

Oesophageal strictures can be classified into benign and malignant types.

1. Benign strictures

2. Malignant strictures-

Commoner causes of oesophageal strictures are listed below

I. Benign

I.BENIGN	SITE	FEATURES
● Peptic		
- Reflux oesophagitis	Distal, near GOJ, above a hernia	Smooth, tapering
- Barrett's oesophagus	More proximal	Deep ulcer, reticular mucosa
● Nasogastric intubation	Distal	Long stricture, history
● Schatzki's ring	Gojunction	Symmetrical, 2-4 mm long
● Caustic ingestion	Single or multiple, long stricture	History
● Radiation	Related to the portal	Tapered stricture, history
● Skin disease	High in the oesophagus	Strictures or webs, bullous diseases
● Drug ingestion	Above left atrium	History of drug ingestion (enteric KCl)
● Post infective	Usually in mid part	Candida, TB
● Benign tumour	Variable	Submucosal lesion. Smooth muscle tumour content

II. Malignant

- Carcinoma
- Leiomyosarcoma
- Lymphoma
- Extrinsic carcinoma

Barium studies:

Biphasic double contrast radiography is the method routinely used for examining upper gastrointestinal tract. High density barium, gas producing granules and hypotonic agent (glucagon) are used. Double contrast views are best for evaluating mucosal abnormalities, where as the single contrast views are best for evaluating oesophageal and gastroduodenal motility, and for demonstrating structural abnormalities restricting wall expansion.

Oesophageal motility is assessed by fluoroscopic observation after a single swallow of barium taken by a patient in the prone oblique position. 3 to 5 successive single barium swallows are recommended as necessary to demonstrate incidence of peristalsis.

Difference between benign and malignant stricture on barium study

BENIGN	MALIGNANT
1. Multiple	1. Single
2. Sites of normal constriction	2. Middle $\frac{1}{3}^{rd}$ or anywhere
3. Regular mucosa	3. Irregular mucosa
4. Marked proximal dilatation	4. No proximal dilatation
5. Corrosive burns is the commonest cause	5. Carcinoma due to chronic irritation is the cause

Endoluminal ultrasonography (EUS)

Endoluminal ultrasonography is often used in conjunction with fibre-endoscopy. For exploration of the oesophageal and rectal wall, a water-filled balloon covering the ultrasonic probe is used. Due to its high resolution properties, EUS readily identifies the different layers of gut wall.

By means of the high frequency EUS beam intramural tumour growth is classified, as is the existence of spread to local lymphnodes. Thereby the evaluation of tumour resectability is facilitated. Malignant mucosal lesions are hypoechoic and in most instances clearly defined.

RETROPHARYNGEAL ABSCESS

The diagnosis of a retropharyngeal abscess can be made by:

1. Marked increase in the prevertebral space area, it being more than three-fourth of the size of the vertebra.

2. Air-fluid level. Normally the pharynx is a collapsed structure, not containing any air.

3. Loss of normal curvature of the spine leading to straightening of the cervical spine.

   The vertebrae should be carefully seen for any destruction or presence of a foreign body (mutton bone). Commonest cause of retropharyngeal abscess is Koch's spine and foreign body in the pharynx (adults), dental and tonsillar infections in children.

SECTION - VI

ANAESTHESIA

- Dr. Vandana Lehiri
- Dr. Prerna Shroff

≪ GENERAL PRINCIPLES ≫

Cooperation between ENT surgeon and anaesthesiologist is essential as both of them work in the same field. Other principles to be followed are:

- Secured airway
- Deep level of anaesthesia
- Rapid recovery

PREOPERATIVE ASSESSMENT

- General examination
- Systemic examination
- Medical diseases
- Drug allergy
- Previous history of anaesthesia (especially difficult intubation)
- Airway assessment: nasal passages, neck mobility, dentition, mouth opening
- Indirect laryngoscopy, if required

INVESTIGATIONS

- Complete blood count
- Bleeding time, clotting time
- X-ray chest
- Electrocardiogram*
- Blood sugar (fasting and post-prandial)*
- Others depending on medical problems and surgical procedures to be performed

    *For more than 35 years of age and if history suggests the need to do in patients less than 35 years of age.

CONSENT

- Written, informed, valid consent for anaesthesia and for surgery
- Special consent for medical problems due to medical diseases and for tracheostomy, if difficult intubation or airway pathology is suspected

PREOPERATIVE FASTING

- For solids: not less than 6 hours
- For liquids: not less than 4 hours

MONITORING

- Pulse
- Blood pressure
- ECG
- Pulse oximetry*
- End tidal CO_2*
- Others depending on medical problems and surgical procedures to be performed e.g., Central venous pressure (CVP), input / output, blood loss, temperature, air entry, airway patency etc.

    *If available, makes it easy to diagnose hypoxia, vasoconstriction, circuit disconnection, oesophageal intubation, inadequate ventilation and many such events

PREMEDICATION

Aim: To allay anxiety, make the patient calm and co-operative and to prevent nausea and vomiting

DRUGS FOR PREMEDICATION

A. ANTISIALOGOGUES	B. ANTIEMETICS	C. ANXIOLYTICS / SEDATIVES / TRANQUILIZERS	D. OPIOIDS
Atropine Glycopyrrolate	Metoclopramide Ondansetron	Midazolam Diazepam* Promethazine	Pentazocine Pethidine* Tramadol Fentanyl
	*Long acting, hence to be used for major / long lasting surgery		

GENERAL ANAESTHESIA (G.A.)

The following steps are followed in an orderly manner:

A. PREOXYGENATION

100% O_2 is given under mask for 3-5 minutes. It is given prior to any general anaesthetic to take care of respiratory depression or apnoeic episodes during anaesthetic induction (effect of anaesthetic drugs)

B. INDUCTION

1. Intravenous (Faster and pleasant induction)

2. Inhalational (Slow induction but useful in children and in patients with difficult airway)

1. Intravenous:

Any one of the following agents + any one muscle relaxant for intubation

INTRAVENOUS AGENTS	MUSCLE RELAXANTS:	DRUG	DOSE
Pentothal - 5-7 mg/kg. Propofol - 1-2 mg/kg. Ketamine - 1-2 mg/kg.	Depolarizing Nondepolarizing	Scoline* Pancuronium** Vecuronium** Atracurium**	1-2 mg/kg. 0.08 mg/kg 0.08 mg/kg 0.5 mg/kg

*Short acting   **Long acting

2. Inhalational:

O_2+N_2O+Inhalational agent (Halothane / Isoflurane / Sevoflurane / Ether / Trilene)

- Muscle relaxant is not mandatory for intubation.
- When patient is deeply anaesthetized, he/she can be intubated on spontaneous breathing during the inspiratory phase when vocal cords are most apart.
- If airway obstruction occurs while patient is being anaesthetized (despite chin lift, jaw thrust and oro-pharyngeal airway), the process can be reversed by administering 100% O_2 and other methods of intubation can be tried,   especially when difficult airway is suspected.

If difficult intubation is anticipated, following things should be kept ready:

- Extra large blade laryngoscope, flexitip blade larynogscope and endotracheal tube stylet
- Endotracheal tubes of various sizes (especially small sized tubes)
- Endotracheal tube guide and tube exchangers
- Oesophageal bougie, light wand or lighted stylet
- Laryngeal mask airway (LMA)
- Intubating LMA, if available
- Cricothyrotomy set
- Tracheostomy set

Once intubation is done, confirm correct placement of endotracheal tube

Throat packing is to be done in nasal and oropharyngeal surgery soon after induction

C. MAINTENANCE

Any one of the following methods can be used to maintain anaesthesia:

1. Intravenous agent + N_2O and O_2 ± Muscle relaxant
2. Inhalational agent + N_2O and O_2 ± Muscle relaxant
3. Intravenous agent + Inhalational agent + N_2O and O_2 ± Muscle relaxant

During maintenance of anaesthesia, following things should be taken care of:

- Adequate oxygenation and ventilation (removal of carbon dioxide)
- Maintenance of adequate circulation
- Maintenance of normothermia
- I.V. Fluids: 2ml/Kg/hour of 5% Dextrose / Ringer Lactate / DNS and
- Replacement for insensible loss + expected or actual urine output + blood loss

  Induced hypotension may be used for microscopic surgeries or vascular tumours with either judicious use of inhalational agents or propofol alone or in combination with β blockers like Esmolol (short acting) or Metoprolol (long acting)

D. REVERSAL AND EXTUBATION

- Shut off inhalational agent and N_2O
- Continue giving 100% oxygen
- If non-depolarizing muscle relaxant is used, reverse it with anticholinesterase like neostigmine or prostigmine (only after patient shows signs of attempting breathing). An anticholinergic drug like atropine or glycopyrrolate is administered along with an anticholinesterase to counteract the muscarinic side effects like bradycardia, profuse salivation, bronchospasm and at times arrhythmias.
- With return of airway reflexes, remove the throat pack, if inserted, and deflate the endotracheal tube cuff
- With the return of consciousness, protective airway reflexes and muscle power (sustained head lift for > 5 seconds), extubate the patient
- Keep the patient nil by mouth for atleast 6 hours

E. POST-OPERATIVE PAIN RELIEF

- Any suitable analgesic which is not a respiratory depressant or a strong sedative e.g., Diclofenac sodium 2-3mg / Kg. I.M. half to one hour before the end of surgery or Tramadol 1-2mg / Kg. I.V. / I.M. prior to extubation is to be given.

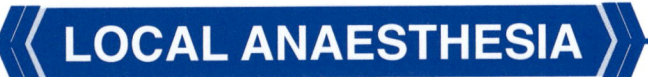

LOCAL ANAESTHESIA

A. Topical (surface)*   **B.** Infiltration*   **C.** Conduction (various nerve blocks)

* Practiced extensively by ENT surgeons.

Commonly used nerve blocks in ENT practice, especially for awake intubation are:

BLOCK	ANAESTHETISED AREA	DOSE
Superior laryngeal nerve block	Anaesthetizes the area from inferior aspect of epiglottis to the vocal cords	• Patient in supine position with neck extended • Displace the hyoid bone laterally to the side to be blocked • Insert the needle so as to walk off the

BLOCK	ANAESTHETISED AREA	DOSE
		greater cornu of the hyoid bone inferiorly and advance the needle 2-3 mm • As the needle passes through the thyro-hyoid membrane, a slight loss of resistance is felt • The block is repeated on the other side
Translaryngeal block: (Transtracheal injection)	Anaesthetizes the trachea below the vocal cords	• Avoid in patients in whom coughing is undesirable • Patient in supine position preferably with neck extended • Locate the criciothyroid membrane in the midline and introduce the needle to puncture it • Aspiration of air confirms the placement of needle in trachea • Inject 3-5 ml of local anaesthetic solution rapidly, resulting in coughing which aids in spread of the solution within the trachea
Glossopharyngeal nerve block: (Intraoral approach)	Anaesthetizes posterior $\frac{1}{3}^{rd}$ of tongue, pharynx and superior surface of the epiglottis	• Inject 5ml of local anaesthetic solution at the base of each posterior tonsillar pillar

Surgical procedures that deserve special mention are:

1. **Post tonsillectomy bleeding:**

   Problems:
   - Hypovolemia
   - Hypotension
   - Full stomach (swallowed blood)
   - Airway obstruction

   Management:
   - Intravenous fluids
   - Blood transfusion
   - Ryle's tube suction prior to induction
   - Awake intubation or inhalational technique without using muscle relaxant
   - If muscle relaxant is used for intubation then rapid sequence intubation with cricoid pressure is done
   - Extubate only after proper haemostasis and return of protective airway reflexes
   - Observe the patient for signs of hypovolemia and anaemia

2. **Endoscopies: (D.L. Direct laryngoscopy, M.L. Microlaryngoscopy, Cricopharyngoscopy, Nasopharyngoscopy, Bronchoscopy and Oesophagoscopy)**

   Aim : To give the surgeon a clear immobile view and sufficient space to work despite difficulty in maintaining a clear airway, adequate oxygenation and adequate ventilation

   Anaesthetic implications:
   - Airway protection

- Difficult airway
- Antisialogogues to reduce secretions
- Steroids to reduce airway oedema
- Adequate oxygenation and removal of CO_2
- Deep level of anaesthesia
- Rapid awakening and return of reflexes

Methods:

- Small size endotracheal tube for all endoscopies (except bronchoscopy)
- Ventilating bronchoscope or jet ventilation (venturi principle) or insufflation technique (apnoeic oxygenation for bronchoscopies).
- Muscle relaxant to be avoided if vocal cord movement is to be seen.

COMPLICATIONS

There can be innumerable complications following general or local anaesthesia. However, those related to ENT surgery that deserve mention are:

General anaesthetic:

AIRWAY OBSTRUCTION	BRONCHOSPASM	HYPOTENSION
• Trauma / oedema • Airway pathology • Post instrumentation • Bleeding / secretions	• Irritation of airway • Patients with allergy • Patients with COPD / asthma	• Allergic reaction • Dysrrhythmias • Blood loss

Local anaesthetic: mostly as a result of toxicity (higher dose) or intra-vascular injection (since the area is highly vascular and many prolonged procedures are done under local anaesthesia)

CVS	CNS
• Dysrrhythmias • Hypotension	• Tingling • Circumoral numbness • Dizziness • Convulsion

Treatment:

- Maintain airway
- 100% oxygen under mask
- Maintain blood pressure (fluids) and heart rhythm (xylocard)
- I.V. diazepam / midazolam / thiopentone sodium (pentothal)

CARDIO PULMONARY RESUSCITATION (CPR)

Since many ENT surgeries are done under local anaesthesia in the absence of an anaesthesiologist, the operating surgeons must be well versed with the prompt diagnosis of a cardiac arrest and its management as prompt recognition and treatment is the key to favourable outcome.

Pale surgical field or sudden cessation of bleeding should raise the suspicion of a cardiac arrest to the operating surgeon. Dark coloured blood suggests airway obstruction due to the drapes or inadequate breathing due to over-sedation, which if ignored, may ultimately lead to hypoxia and cardiac arrest.

MANAGEMENT

To call for help but do not leave the patient

1. PRIMARY SURVEY

A. Airway	:	Open airway by jaw thrust, chin lift and give head tilt
B. Breathing	:	Positive pressure ventilation - mouth to mouth or via resuscitation bag
C. Circulation	:	Closed chest compression (external cardiac massage)
D. Defibrillation	:	In pulse-less patients with ventricular tachycardia or ventricular fibrillation

2. SECONDARY SURVEY

A. Airway	:	Endotracheal intubation
B. Breathing	:	Assess adequacy of ventilation via endotracheal tube and continue IPPR
C. Circulation	:	I.V. access for fluid + medication. Appropriate cardiovascular drugs for correction of rhythm while continuing cardiac massage
D. Diagnosis	:	Differential diagnosis of cause of arrest - especially reversible causes and the Remedial measures.

External cardiac massage :

It is given by compressing the lower sternum and xiphoid process by about 1½ to 2 inches by the palms of both hands without flexing the elbows. External cardiac massage to IPPR ratio or chest compression to ventilation ratio should be 15:2 in case of one rescuer and 5:1 when two rescuers are present.

Defibrillation	:	It is given in a pulse-less patient having ventricular tachycardia or ventricular fibrillation
		Begin with 200 joules, repeat with 300 joules and 360 joules i.e. 3 shocks
		If no response, continue CPR for 1 min.
		If no pulse, repeat shocks: 3 of 360 joules each
		If no response, continue CPR for 1 min. and again repeat 3 shocks
		Continue the above sequence till the rhythm comes back
Drugs	:	(to be combined with CPR and defibrillation in Drug-Shock-Drug-Shock....Pattern)
Adrenaline*	:	1 mg to be pushed I.V., to be repeated every 3-5 minutes
Sodabicarb	:	1 mEq./Kg., only if hyperkalemia or metabolic acidosis is documented or suspected
Lignocaine	:	1-1.5mg/kg. I.V., to be repeated after 3-5 min. upto maximum of 3mg/kg
		* Defibrillation to begin within 30-60 seconds of adrenaline injection
If asystole occurs:		(confirmed by more than 1 lead) → Continue CPR, No defibrillation
Treat cause	:	Hypoxia, hyperkalemia, hypokalemia, hypothermia, acidosis, drug over-dosage
Drugs	:	Adrenaline : 1mg to be pushed I.V., to be repeated every 3-5 minutes
		Atropine : 0.6-1mg to be pushed I.V., to be repeated upto 0.03-0.04mg/kg.

Consider transcutaneous pacing

If pulse-less electrical activity	:	Continue CPR, No defibrillation
Treat cause	:	Hypoxia, hyperkalemia, hypokalemia, hypothermia, acidosis, drug overdosage, hypovolemia, cardiac tamponade, tension pneumothorax, pulmonary embolism, acute myocardial infarction
Drugs	:	Adrenaline: 1mg to be pushed I.V., to be repeated every 3-5 minutes
If H.R. < 60/min	:	Atropine: 0.6-1mg to be pushed I.V., to be repeated upto 0.03-0.04mg/kg.

⟪ ANAESTHETIC DRUGS ⟫

DRUGS	USES	DOSAGE	EFFECTS

I. PREMEDICANTS
A. Antisialogogues:
  1. Atropine:
   - It is an anticholinergic drug
   - Available as 0.6mg/ml.
	• Premedication: used to decrease oropharyngeal secretions
	• During reversal of non-depolarizing muscle relaxant to antagonize the muscarinic effects of anticholinesterase
		Dosages:
		Premedication: 0.01mg/kg, I.M./I.V.
		Reversal of muscle relaxant: 0.02mg/kg. I.V.
			• Tachycardia
			• Decreased secretions
			• Pupillary dilatation
			• Bronchodilatation
			• Crosses blood brain barrier

2. Glycopyrrolate:
   - It is a synthetic anticholinergic drug producing less tachycardia than atropine
   - Available as 0.2 mg/ml.
	• Premedication: used to decrease oropharyngeal secretions
	• During reversal of non-depolarizing muscle relaxant to antagonize the muscarinic effects of anticholinesterase
		Dosage:
		Premedication: 4μg/kg, I.M./I.V
		Reversal of muscle relaxant: 8μg/kg I.V.
			• Mild tachycardia
			• Decreased secretions
			• Does not cross blood brain barrier

B. Anxiolytics/Sedatives/Tranquilisers
  1. Midazolam:
   - Available as 1 mg/ml. or 5 mg/ml.
   - Water soluble, less irritant and hence no pain on injection
   - Action lasts for 1-4 hours
	• Premedication
	• Conscious sedation
	• Induction of anaesthesia
	• Supplementation of anaesthesia
		Dosages:
		Induction: 0.15-0.3 mg/kg.
		Sedation:
		• **I.V.:** 0.03-0.05 mg/kg.
		• **I.M.:** 0.1-0.15 mg/kg.
		• **Oral :** 0.5-0.75 mg/kg.
		• **Nasal:** 0.2 -0.3 mg/kg.
			• Anxiolytic
			• Hypnotic
			• Amnesic
			• Anticonvulsant

2. Promethazine (Phenargan) - Available as 25 mg/ml. or 50 mg/ml.	• Premedication • Sedative • Antiemetic	**Dosages:** 0.5-1.0 mg/kg I.V.	• Hypnotic • Antihistaminic • Antiemetic • Antishivering • Bronchodilator • Antanalgesic

C. Opioid analgesics (Narcotics):
  1. Pentazocine (Fortwin):
   - It is a synthetic Benzomorphinian opioid
   - Available as 30 mg/ml.
	• Premedication
	• Analgesic
	• Sedative
		Dosages:
		0.6 mg/kg I.V.
			• Sedation
			• Analgesia
			• Tachycardia
			• Raised B. P.
			• Nausea
			• Vomiting

2. Pethidine:
   - It is a synthetic opioid agonist
   - Available as 50 mg/ml. or 100 mg/ml.
	• Premedication
	• Analgesic
	• Sedative
	
	• Premedication
		Dosages:
		0.5 mg/kg I.V./I.M.
			• Sedation
			• Analgesia
			• Tachycardia
			• Orthostatic hypotension
			• Vomiting
			• Dependence

                                                             Clinical ENT

DRUGS	USES	DOSAGE	EFFECTS
3. Tramadol: - It is a synthetic opioid agonist - Available as 50 mg/ml.	● Analgesic ● Sedative ● Premedication	**Dosages:** 0.5-2 mg/kg I.V./I.M.	● Sedation ● Analgesia ● Tachycardia ● Vomiting
4. Fentanyl: - It is a phenylpiperidine opioid - It has a rapid onset and short duration of action (30-60 minutes) - Available as 50 μg/ml.	● Analgesic ● Induction of anaesthesia	**Dosages:** 0.5-2 mcg/kg I.V.	● Sedation ● Analgesia ● Bradycardia ● Hypotension ● Bradypnoea ● Muscle rigidity ● Nausea, vomiting ● Pruritus
D. Antiemetics: **1. Metoclopramide** - Available as 5 mg/ml.	● Antiemetic	**Dosage:** 10 mg I.V./I.M. either soon after induction or 15-30 min. prior to extubation	● Accelerates gastric emptying and intestinal transit ● Inhibits chemoreceptor trigger zone mediated vomiting ● Minimal sedation ● Occasionally extrapyramidal reaction
2. Ondansetron - Available as 2 mg/ml. or Syrup 4 mg/5 ml.	● Antiemetic	**Dosage:** 4 mg (50-150 μg/kg.) slow I.V. (over 1-5 min.) just before/after induction or just prior to extubation	● Antagonizes 5-HT$_3$ receptors on vagal nerve endings and in chemoreceptor trigger zone ● Transient increase in hepatic transaminase levels ● Constipation ● Crosses placenta and is excreted in breast milk
II. I. V. INDUCTION AGENTS: **1. Thiopentone Sodium (Pentothal):** - It is an ultrashort acting thiobarbiturate - It is also an anticonvulsant - It is available as 0.5 or 1.0 gm vial in powder form - It is to be diluted with normal saline or distilled water to make a 2.5%		**Dosage:** 5-7 mg/kg.	● Hypnosis ● Unconsciousness ● Hypotension ● Antanalgesia ● Respiratory depression if given too fast ● Bronchospasm in susceptible people ● Laryngospasm in lighter plane of anaesthesia ● Pain on injection if extravasates

DRUGS	USES	DOSAGE	EFFECTS
solution (25 mg/ml.) **Absolute contraindication: Acute intermittent porphyria**			
2. Propofol: - It is a diisopropylphenol - It is available as an emulsion: 10 mg/ml. - It should be protected from light - It should be shaken well before use **It is contraindicated in patients allergic to eggs or soyabean oil**	• Sedation: • Induction: • Maintenance: • Antiemetic:	I.V. Bolus -0.5-1.0 mg/kg. Infusion - 20-75 µg/kg/min. I.V.-2.0-2.5 mg/kg slowly I.V. Bolus-25-50 mg Infusion -100-200 µg/kg/min. I.V.-10 mg	• Rapid induction • Rapid recovery • Hypotension • Bradycardia • Pain on injection • Allergic reaction in the form of anaphylaxis
3. Ketamine: - It is a phencyclidine derivative - It is available as 10 mg/ml or 50 mg/ml - To reduce secretions, antisialogogue premedication is necessary - To reduce hallucinations it is generally combined with diazepam or midazolam **It is contraindicated in patients with intracranial hypertension or raised intraocular tension**	• Sedation: • Analgesia: • Induction: • Maintenance:	I.V.-0.5-1.0 mg/kg. or 2.5-10 IM mg/kg. Oral-6-10 mg/kg. Nasal - 3-6 mg/kg 1.0-2.5 mg/kg Infusion-15-80 µg/kg/min	• Dissociative anaesthesia • Increased salivation • Slightly enhanced laryngeal and pharyngeal reflexes • Hallucinations, delirium • Bronchodilatation • Increase pulse, blood pressure. Intra ocular pressure, intra cranial pressure and blood sugar • Nystagmus, convulsion
III. INHALATIONAL AGENTS: **1. Halothane** - It is noninflammable halogenated volatile liquid - Used for induction as well as maintenance of anaesthesia - Available in amber coloured 250 ml bottles. - It is to be used in vaporisers meant for Halothane e.g. Goldman or Fluotec			• Hypotension • Bradycardia • Arrhythmias • Bronchodilatation • Myocardial depression • Respiratory depression • Sensitizes myocardium to the action of adrenaline • Hepatic dysfunction

DRUGS	USES	DOSAGE	EFFECTS
2. Isoflurane: - It is noninflammable volatile liquid - Used for induction as well as maintenance of anaesthesia - Available in amber coloured 100ml. bottles. - It is to be used in vaporizers meant for Isoflurane			• Hypotension • Tachycardia • Arrhythmias • Peripheral vasodilatation • Respiratory depression
3. Nitrous oxide: - It is a noninflammable anaesthetic gas, but supports combustion. - It is a strong analgesic, but a weak anaesthetic. - Used for supplementation of anaesthesia - Supplied in blue coloured cylinders (liquid + gaseous form)			Diffuses into air-containing cavities faster (34 times more soluble) than nitrogen, causing potentially dangerous pressure acumulation e.g.: • Diffusion hypoxia • Middle ear abnormalities (serous otitis media, transient postoperative hearing loss) • Bowel obstruction • Pneumothorax • Increased endotracheal cuff volume and pressure (resulting in glottic and subglottic trauma)
IV. MUSCLE RELAXANTS: **1. Succinyl choline (Suxamethonium, Scoline)** - A depolarising muscle relaxant - Available as 50 mg/ml. solution or 100 mg/vial powder - Solution is to be refrigerated, powder is stable at room temperature - Generally used for intubation (1-2 mg/kg) - Quick and short acting - Intubation can be done between 60-90 seconds			• Fasciculation • Hyperkalemia • Bradycardia (with second/repeated doses) • Increased intraocular pressure • Increased intracranial pressure • Increased intragastric pressure

DRUGS	USES	DOSAGE	EFFECTS
- Action lasts for 3-5 minutes - Can be used for maintenance in short surgical procedures e.g. scopies - Does not require reversal			
2. Pancuronium (Pavulon): - A non-depolarising muscle relaxant - Available as 2 mg/ml. - Can be used for intubation (0.08 mg/kg) - Takes time to act-intubation can be done between 150-180 seconds - Long acting, action lasts for 45-60 minutes - Generally used for maintenance in surgical procedures, lasting more than 40 minutes - Maintenance dose:- 0.01-0.05 mg/kg - Requires reversal at the end of surgery			• Increased heart rate • Increased blood pressure • No fasciculation • Histamine release- rarely
3. Vecuronium (Norcuron): - A non-depolarising muscle relaxant - Available as 4 mg/vial in powder form - Requires reversal at the end of surgery	• Can be used for intubation (0.08 mg/kg) • Takes time to act-intubation can be done between 120-150 seconds • Long acting, action lasts for 25-30 minutes • Generally used for maintenance in surgical procedures lasting more than 30 minutes	• Maintenance dose:- 0.01- 0.05 mg/kg	• No change in heart rate or blood pressure • No fasciculation
4. Atracurium (Tracrium): - A non-depolarising muscle relaxant - Available as 10 mg/ml., to be refrigerated - Requires reversal at the end of surgery - Metabolised by Holfman degradation and ester hydrolysis, hence useful	• Can be used for intubation (0.5 mg/kg) • Takes time to act-intubation can be done between 150-180 seconds • Long acting, action lasts for 10-20 minutes • Generally used for	Maintenance dose:- 0.1-0.2 mg/kg.	• Hypotension • Increased heart rate (>0.5 mg/kg. doses) • No fasciculation • Histamine release (>0.5 mg/kg. doses)

DRUGS	USES	DOSAGE	EFFECTS
in patients with renal and hepatic disease	maintenance in surgical procedures lasting more than 20 minutes		
V. LOCAL ANAESTHETIC AGENTS: **1. Xylocaine (Lignocaine):** - It is an amide group of local anaesthetic - It is available as: 0.5, 1.0, 1.5 and 2.0% solutions without/with adrenaline (1:50,000, 1:100,000, 1:200,000) 4.0% solution and 10% spray for use in ENT surgery - It has antiarrhythmic effects - 1.0-1.5 μg/kg I.V. and then 15-50 mg/kg/min. I.V. - It attenuates the pressor response (tachycardia and hypertension) to intubation - 1.5-2.0 mg/kg I.V. given 2-3 min. prior to laryngoscopy		**Maximum safe dosages:** ● Without adrenaline 4 mg/ kg. ● With adrenaline (1:200,000) (5 mcg per kg) (1 ml of adrenaline in 200 ml solution) 7 mg/kg **Duration:** 45 min. to one hour One to one and half hour **Route of administration:** ● Topical ● Infiltration ● Superior laryngeal nerve block ● Transtracheal	
2. Bupivacaine (Marcaine) - It is an amino amide local anaesthetic - It is available as: 0.25 and 0.5 % solutions without/with adrenaline (1:200,000) - If the dose exceeds the maximum safe level, it can cause refractory cardiac arrest and death		**Maximum safe dosage:** ● Without adrenaline: 2 mg/kg (<150 mg for infiltration/nerve block) ● With adrenaline: 3 mg/kg (<225 mg) - It improves quality of analgesia and not duration ● Do not exceed rate of injection to more than 10 mg/min of the drug **Duration: 2 to 6 hours**	
VI.OTHER DRUGS: **1. Adrenaline** - An ionotropic agent that activates both α and β-adrenergic receptors - Available as 1 mg/ml. (1:1000) - Used with local anaesthetics to reduce their absorption and			**Therapeutic doses** Effect on β-receptors ● Increased myocardial contractility ● Increased heart rate ● Increased blood pressure ● Relaxation of bronchial smooth muscles

DRUGS	USES	DOSAGE	EFFECTS
thereby lessening the potential for systemic toxicity and to prolong their duration of action and to reduce blood loss - The concentration should not exceed 5-10 μg/ml or 0.5-1.0 mg/100 ml (1:2,00,000 - 1:1,00000) - The dose should not exceed 100 μg (10 ml of 1: 1,00,000) over a 10 min. period or 300 μg (30 ml. of 1:1,00,000) over any 60 min. period in adults. - If used along with inhalational agents like halothane; can give rise to arrhythmias			• Dilatation of skeletal muscle vasculature **Higher doses:** Effect on α-receptors • Increased total peripheral resistance • Decreased renal blood flow • Decreased urinary output • Ventricular arrhythmias • Angina
2. Neostigmine/ Prostigmine - An anti-cholinesterase - Available as 0.5 mg/ml or 2.5 mg/ml - Used for reversal of nondepolarising muscle relaxants (0.05 mg/kg, max. of 5 mg) - It is used along with atropine/glycopyrrolate to avoid muscarinic actions			• Increased secretions - oral and bronchial • Bronchospasm • Respiratory depression • Bradycardia • Hypotension • Arrhythmias

⟪ ANAESTHETIC INSTRUMENTS ⟫

1. MASK

- It is an integral part of any anaesthetic breathing system or circuit during the induction phase (beginning) of anaesthesia or any resuscitation procedure
- Allows administration of gases from the breathing system or from the resuscitation bag without introducing any invasive apparatus (e.g. an endotracheal tube) into the patient
- It is placed on the patient's face covering his mouth and nose (face mask) or only the nose (nasal mask)
- Nasal masks are smaller in size than face masks and generally used only for conservative dentistry for dental chair anaesthesia

Parts : Connector or mount
- Body
- Edge or seal

Sizes: 1, 2, 3, 4, 5

2. AIRWAY

- Prevents fall of tongue on posterior pharyngeal wall and helps to maintain airway
- Made up of metal / rubber / plastic

Uses:

- To maintain airway in unconscious or heavily sedated patient
- To obtain a better mask fit
- To prevent a patient from biting and occluding an orotracheal tube
- To protect the tongue from being bitten
- To facilitate oropharyngeal suctioning through the air or suction channel
- To provide oxygen through air or suction channel

ORAL   :   Lies from lips to pharynx

Parts: Flange, bite portion, air / suction channel (curved portion)

Sizes: 1, 2, 3, 4

Method of insertion: After lubrication, it is held with concave side facing upper lip, advanced and rotated through 180^0 so that it lies posterior to tongue.

- Pharyngeal and laryngeal reflexes should be depressed before placement of an oral airway to avoid coughing or laryngospasm.
- Selection of the correct size is very important as too small an airway may cause the tongue to kink and push part of it against the roof of the mouth, causing obstruction, and too large an airway may cause obstruction by displacing the epiglottis posteriorly and may traumatize the larynx.

NASOPHARYNGEAL: Lies from nose to pharynx

Parts :   Flange or a movable disc at proximal end to prevent migration to nose. A safety pin can also be used as a flange.

Sizes (diameter)   :   - 7.0 / 7.5 for adult males
- 6.5 / 7.0 for adult females
- same / one size smaller than an appropriate endotracheal tube for children
- Resembles a shortened endotracheal tube
- Better tolerated in the patient with intact airway reflexes than an oral airway
- The flanges lies outside the nostril and the tube in the nasal cavity
- The pharyngeal end of the tube may be straight or beveled and it lies below the base of the tongue but above the epiglottis

Method of insertion: After lubricating thoroughly along its entire length, it is passed through the patent nostril (vasoconstrictor may be applied before insertion to reduce bleeding) with the bevel against the septum and inserted perpendicularly, in line with the nasal passage. It is then gently advanced posteriorly. If resistance is felt during insertion, the other nostril or a smaller size should be used.

- The airway length may be adjusted by sliding it in or out till the pharyngeal end rests below the base of the tongue but above the epiglottis
- If it is inserted too inside, laryngeal reflexes may be stimulated and if it is too outside, airway obstruction may not be relieved

Contraindications to the use of a nasopharyngeal airway:

- Patients with haemorrhagic disorders
- Coagulopathy
- A history of epistaxis requiring medical treatment
- Patients on anticoagulants
- Patients with basilar skull fracture
- Sepsis or deformity of the nose/nasopharynx

3. LARYNGEAL MASK AIRWAY (LMA)

- A device which is midway between mask and endotracheal tube
- Makes an airtight low-pressure seal around laryngeal inlet after inflation of the cuff

Versions: Plain, Reinforced, Intubating and Proseal

Parts : Mask, tube at an angle of 30 degrees, black line on tube to face upper incisors and pilot balloon.

Sizes : 1, 1.5, 2, 2.5, 3, 4, 5
  - To be autoclaved before every use
  - Deeper level of anaesthesia is required for insertion to avoid laryngospasm
  - Can be passed with / without use of muscle relaxants

Method of insertion: With patient in position as for laryngoscopy and with cuff deflated it is held like a pen and with its aperture facing anteriorly it is pressed against hard palate and advanced till it goes beyond the base of the tongue. Cuff is inflated and then connected to the breathing circuit.

Advantages : - No laryngoscopy is required
  - Less postoperative sore throat
  - Useful in failed intubation to ventilate the patient
  - Intubating LMA is useful (endotracheal tube can be passed through it) in intubating patients with difficult airway

Disadvantages: - Does not prevent aspiration
  - Can cause gastric distension

4. ENDOTRACHEAL TUBES

Types

- Red rubber (reusable) / PVC (disposable)
- Oral / nasal
- Plain / cuffed - High volume low pressure cuff (PVC)
  - Low volume high pressure cuff (red rubber)

Sizes: 2, 2.5, 3, 3.5, 4,......... 10, 10.5 (internal diameter in mm.)
  - Bevel at patient end
  - Connector to be placed at machine end
  - Passed with direct laryngoscopy under vision after anaesthetising the patient

Uses:

- Procedures in which it is not feasible to administer anaesthetic gases via mask
- Procedures which are long lasting
- Procedures in which there are chances of having blood, secretions, pus, vomitus etc. in the oral cavity
- Procedures in which patients need to be given muscle relaxants and controlled breathing

Special tubes: Oxford (L-shaped), Tehran (S-shaped), Precurved e.g., Ring Adair Ellwyn (RAE) Nasal (North Pole) / Oral (South Pole), Reinforced (armoured / flexometallic) etc.

- For laser surgery various 'laser-resistant' tubes are available. Each has its own advantage and disadvantage.
- Nasal tubes are characterized by a longer bevel, a softer tip, a streamlined cuff and no side port

5. LARYNGOSCOPE

It is designed for direct laryngoscopy and to pass an endotracheal tube into the larynx under vision

Parts : Handle, blade with light bulb

Sizes (for the blades) : neonate (infant), paediatric (child), adult and extra large

Method of insertion:

1. Patient supine with flexion of the lower cervical spine and extension of the head at the atlanto-occipital level.

2. Head should rest on a small pillow or a ring:- 'sniffing the morning air position'

3. Mouth of the patient is then opened by the right hand of the operator

4. Laryngoscope is introduced

5. The tip of the curved blade is advanced up to the junction of the base of the tongue with the epiglottis and the blade then lifted upwards and forwards along the axis of the handle so as to carry the base of the tongue and the epiglottis forwards

6. The tip of the straight blade is passed posterior to the epiglottis so as to pick up the epiglottis with the tip of the blade and the blade is then lifted anteriorly, thereby elevating the epiglottis directly to expose the laryngeal inlet

6. MAGILL'S FORCEPS

It is L-shaped and it has no catch

Sizes: Adult and Paediatric

Uses:

1. Guiding an endotracheal tube from the pharynx into the larynx during nasal intubation

2. To pack the throat with a roller gauze during oral and pharyngeal surgery

3. To pick up a broken or dislodged tooth / foreign body lying in the oral cavity

4. To pass a ryles (naso gastric) tube

7. BITE BLOCK (Mouth Bite / Gag / Prop)

It is placed between the molar teeth or gums to prevent them from occluding an endotracheal tube and to keep the mouth open for suctioning. It does not extend into the pharynx and is therefore less irritating than an oral airway

8. ANAESTHESIA MACHINE

It consists of a metallic frame having a facility to connect central pipelines as well as cylinders of gases like oxygen, nitrous oxide, air etc., flow meters, vaporizers and a facility to deliver high flow of oxygen (oxygen flush or emergency oxygen knob) in the event of any leak or an emergency situation. It also has a working platform to keep various drugs and small equipment, and at times a tray on the top to keep various monitors. The gas flow can be either intermittent (gases flow only on demand by the patient e.g. Walton 5) or continuous gases flow by using flow meter continuously e.g. Boyle machine. In continuous flow machines oxygen, nitrous oxide, air etc. have individual flow meters for setting desired flow of each gas. Vaporizers are for setting desired percentage output concentration of the liquid anaesthetic agents like halothane, isoflurane, sevoflurane etc (ether and trilene in older models of the machines). Flow meters for gases and vaporizers for liquid anaesthetic agents are gas/agent specific and the one meant for a particular gas or anaesthetic agent cannot be used for the other. Most of the newer anaesthesia machines have devices which in the event of delivery of a hypoxic gas mixture activate an alarm, either auditory or visual which tells the operator that a hypoxic gas mixture is being delivered so that immediate action can be taken. Anaesthesia machines have been evolved from simple pneumatic devices to complex computer based integrated systems with numerous controls, displays, indicators and alarms. The prevailing trend is to incorporate and integrate ventilators and vigilance aids such as airway pressure monitors, respiratory gas monitors, pulse oximeters, electrocardiograms and automatic blood pressure monitors into the machine

9. BREATHING SYSTEM (CIRCUIT)

It is an assembly of equipment, that not only carries anaesthetic mixture from the outlet of anaesthesia machine to the patient, but also allows to monitor and control patient's breathing.

Components: (in addition to various connectors and adaptors)

1. A bag mount with a reservoir bag (1.5 to 2 litre capacity)

2. Long (one meter) corrugated rubber or plastic tubing/s (breathing tube/s)

3. Expiratory valve, ordinary spring loaded/non re-breathing valve

Types:

1. Breathing system can be re-usable or disposable
2. It can have a single simple corrugated tubing (e.g., Magill's system) or can have a co-axial tubing i.e. one tubing within the other (e.g., Bains System) or can have double tubing, inspiratory and expiratory (e.g., closed circuit)
3. It can allow entire exhaled gases to vent to the atmosphere (e.g., Magill's system with NRV) or allow minimal / partial rebreathing (e.g., Magill's system with Heidbrink valve or Bain System) or it can allow exhaled gases from the patient to be re-used (re-breathed) after getting rid of carbon dioxide from the exhaled gases (e.g., circle absorber / carbon dioxide absorber / closed system)

OPEN SYSTEM (MAGILL'S)	CLOSED SYSTEM
1. Less economical	1. Economical as low flow of anaesthetic gases are required
2. Increase heat and moisture loss from patient's body	2. Less heat and moisture loss from patients body
3. Increased theatre pollution which can be reduced by using scavenging system that gets rid of exhaled gases entering into the operation theatre atmosphere.	3. Operation theatre pollution is almost nil.

RESUSCITATION AND OXYGENATION EQUIPMENT

1. RESUSCITATION BAG

- An assembly of equipment consisting of a self-inflating bag with a nipple for connecting an oxygen source, a non-rebreathing valve and a facemask
- Useful for ventilating a patient in an emergency situation / during transport
- Can also be used for administering anaesthesia in the absence of an anaesthesia machine e.g., in rural setup or field situations
- They are generally re-usable, but even disposable resuscitation bags are available

Sizes: Three sizes are available; for infants, children and adults.

Method of use:

After proper positioning of the patient, the mask has to be placed on the patient's face and the bag can be intermittently compressed and released while watching the inflation and deflation of the patient's chest. The exhalation blast can be heard or felt from the expiratory port of the non-rebreathing valve

2. OXYGEN CYLINDER

- Oxygen cylinders are available in various sizes
- They are black in colour with a shoulder painted white
- Those meant to be used on anaesthesia machines have a flushed valve and it is not possible to use a flushed valve cylinder in the wards
- Those meant for ward use have a bull-nose valve
- On the ward cylinder, oxygen flow meter can be attached and there is also a facility to attach a humidifier to the flow meter

3. OXYGEN FLOWMETER

- It allows the operator to deliver a desired flow of oxygen to the patient
- Generally, 3 to 4 liters per minute of flow is given but it varies from patient to patient depending upon:
  Type of oxygen delivery system (poly mask, venti mask, nasal cannula, nasal catheter, T-piece etc.)
  Type of surgery done, age of the patient and general condition of the patient

4. OXYGEN MASK

- These are generally facemasks of different varieties
- **Poly mask** is a semi oval shaped mask, available in two sizes, for children and for adults. It is a loosely fitting mask around the mouth and nose through which moderate flows of oxygen (3 to 6 liters) can be delivered. Too little oxygen flow will allow rebreathing and too high flow may obstruct exhalation. Oxygen percentage cannot be judged and not more than 35% can ever be given
- **Venti masks** are designed to work on venturi principle. Here the delivered oxygen flows through a jet and entrains room air from the surrounding entrainment port while it approaches the patient. Various flow rates of oxygen with its approximate delivered oxygen concentrations are written on the device and hence it becomes easy for the operator to choose the mask and deliver the desired concentration of oxygen
- There are some oxygen facemasks that have a reservoir bag for oxygen, and some have even directional valves. Recommended flow rates are 10-15 liters/min. of oxygen. With reservoir bag, one can deliver up to 65% oxygen and if they have directional valves also, then one can deliver even up to 90% oxygen

5. NASAL CATHETER / PRONGS

- These are the most simplest, most commonly used and easily available devices
- Not more than 1 to 3 liters of oxygen per minute can be delivered as high flows make the patient uncomfortable due to wheezing sound and a feeling of dry mouth
- Concentration of delivered oxygen is generally low and can never be judged
- Generally with oxygen flow rate of 1-2 liter/min., these devices provide 24-28% oxygen.
- If a nasal catheter is used, its tip should be advanced up to the fold of the soft palate. If it is introduced too far, it can produce gaseous distension of the stomach
- Nasal prongs (two short plastic prongs that fit into the external nares) are preferred by some as they are comfortable for the patients

USEFUL MONITORS

1. BLOOD PRESSURE MONITOR

It is necessary to monitor patient's blood pressure as most of the anaesthetic agents are vasodilators and / or myocardial depressants, giving rise to hypotension.

It is available in various forms:

1. Simple sphygmomanometer/anaeroid dial
2. Non-invasive automatic blood pressure monitor (NIBP)
3. Invasive direct arterial blood pressure monitor (IABP)

2. CARDIOSCOPE

Drugs used for anaesthesia have effects on rate, rhythm and contractility of the heart and hence it is a vital monitor. Cardioscope with a defibrillator is useful as it allows to defibrillate the heart on the spot, if the need arises.

Uses:

1. To monitor the electrocardiogram (E.C.G.) of the patient
2. To monitor patient's heart rate, rhythm, the type of arrhythmias and ST-segment changes (important to diagnose myocardial ischaemia)
3. To alarm the anaesthesiologist about cardiac arrest well in advance as generally slowing of the heart rhythm or intractable arrhythmias occur before cardiac arrest

3. PULSE OXIMETER

It is a non-invasive equipment that allows to monitor the oxygen saturation of the patient and also the heart rate continuously. It has a small probe which can be attached on any of the fingers or toes or on the ear lobule.

Uses:

1. To detect hypoxia (breathing of hypoxic gas mixture or circuit disconnection)
2. To detect hypotension / peripheral vasoconstriction

4. CAPNOMETER / CAPNOGRAPHS (End Tidal CO_2 - $ETCO_2$ Monitor)

It continuously records the carbon dioxide tension (in mm Hg or %) of the expired gas mixture (only numerical values as in capnometer or numerical value with graphical recording as in capnograph). A non-invasive monitor having a probe or an adaptor that can be attached to an endotracheal tube, a facemask or a nasal catheter. It allows the anaesthesiologist to monitor whether the patient is breathing adequately (if on spontaneous breathing) or whether the patient is being ventilated adequately (if he is on controlled breathing)

Also allows the anaesthesiologist to know:-

1. Inadvertent oesophageal intubation
2. Breathing circuit disconnection / function (e.g., re-breathing)
3. Adequacy of fresh gas flow from anaesthesia machine
4. Pulmonary air embolism

5. RESPIRATORY GAS MONITOR

It allows the anaesthesiologist to monitor the contents and the concentration of the inspired as well as expired gas mixture and thereby the concentration of the anaesthetic gases (Inhalational agent), oxygen and carbon dioxide of the inspired gases. It is a non-invasive monitor having a probe or an adapter that can be attached to an endotracheal tube, a facemask or a nasal catheter. It helps preventing delivery of a hypoxic gas mixture and also concentration of anaesthetic gases.

SECTION - VII
AUDIOLOGY

- Mrs. Geeta B. Gore
- Mrs. Deepa A. Valame

PURE TONE AUDIOMETRY

INTRODUCTION

Audiology is built on the foundations of physical, biologic and social sciences.

Hearing is one of the vital senses used by all of us in our every day life. However, nature of "hearing" is elusive in the sense that it cannot be seen, but only be "experienced". It is obligatory i.e. occurs constantly. The process of quantification of "hearing" is even more elusive, in that it encompasses the quantification of various facets of hearing like detection, discrimination, recognition, auditory memory, loudness perception, localisation, comprehension etc

"Hearing" takes place at all these levels simultaneously and each can be tested using different materials and methods.

The present chapter focuses on the most basic element of "hearing" i.e the stage of detection, absolute sensitivity.

Detection refers to the capacity of the auditory system to discern the presence or absence of sound. The procedure carried out routinely for measuring person's ability to detect sound is "pure tone audiometry." Thus, PTA is a test of "hearing sensitivity" & not a test of hearing. The quantification of sensitivity can be done by determination of threshold of audibility or threshold of detection of change.

HOW CAN THE HEARING SENSITIVITY BE MEASURED?

To answer this question we must first look at what is SOUND and its characteristics. Here we are concerned with the response of the human ear to auditory stimuli. Hence it is necessary to study the physical nature of sound.

Sound is a form of energy, which is propagated in a medium in the form of longitudinal waves comprising of alternating condensations & rarefactions. Whenever a force acts on an elastic medium, the particles of that medium move to and fro causing alternating compression & rarefaction. This results in a pressure wave that emanates from the source. When these pressure variations are within the range of human sensitivity, one can perceive the presence of "sound"

Sound can be characterised by two main features viz. frequency and intensity.

FREQUENCY

Humans can "hear" frequencies in the sonic range of 20Hz-20,000Hz.

Frequencies below this range are called infrasonic and those above this range are known as ultrasonic.

In PTA the hearing sensitivity is determined for the range of frequencies from 250 Hz to 8000Hz in Octave intervals (An Octave is a band of frequencies F2-F1 such that F2 = 2 F1) because most of the speech sounds occur in this range.

INTENSITY

The human ear is responsive to a wide range of sound pressures. The difference between the pressures of the quietest sound which can be heard and the loudest sound that can be tolerated is several million-fold. To accommodate this vast range of values on a convenient scale, a logarithmic scale is used with its unit "the decibel".

Figure : The decibel Scale

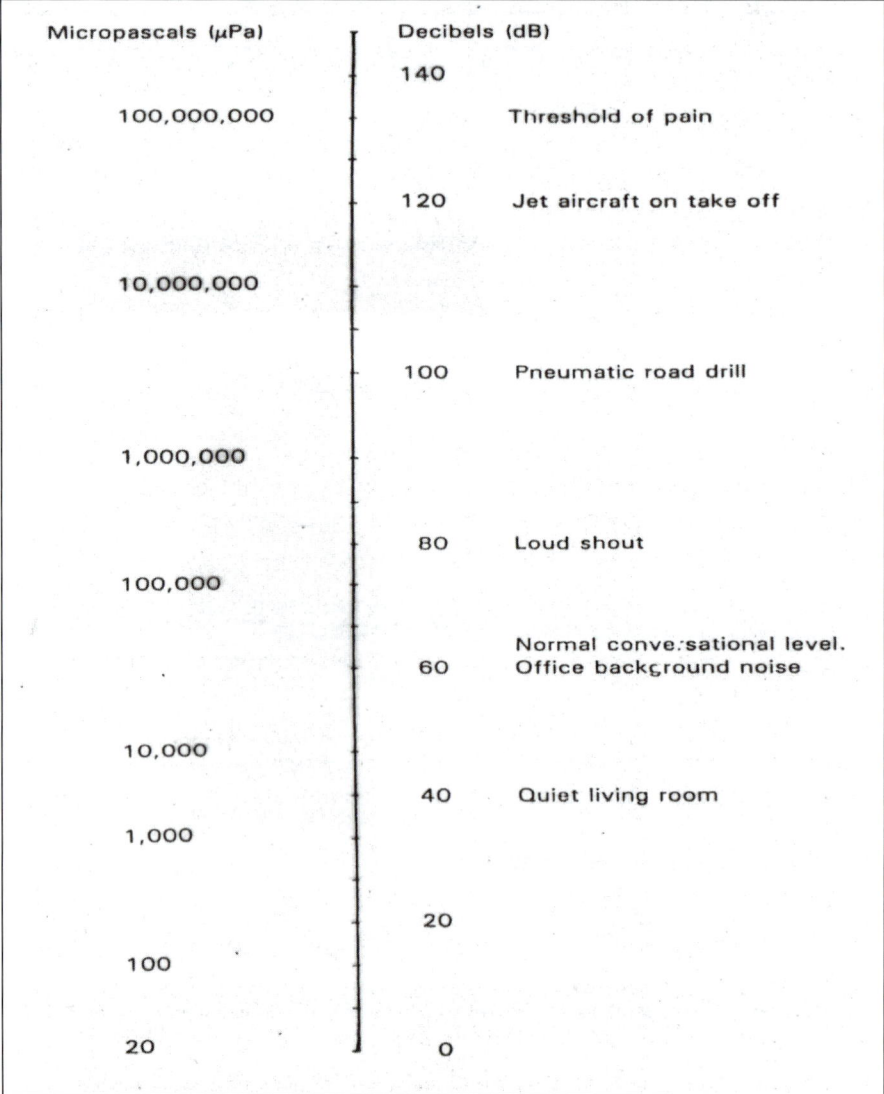

Screening for hearing impairment in young children Barry Mccormick Croom Helm Land 1988

The decibel is a logarithmic ratio of two quantities. Say for dBSPL, it is the ratio of the reference sound pressure (P2) and the sound pressure of interest (P1), Here the reference is the sound pressure required by normal hearing adults to perceive the presence of sound.

P2 = 0.0002 dynes/cm2 or 20 u Pa.

n dBSPL = 20 log (P1/ P2)

Thus, if P1 = P2 = 20 u Pa

n dB SPL = 20 x log (1)

= 0

Thus 0 dBSPL means that the sound pressure is equal to the reference pressure.

The dB sound pressure level scale is a logarithmic scale that compresses the million to one pressure values in the audible range into a 0- 120 dB SPL range..

The unit decibel should always be used w.r.t. its reference, otherwise it is meaningless. e.g. 'A sound is 20dB in intensity' is a meaningless sentence. It means "A sound is 20 times. Unless the reference is stated, the phrase 20 times has no meaning. Various references are used w.r.t. the decibel scale Viz. dBSPL, dBIL, dBHL, dBA etc.

Nature of Hearing Sensitivity

Absolute hearing sensitivity varies as a function of numerous factors such as the psychophysical method used, whether testing is done in sound field conditions or under earphones, type of earphone etc.

The graph of audibility of pure tone signals is called the "minimum audibility curve". It is a graph of the SPL required by normal hearing individuals to reach audibility as a function of frequency. The minimum audibility curve is not a straight line indicating that hearing sensitivity varies as a function of frequency. It is clearly seen that more SPL is required to reach "threshold" in low and high frequency ranges as compared to mid frequencies, thus the ear is most sensitive to mid frequencies.

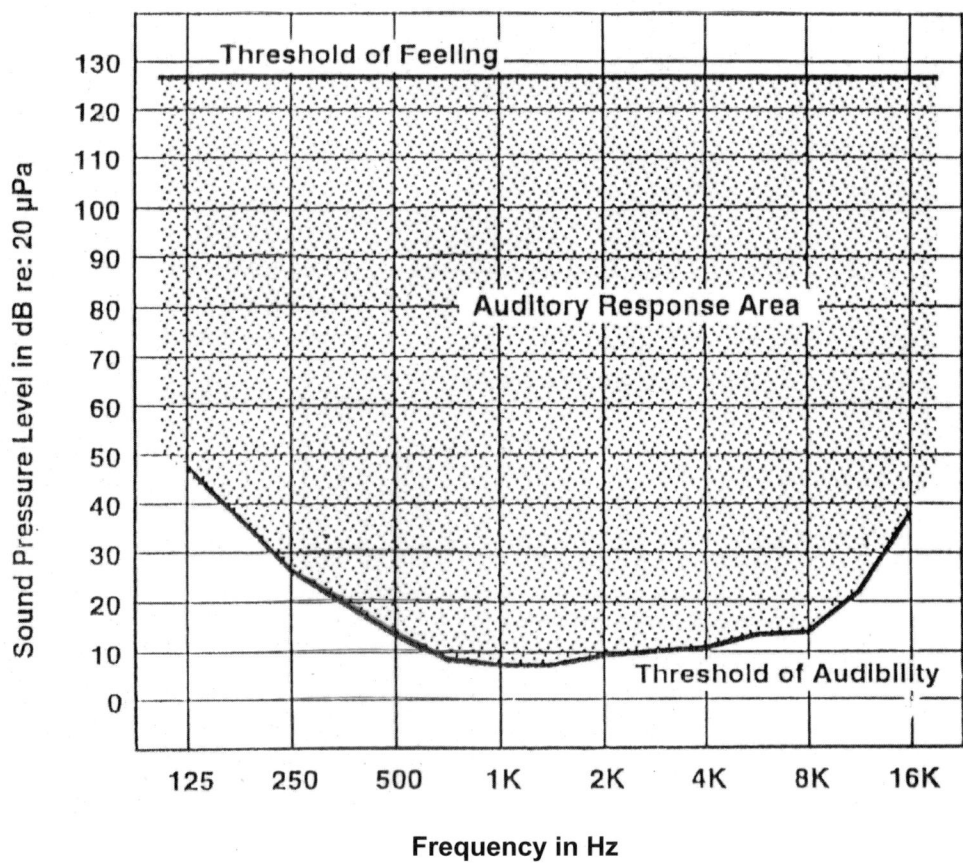

Frequency in Hz

Figure. Auditory response area from the threshold of audibility to the threshold of feeling across the frequency range that encompasses most of human hearing.

The MAP curve serves as the basis for PTA in which a patient's thresholds of audibility is measured and compared to this normal curve. For clinical purpose, this curve is converted into "straightened" graph using a unit - the dB hearing level. This straight line is the "Audiometric zero".

Thus "Audiometric zero" is the SPL at which the threshold of audibility occurs for normal listeners i.e. at each frequency, the sound pressure level (in dB SPL) required for normal listener to achieve audibility is designated as 0 dB HL for that frequency. This is shown in the figures given below:

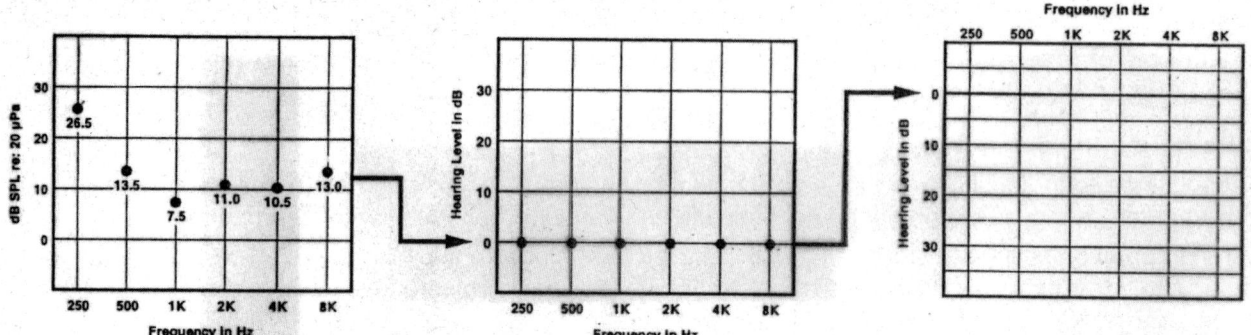

Figure : The conversion from sound pressure level to hearing level to an audiogram.

The conversion from sound pressure level to hearing level to an audiogram

Audiogram is a graph of auditory sensitivity as function of frequency. It uses the "dBHL" scale.

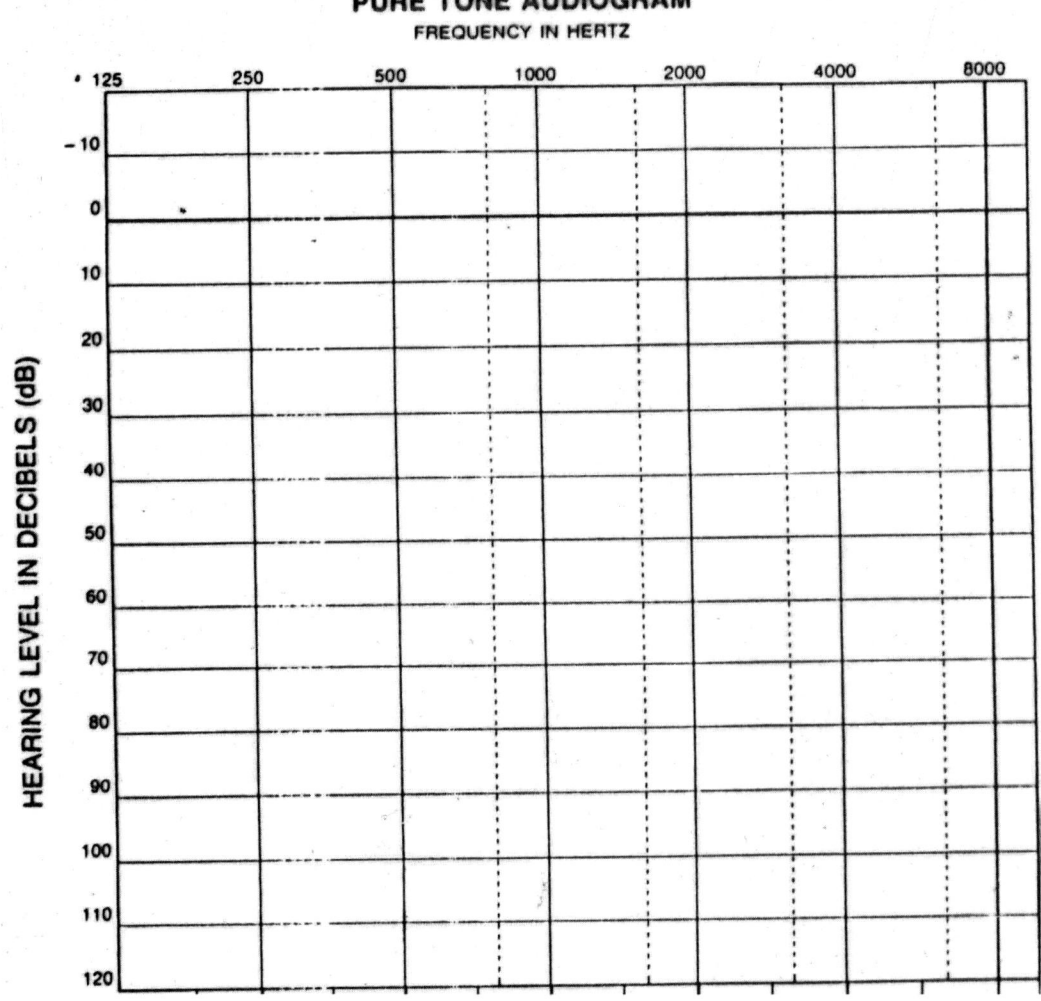

Audiogram recommended by the American Speech-Language-Hearing Association 1990.

PURE TONE TESTING

The basic audiologic evaluation has several purposes, such as diagnosis, determining the need for non-surgical rehabilitation, deciding subsequent audiological test battery approaches and determining disability and compensation. One of the tests in a basic evaluation is PTA, which is a test of hearing sensitivity as a function of frequency.

Obtaining Pure Tone Audiometry (PTA).

A. Preparation

1) Case history: - A detailed case history is mandatory before obtaining a PTA. It covers the following points:

    i)   Hearing loss - in which ear, since when, progression, etc.

    ii) Otorrhoea

    iii) Otalgia

    iv) Tinnitus

    v)   Giddiness and vertigo

    vi) Family history

    vii) Medical history

    viii)History of noise exposure etc.

    Above information is useful

    i)   To estimate the patients approximate hearing difficulty so as to determine at what level to start testing.

    ii) To determine mode of communication needed to give instructions for audiometry .

    iii) To validate audiometric findings

2) Otoscopic Examination:

    Prior to audiometric testing, Otoscopic examination is a must in order to rule out presence of wax or cotton in the ear which if unnoticed can lead to an apparent conductive hearing loss on the pure tone audiogram. Further an Otoscopy can also reveal presence of collapsible ear canals. This is very important because it can cause a spurious conductive hearing loss esp. in the high frequencies.

3) Seating the patient

    The patient should be seated is such a way that - he/she cannot see the face of the audiometer & he/she cannot see the clinician's movements. These visual cues must be avoided as they can lead to false responses by the patient. It would be ideal if the patient's face were visible to the clinician (at least in profile so as to observe his/her reactions to presentation of the stimulus.

4) Instructions

    The patient should be given clear instructions to raise his hand in response to the tone and to lower his hand as soon as he stops hearing the tone. The client should respond to the softest audible tone. At times during case history taking, it may be seen that the patient appears not to hear even very loud sounds. In such cases the instructions can be given either using gestures or in written form (if patient can read).

5) Placement of Transducers

    Transducers used during audiometry are:

    1. Earphones during air conduction testing

    2. Bone vibrator during bone conduction testing.

    To get valid thresholds, proper placement of transducers is mandatory.

    Earphone placement

    - By convention, the earphone marked in red must be placed over the right ear and the one marked in blue must be placed over the left ear. By adjusting the swivel joints earphones must be placed on the client so that he/ she is comfortable. Ensure that the diaphragm of the earphone lies in front of the opening of the EAC. Client must be asked to remove glasses, earring, headbands or any such thing which can cause discomfort and comes in the way of proper placement.

Bone Vibrator Placement

- It is conventionally placed on the mastoid process of the ear with better air conduction hearing. However, vibration of the BC vibrator will stimulate both the cochlea simultaneously, hence vibrator can be placed on any mastoid process.

- Care must be taken to avoid the BC vibrator touching the pinna or sound transmission may occur via the air conduction route.

C. TESTING

After preparing the patient, actual testing can be undertaken.

The testing can be divided into 2 parts:

- AC testing: - First AC testing is attempted in which the pure tone is presented via the earphones. The tone travels from the outer ear to middle ear to the cochlea and thus AC testing provides an overall estimate of the peripheral hearing sensitivity.

After AC testing, BC testing is undertaken using the BC vibrator. Here the assumption is that the BC presented tone directly stimulates the cochlea bypassing the outer and middle ears and thus provides an estimate of the cochlear reserve.

Which ear to test?

One should always start testing the patient's better ear as suggested in case history. In absence of ear difference, any ear can be tested first.

Frequency sequencing

Testing is begun at 1000 Hz except in case of profound losses when patient doesn't respond at 1000 Hz even at maximum audiometric output, testing can begin with 500 Hz. The sequence of testing is 1000 Hz - 2000 Hz – 4000 Hz - 8000 Hz. Then recheck at 1000 Hz, The obtained threshold should be within +/- 5 dB of threshold obtained earlier. Then proceed to 500 Hz and 250 Hz. After this, the other ear can be tested.

For BC testing, the same sequence is followed except that BC testing is not carried out at 8000Hz.

Note: If the thresholds at adjacent octaves differ by greater than 20dB, mid octaves should be tested.

Method Used

PTA can be carried out using various methods such as

- Ascending method
- Descending method
- Bracketing method

The procedure routinely used to determine thresholds of hearing

Sensitivity is the Hughson-Westlake Ascending technique modified by Carhart & Jerger, 1959. The important features of this approach are:

1. The starting level

    During the case history interview, the audiologist can make some estimate of the patient's hearing capacity; based on which the starting level can be decided.

If the patient appears to have	Start at
Normal hearing sensitivity	30-40 dBHL
- Moderate hearing loss	70 dBHL
- Severe hearing loss	100 dBHL

2. After the initial response :-

    Decrease the intensity in 10-15 dB steps until no response is obtained i.e. inaudibility is reached.

    It is important to remember that the tone duration should be 1 to 2 seconds and the interstimulus interval should be no shorter than the duration of the test tone.

3. Once inaudibility is reached:

    We can begin the threshold search using ascending technique. Increase the intensity of the signal in 5dB steps, until the patient responds i.e. the threshold of audibility. When the patients responds again carry out the 5 dB up, 10 dB down procedure till threshold is obtained.

Criterion for Threshold

As per ANSI (1978, 1986) standards:-

Threshold is the lowest hearing level at which responses occur in at least one-half of a series of ascending trials, with a minimum of two responses out of three required at a single level".

Examples:

1. Presentation level (dBHL)   Response/ No response (R/NR)

70	R
55	R
40	NR

_____ Threshold search begins

45	NR
50	NR
55	R —— (i)
45	NR
50	NR
55	R — (ii)

Therefore Threshold is 55dBHL

2.

40	R
25	NR

_____ Threshold search begins

30	NR
35	R

(i) response. at 35 dBHL

25	NR
30	R

(i)response at 30dBHL

20	NR
25	NR
30	NR
35	R

(ii) Response at 35 dBHL

Therefore Threshold is 35 dBHL.

RECORDING OF RESULTS

The pure tone thresholds obtained during air conduction and bone conduction testing is recorded graphically on the "audiogram".

The audiogram is a graph of a patient's hearing thresholds across the frequencies in octaves from 250 Hz to 8000 Hz.

This graph has on its abscissa - the frequencies (in Hertz) plotted on an Octave (i.e. logarithmic) scale and on its Ordinate - intensity level in dBHL (i.e. logarithmic scale). Thus an audiogram is graph of log-log nature.

The symbols for thresholds as recommended by ASHA (1990) are:

			Right	Unspecified	Left
Ac.	-	Earphones			
		Unmasked	O		**X**
		Masked	Δ		❑
Bc	-	Mastoid	<	^	>
	-	Unmasked			
	-	Masked	[	]	]

Note:

< = Bc threshold obtained with vibrator on R. Mastoid

Not necessarily response of R. ear

> = Bc threshold obtained with vibrator on Left Mastoid

Not necessarily response. of Left ear

^ = Common/Unmasked bone conduction i.e. response of the better cochlea.

INTERPRETATION

The audiogram provides us with both qualitative and quantitative information about patient's hearing loss.

Quantitative - Degree of loss

Qualitative - Type of hearing loss

Quantitative -The degree of hearing loss is calculated based on the PTA (PTA is the average of the patient's threshold at the frequencies 500 Hz, 1000Hz and 2000Hz).

PTA (dBHL)	Description
- 10 to 15	Normal Hearing Sensitivity
- 16 to 25	Mild Hearing Loss
- 41 to 55	Moderate hearing loss
- 56 to 70	Moderately severe hearing loss
- 71 to 90	Severe hearing loss
- > 91	Profound hearing loss

Qualitative: Helps in topological diagnosis

The type of hearing loss can be determined using

- AC PTA
- BC PTA

Air bone gap (AC PTA - BC PTA)

Conductive hearing loss

Here the lesion lies in the outer/middle ear or both i.e. in the AC pathway

Therefore Due to lesion in the AC pathway, patient's AC threshold is worse than normal i.e. 25 dBHL However, BC thresholds will be normal because the inner ear is intact.

Therefore in conductive loss

- BC threshold- Within normal limits
- AC threshold-Worse than normal
- Presence of airborne gap (> 10dB)

Sensorineural hearing loss

Here, the lesion is in the inner ear and / or the auditory nerve

As seen above as the inner ear has a lesion, transmission of sound is affected in both the AC as well as the BC pathway. Therefore in SN Loss,

- the BC threshold is worse than normal i.e. worse than 25 dBHL,

- the AC threshold is worse than normal i.e. worse than 25dBHL

Therefore A-b gap < 10 dB.

Mixed Hearing Loss.

Here the lesion lies in O.E/M.E and I.E./nerve .

Thus, AC pathway has 2 lesions. Therefore AC threshold is worse than that in normal i.e. worse than 25 dBHL. BC threshold will also be worse than that in normal hearing. However, to a lesser extent as compared to AC thresholds. Therefore there is presence of an air bone gap> 10dB.

NOTE

The validity of results obtained in pure tone Audiometry depend upon various factors, of which, the test environment is very important.

Test Environment

An ideal test environment must meet the requirements of

- Sufficient space

- Adequate comfort to the patient

**- Adequate quiet

This is most important as ambient noise levels can cause serious errors in interpretation. Noise levels that are greater than those permissible can lead to an apparent hearing loss since noise will mask the tone.

TABLE 1. Octave and one-third octave band maximum permissible ambient noise levels for three test frequency ranges specified in ANSI S3.1-1999 for ears not covered

Center Frequency	Octave Band			One-Third Octave Band		
	125 to 8000 Hz	250 to 8000 Hz	500 to 8000 Hz	125 to 8000 Hz	250 to 8000 Hz	500 to 8000 Hz
125	29.0	35.0	44.0	24.0	30.0	39.0
250	21.0	21.0	30.0	16.0	16.0	25.0
500	16.0	16.0	16.0	11.0	11.0	11.0
800				10.0	10.0	10.0
1000	13.0	13.0	13.0	8.0	8.0	8.0
1600				9.0	9.0	9.0
2000	14.0	14.0	14.0	9.0	9.0	9.0
3150				8.0	8.0	8.0
4000	11.0	11.0	11.0	6.0	6.0	6.0
6300				8.0	8.0	8.0
8000	14.0	14.0	14.0	9.0	9.0	9.0

Note : Values are in dB re : 20 µPa to the nearest 0.5 dB and have been reprinted by permission of the Acoustical Society of America, New York, U.S.A.

TABLE 2. Octave band ears covered maximum permissible ambient noise levels for three test frequency ranges as specified in ANSI S3.1-1999 for ears covered testing is done using a supra-aural or insert earphone

Octave Band Intervals	Supra-aural Earphone			Insort Earphone		
	125 to 8000 Hz	250 to 8000 Hz	500 to 8000 Hz	125 to 8000 Hz	250 to 8000 Hz	500 to 8000 Hz
125	35.0	39.0	49.0	59.0	67.0	78.0
250	25.0	25.0	35.0	53.0	53.0	64.0
500	21.0	21.0	21.0	50.0	50.0	50.0
1000	26.0	26.0	26.0	47.0	47.0	47.0
2000	34.0	34.0	34.0	49.0	49.0	49.0
4000	37.0	37.0	37.0	50.0	50.0	50.0
6000	37.0	37.0	37.0	56.0	56.0	56.0

Note : Values are in dB re : 20 μPa to the nearest 0.5 dB and have been reprinted by permission of the Acoustical Society of America, New York, U.S.A.

Remember:

- To compensate for high ambient noise levels in the Test rooms, some people use correction factor. This is completely erroneous because

1. Noise is not constant. It varies from time to time and affects different frequencies to varying degrees.

2. Effects of noise also depend upon the patient's hearing sensitivity. A particular noise level may affect the threshold of a person with mild loss but may be insignificant to testing of a severely hearing impaired person. Therefore use of a common correction factor is erroneous.

SECTION - VIII
TIPS FOR DNB PRACTICALS

TIPS FOR DNB PRACTICALS

The DNB practical exam is based on day-to-day clinical practices and evaluates your efficiency in performing routine clinical tasks as well as your skills in interacting with patients. The DNB OSCE questions also evaluate some amount of theoretical knowledge of the candidates (e.g classifications, grading systems, etc.) Although it is not possible to include detailed descriptions and answers in this chapter, a few sample questions based on previous DNB practical exams have been provided to give a general idea about the exam process. Most of the topics have been covered in the previous sections of this book. Also suggestions about extra reading have been provided.

The DNB practical examination comprises of

- OSCEs
- Table Vivas (4 tables): The viva tables are kept as a part of the OSCE rounds with a specific time allotted at each table: Measurements/Dimensions, Recent advances, Rhinology, Throat
- 2 clinical case presentations

SAMPLE CASES

Ear

- CSOM
- Serous otitis media
- Adhesive otitis media
- Acute suppurative otitis media
- Aural polyp
- Otosclerosis
- Facial palsy

Nose

- Deviated nasal septum
- Nasopharyngeal angiofibroma
- Other Nasal Tumors: Benign & Malignant
- Nasal Polyps
- Complications of sinusitis

Larynx & Head and Neck

- Vocal Nodules
- Vocal Polyps
- Laryngeal Papilloma
- Vocal Cord Paralysis
- Laryngeal web
- Laryngocele
- Carcinoma larynx & laryngopharynx
- Cleft lip / palate

- (Malignancies of Larynx, Hypopharynx, (Nasopharynx, Oropharynx)
- Neck swellings
    - Lymphadenopathy
    - Secondaries neck with unknown (primary)
    - Parotid/ Submandibular (salivary gland (swelling)
    - Thyroid (swellings)
    - Thyroglossal cyst
- Thyroglossal fistula
- Branchial sinus
- Tuberculous lymphadenopathy with sinus

OSCEs:

The OSCE stations may be broadly divided into the following stations:
- Clinical examination
- Patient interaction e.g.: Patient counselling
- Demonstrating clinical procedures / performing clinical tests
- Questions based on hypothetical clinical case scenarios
- Clinical photographs
- Videos of procedures
- Photographs of CT scans/ MRI / X-rays or actual films
- Microbiology/ Pathology
- Instruments
- Drug vials

General points to remember:

- Every OSCE is allotted a specific time. Immediately switch over to the next OSCE as soon as the alarm sounds.

- In the OSCEs based on clinical examination or procedures to be performed, marks are also allotted to how you conduct yourself during examination / performing the procedure, in addition to the actual task to be performed.

- At any station where you have to examine, counsel or interact with a hypothetical patient, always remember to greet the patient and introduce yourself. Enquire about the patient's name and age before you proceed further.

- Certain OSCE stations may be based on the previous OSCE station e.g. You may be asked to perform only a clinical examination at an OSCE station with the examiner observing how you carry it out. The following OSCE may have questions based on this examination.

Clinical Examination

Sample OSCEs:

Q. Examine the patient's ear / nose / throat
- Greet the patient and introduce yourself to the patient.

- Ask the patient his/her name and age (The next OSCE station may have a question such as 'What was the name of the patient you examined at the previous station?')

- Ask the patient if he has any specific complaint in brief (ear/nose/throat – as per the OSCE). Do not spend too much time on this as the examination has to be performed within the limited time.

- Make sure you accurately adjust the headlight / head mirror / Bull's lamp.

- The examiner and the patient have to be positioned properly

- Perform a complete examination including inspection and palpation first followed by examination with instruments.

Q. - Examine the patient's neck and describe your positive findings.
- What is the level of lymph nodes that are palpated.
- What investigations will you advise the patient?
- Give 4 differential diagnoses of the lesion palpated?

Q. Perform an indirect laryngoscopy examination. Describe your findings.

Q. Perform a posterior rhinoscopy. Describe your findings.

Clinical Tests

Q. Demonstrate clinical tests for hyperthyroidism.
(Note: While demonstrating measurement of resting pulse rate, inform the examiner that ideally the patient should be sleeping and not just lying down.)

Q. Check for thyroid eye signs

Q. Demonstrate Dix-Hallpike test

Q. Demonstrate Epley's manoeuvre (Remember to tell patient about post-Epley's precautions)

Q. Perform cranial nerve examination.

Q. Perform tuning fork tests.

Q. Demonstrate Brandt Daroff exercises

Q. Perform Cottle's Test

Q. Perform distraction test.

- Tell the examiner before starting the test, that you will require a distractor. The examiner may tell you to proceed without the distractor.

Q. Test bone conduction / air conduction levels in the right ear of this patient by performing pure tone audiometry. OR Demonstrate masking in the left ear.
(Start by saying that you would like to perform a TFT before the actual PTA).

Q. Demonstrate myringotomy.

- Begin by telling the examiner that you would like to wash-up, wear gloves, clean and drape the ear and inject local anesthesia. Then proceed to perform the actual procedure.

Q. Demonstrate ligation of the lower pole in the tonsillar fossa.

Q. Demonstrate one finger/ two finger/ three finger knots.

Q. Demonstrate bronchoscopy in the provided dummy.

- Begin by telling the examiner that you would like to wash-up, wear gloves, clean and drape. Give the appropriate position. Then proceed further.

Q. Demonstrate PMMC flap on a dummy. (Any other flap may be asked).

Q. A person sitting in your OPD waiting room suddenly holds his own neck and collapses. What will you do? The emergency team number is 3030. Assume that the dummy provided is the patient. (Inform the examiner that you will first call for help on 3030 and then proceed to demonstrate the CPR).

Patient Counselling

Q. Counsel a 2nd year medical student who complains about burning sensation in throat, bloating, dry cough on lying down.

- Begin by telling the patient 'You are most likely suffering from gastro-esophageal reflux'
- Include the following in your counseling:
  - Diet: Diet modification, small frequent meals, drinking plenty of water, etc.
  - Sleeping habits: e.g Not lying down immediately after meals, Keeping head end of bed raised (and not just using pillows to lift up head)
  - Stress relief, Avoid staying up late nights
  - Anti-reflux medications

Q. Counsel a patient scheduled to undergo total laryngectomy.

Include the following points:
- Explain structure of larynx in brief
- Nature of disease, stage of disease
- Pre-op investigations
- Anesthesia, Surgical procedure, Post Op Care, Hospital Stay
- Complications / Recovery course (Loss Of Speech, Fistula, Leak, Anosmia , Chylous Leak, etc)
- Nutrition (Dietician referral)
- Psychological counseling (You may need to see our psychologist)
- How surgery may affect routine activities (e.g. No swimming)
- Post Op Radiotherapy / chemotherapy
- Voice Rehabilitation
- Family counseling

Q. Counsel a patient undergoing surgery (e.g.: myringotomy, FESS, stapedectomy, etc.)

Q. Counsel a $T_1N_0M_0$ Ca Larynx patient scheduled for radiotherapy.
(Remember to include risk of recurrence, options in case of recurrence. Discuss surgical option)

Q. Counsel a tracheostomy patient. (Include counseling about tracheostomy tubes with speaking valves)

Q. Counsel the mother of a child with bilateral severe-profound sensorineural hearing loss.

Q. Counsel a patient with sudden sensorineural hearing loss.

Clinical photographs

e.g. Tracheo-esophageal fistula, exophthalmos, facial palsy, herpes zoster, battle sign, perichondritis, Ca vocal cords, rhinosporidiosis, etc.

Videos

Balloon sinuplasty, Eustachian tube balloons, Heimlich's manoeuvre, Virtual bronchoscopy, etc.

Radiology

CT scans / MRI / X-ray
Remember to look for the patient's name, age, sex, thickness of CT scan cuts. You may be asked these at the subsequent OSCE station.

- **Q:** HRCT Temporal bone with fracture line (longitudinal fracture). Which segment of the facial nerve is likely to be damaged in this kind of a fracture? How will you manage it?

- **Q:** MRI neck: Identify the highlighted neck space. Identify the pathology. What are the contents of this neck space?

- **Q:** X-ray mastoid Schuller's view: Explain patient positioning for this view. What structures are visible in the X-ray? What other views can be taken to visualize the mastoid?

Drug vials

General tips

- Check the expiry date of the vial. If you have been asked indications for use and the vial is past its expiry date, mention that it cannot be used in a patient as it is an expired vial! Then mention that if not expired, it could have been used for the following indications.....
- Read about Anti-tuberculous therapy, anti-retroviral therapy in addition to other routinely used drugs.
- Vaccines

Instruments

Remember to give the full name of the instrument. E.g. Tilley-Henkel's ethmoid punch.

Microbiology / Pathology

Photographs or actual specimens may be kept.

Examples:

- Photograph showing acid fast bacilli:
  - Identify
  - What is the organism most likely to be? (A. Mycobacterium tuberculosis)
  - Staining technique / Culture media
  - Explain steps of sputum collection for Kochs/TB
  - Treatment
- Tests for HIV
- Tests for H_1N_1

Biostatistics / Preventive Medicine

- National Programmes
- Biostatistics: Mean, Median, Mode, Chi Square test, etc.
- Vaccination schedules

Viva Tables

Measurements

Say 'pass' if you do not know the answer to a specific question (E.g.: Volume of the middle ear), or the examiner may not be able to ask you all the questions he/she is supposed to ask within the allotted time.

Dimensions of:

- Tympanic membrane
- External auditory canal
- Internal auditory canal
- Internal auditory meatus
- Round window
- Oval window
- Stapes footplate

Suggested reads:

- Recent advances: e.g. Stem cell therapy, robotics, endoscopic thyroidectomy, sialendoscopy, brainstem implants, etc
- All TNM stagings
- Various classification systems
- SNOT questionnaire
- VHI (Voice handicap index)
- RSI (Reflux index)
- Recent American Academy guidelines for ENT conditions
- Latest OCNAs, journals
- Scott-Brown, Stell Maran, Ballinger's

SECTION - IX

ADDITIONAL CHAPTER

1. RADIOFREQUENCY

Radiofrequency is high frequency alternating current used to cut or ablate tissues.

When radiofrequency is applied to a particular target tissue, the energy travels within and creates a zone of ionization and inflammation which then heals by subsequent fibrosis.

Ablation target tissue in ENT usually comprises of cases of obstructive sleep apnoea where RF is used mainly on the turbinate, palate and tongue base and also the tonsils.

The target tissue is determined by the procedure called DISE-drug induced sleep endoscopy wherein the patient is put to sleep/sedation by artificial means of adequate anaesthetic medication followed by endoscopy (flexible nasoendoscopy). The patient is said to have attained an appropriate sleep / sedation level when apparent snoring during the procedure begins.

After identifying the tissue / structure that leads to snoring, RF is applied to that structure.

Target tissue	DISE Picture	RF output
1) Turbinate	• HIT • Turbinate obstructing • Ass/w DNS • Nasal component of snoring	• Particular power output for each application of 10 msec
2) Palate	• Palatal flutter • Palatal collapse on endoscopy	• Application only on soft palate
3) Base of tongue	Tongue Base Collapse	• Application on post 1/3rd of tongue and beyond

Salient Points

- All RF procedures: can be carried out under LA/GA.
- RF palate: avoid blanching or overapplication as it can result in palatal perforation
- RF tongue base: More likely to have a complication of infection/bleeding hence aseptic precautions are highly warranted.

RADIOFREQUENCY ABLATION FOR SNORING AND SLEEP APNOEA

ABSTRACT

Radiofrequency is high frequency alternating current used to ablate (cut/coagulate) tissues. It can be applied to nasal turbinates, soft palate, tongue base, tonsils etc. It can be used to perform various procedures in the cutting mode to improve obstructive sleep disordered breathing.

Radiofrequency proves to be a useful tool for snoring/ sleep apnoea cases. Its advantages Include relative precision in incision making, relative bloodless fields if used appropriately, decreased postoperative pain and excellent healing with fibrosis which aids in stiffening tissues.

KEYWORDS: Radiofrequency, snoring, obstructive sleep apnoea.

AIM

The objective/aim was to assess efficacy of radiofrequency as a tool for procedures/surgeries related to snoring/sleep apnoea.

The parameters used were selecting all patients with the likelihood of having even symptoms being suggestive of snoring, sleep apnoea / osa clinical examination falling into Friedman and Mallampati classification. Affordable sleep study, sleep endoscopy if possible and then procedures carried out according to reports findings and feasibility.

Intra operative parameters were blood loss and pain if under local anaesthesia and Post procedure parameters assessed were post-op pain, post- op blood loss, reduction in subjective snoring sounds by patients and partner and reduction in AHI (Apnoea Hypopnoea Index) post operatively.

METHODS

The procedures were carried out over a period of three years. All cases that came to us had complaints of snoring, difficulty in breathing and sleep disturbances at the hospital departments and were included in the study.

A total of 25 cases were studied. A thorough history, clinical examination and flexible endoscopy /sleep study were carried out according to the case.

Patient selection was from history, examination, Friedman and Mallampati classification and from those cases wherein a sleep study and endoscopy was feasible. Also post operatively sleep study was done only in affordable and feasible cases.

The radiofrequency SUTTER BM 780 machine was used to treat patients. The power settings used were from 2 - 6 in the cutting and coagulation mode.

The procedures were carried out under local or general anaesthesia with oral intubation and a throat pack.

RF TONSILLECTOMY

Exposing the tonsil on either side with the To-bite radiofrequency forceps or the RF needle was used to incise open the plane for tonsillar dissection. Dissection was carried out with the same achieving haemostasis at the same time. If properly done bleeding was minimal and pain scores were low post operatively. Fossa deepened and stiffened post operatively. RF setting of 2-3 in cutting mode and 5-6 in coagulation mode was used.

RF ADENOIDECTOMY

Can be performed after retracting lower edge of the palate with tongue depressors or touniquets and coagulating the adenoid with bipolar forceps. The lower edge of the adenoid can be dissected using needle or ball point. Bleeding is negligible and wound heals well. There was no case of postoperative haemorrhage. For recurrent adenoids, RF setting of 5-6 in the coagulation mode is used.

RF PALATE

It is temperature controlled RF volumetric reduction of the palate in order to stiffen or scar the soft palate. The Sutter RF-bipolar probe is used to deliver energy to the soft palate at various points. Blanching has to be avoided. The subsequent stiffening occurs over 6 weeks. It is done under local anaesthesia as an outpatient procedure with no bleeding and low pain scores. Subjective decrease in snoring was achieved even in one sitting.

RF TONGUE BASE

It is temperature controlled volumetric tongue base reduction by giving RF energy to multiple sites of post tongue base with Sutter RF bipolar forceps. Three sittings of application gives a significant reduction in tongue base tissue. There was no incidence of tongue base oedema or infection. The procedure could be done under local or general anaesthesia.

RF UP3

It is achieved by uvular and parauvular lateral cuts and trimming of lower edge of soft palate with RF in cutting mode and tonsillectomy with pillar suturing. The postoperative widening contracture/stiffening helps in achieving a good result.

RAUP

For snoring it is done by uvular and lateral cuts, and redefining the post pillars. Tonsillectomy may be combined. It achieves its result due to removal of the redundant mucosa and subsequent healing with fibrosis. Subjective decrease in snoring is achieved by most patients, RF is used in the cutting mode,

RESULTS   (Pain scores from 0 to 5)

Procedure	No. of cases	Pain scores	Bleeding intra op	Postop bleeding
RF PALATE	5	4:2 pts. 1:3 pts	Nil	Nil
RAUP	6	4:1 pt, 3:1pt	Negligible	Nil
RF TONSILS	6	5:2 pt	10 ml: 3 pts, Nil: 3 pt	Nil
RF ADENOIDS	4	0:4 pts	Nil	Nil
RF UP3	2	4-5: both pts	Nil	Nil
RF TONGUE BASE	4	0-1: all pts	Nil	Nil

DISCUSSION

Of the 27 patients who underwent treatment with radiofrequency, of the 5 palate cases 2 patients got a pain score of 4 and 3 patients got a pain score of 0-1. RAUP patients had a varied score of 1 to 4. RF adenoidectomy was relatively pain free and tonsillectomy was between 4-5. Rf tongue base had very low pain scores. There was no postoperative bleeding in any of the cases. Intra operative bleeding was encountered in tonsillectomy when RF was used in the cutting mode. RF Somnoplasty in one sitting can give a reduction in snoring by 50-70%. RF in cutting mode, if used inappropriately, can give rise to bleeding issue otherwise not.

CONCLUSION

RF appears to be an efficient tool for snoring/sleep apnoea procedures because of:

- Ability to cut fast and maintain a relatively bloodless field
- Ability to cut and coagulate at various settings
- Decreased intraoperative blood loss
- Induced fibrosis and stiffening of tissues
- Decreased postoperative pain

Other advantages

- The instrument unit appears dynamic with a unique feel
- Procedures can be performed under local / general anesthesia
- Instruments are autoclavable/recurring cost is lower
- Machine is ambulatory
- Minimally invasive

References

Steward DL Methods and outcomes of radiofrequency ablation for obstructive sleep apnoea. Department of Otolaryngology, Head and Neck Surgery, University of Cincinnati Medical Centre, Cincinnati Ohio.

Pang KP, Blanchard AR, Terries DJ. Surgical treatment of sleep disordered breathing. Department ot Otolaryngology, TanTockSengh Hospital Singapore and Dept. of Otolaryngology, Medical college of Georgia. Augusta. Georgia,USA.

Note: Radiofrequency thyroid ablation untrasound guided radiofrequency ablation in thyroid.

Indications

- Benign thyroid nodules
- Recurrent thyroid carcinomas

New Novel Techique

Under ultrasound guidance
Ablation of nodule by radiofrequency probe
Follow-up to see changes in pathology and size of nodule

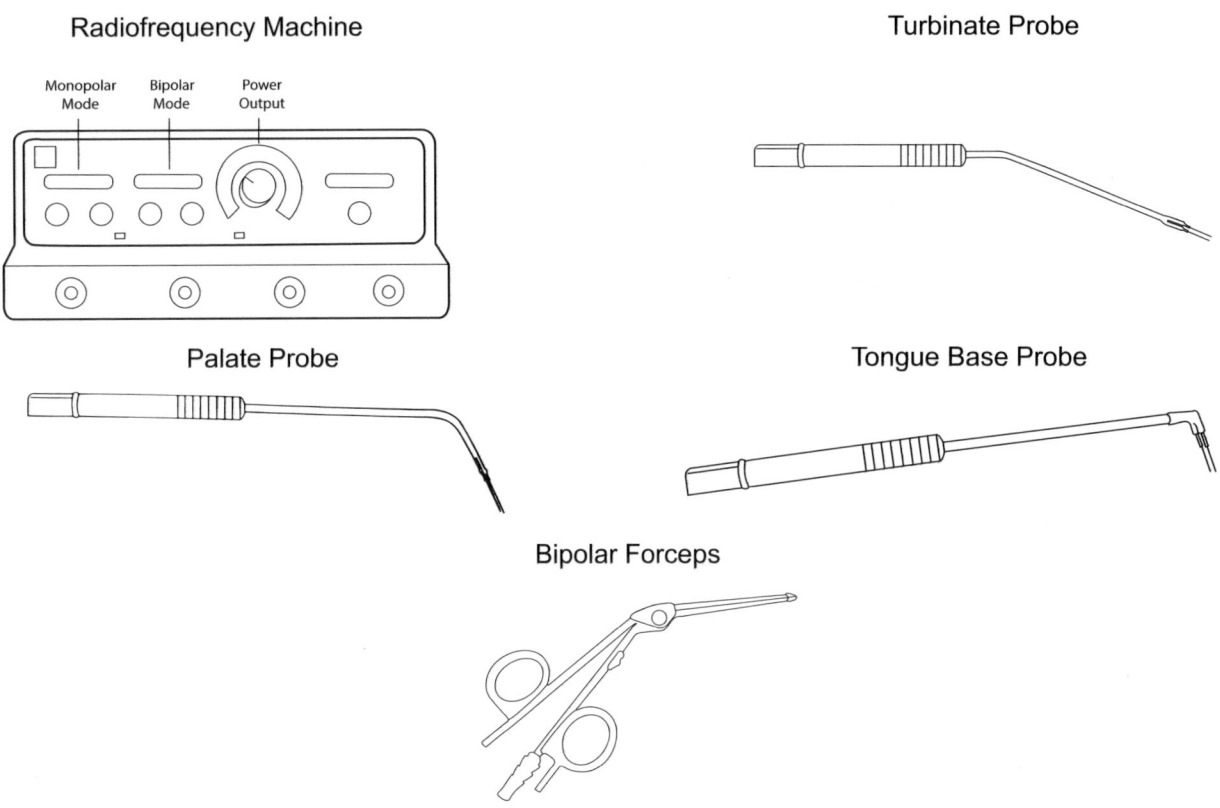

Radiofrequency Machine   Turbinate Probe

Monopolar   Bipolar   Power
Mode   Mode   Output

Palate Probe   Tongue Base Probe

Bipolar Forceps

2. COBLATION

It enables surgeons to precisely dissect and ablate soft tissue while preserving the integrity of surrounding healthy tissue.

The technology uses electrical energy to excite the electrolytes in a conductive medium, such as saline, creating a precisely focused plasma.

The energized plasma particles possess sufficient energy to break organic molecular bonds, resulting in tissue dissection and ablation.

Because the RF current does not pass direclty through the tissue, with Coblation, relatively low temperatures (40°C to 70°C) are generated as a by product of the process.

It dissects or excises tissue while preserving the integrity of surrounding healthy tissue.

Applications:

- Tonsillectomy
- Adenoidectomy
- Reduction of tissues in OSA (turbinates, soft palate, tongue base)
- As a tool in ENT surgeries

Coblation Ward

Sample Coblation Machine

3. FEES

Fibreoptic endoscopic evaluation of swallowing:

It is a procedure used to assess how well you swallow. During the procedure a thin flexible instrument called endoscope is passed through the nose and then parts of the throat are visualized as the patient swallows.

The instrument has a tiny camera and light attached to it. Nose and throat may be sprayed and endoscope is introduced gently through the nose into the pharynx. It sits above the epiglottis for most of the viewing and can be moved down after each swallow so that the vocal folds may be seen.

Observation is made in 2 parts:

1. First part - Structures of pharynx and larynx may be observed. Also how well one swallows saliva prior to giving any food is observed.

2. Second part - It is when food is introduced. Here swallowing will be assessed with different textures and sizes of food and liquid. Different positions and foods are adopted to see the throat and swallowing function. It can show if one is aspirating.

Swallowing movement is a series of actions from muscles of the throat, larynx, pharynx along with coordination with the muscles of breathing, as breathing pauses during a swallow.

The epiglottis acts like a flap and covers the trachea, when a swallow of food or drink occurs. The FEES test can help assess any problem with any part of the process.

INDICATIONS

Dysphagia:

- Sensation of something sticking in throat.
- Dysphagia can be seen in cases of:-
    1. Head and neck cancer
    2. Head injury
    3. Sjogren's Syndrome
    4. Parkinson's disease
    5. Neurological disease
    6. Muscular dystrophies
    7. Oesophageal Obstruction

COMPLICATIONS

- Nose bleed
- Discomfort
- Gagging / vomiting
- Laryngospasm
- Aspiration

4. HEARING AIDS

Hearing aid is a battery powered electronic device meant to improve hearing,

PARTS OF A HEARING AID

1) A **Microphone** picks up sound around you.

2) An **Amplifier** makes the sound louder.

3) A **Receiver** sends these amplified sounds into your ear.

COMMON CAUSES OF HEARING LOSS

- Aging / presbyacusis
- Loud noise / NIHL (noise induced hearing loss)
- Medications
- Diseases

Hearing aid may help people with conductive and/or sensorineural hearing loss. If one has an open ear canal and a relatively normal external ear, a hearing aid can help these patients even if they have ear disease and surgery or medication not being the right or exact correction for them.

Hearing aids are fitted with the help of an audiologist who usually chooses the right device depending on:

1) Severity and type of hearing loss.

2) Age of patient

3) Cost

4) Lifestyle and other factors like management of small devices, family help etc.

TYPES OF HEARING AIDS

1) Analog Hearing aids.

2) Digital Hearing aids.

Analog hearing aids convert sound waves into electrical signals and make them louder.

Digital Hearing aids convert sound waves to computer codes alike and then amplify them. Codes include information on direction, pitch and volume. Sounds are therefore understood better and thereby the results. These are more costly, smaller and more powerful hearing aids.

Styles of Hearing aid

1) Behind the ear (BTE).

2) In the canal (ITC)

3) Completely in the canal (CIC)

Common difficulties with Hearing aids

1) Echo sounds

2) Discomfort

3) Feedback or whistling sounds

4) Background noise

Care of Hearing aids

- Keep away from heat, moisture, pets and children.
- Clean as advised.
- Dead batteries to be replaced immediately.
- Turn off devices when not in use.

In general HA may last for 3 to 5 years and batteries for many days to few weeks.

As the name suggests hearing aid aids hearing and cannot correct it. Most commonly used for sensorineural hearing loss resulting from damage to the hair cells and synapses of cochlear and auditory nerve.

Others

- Spectacle Hearing Aid
- Eye glass aids
- Bone and air conduction spectacles

Principle

> CROS Hearing aid is HA that transmits sound from one side of the head to the other.

> Occlusion effect is when an object fills outer portion of the ear canal and the person perceives hollow or booming echo-like sounds of their own voice.

> BAHA is a surgically implanted auditory prosthesis based on bone conduction. Option for patients without ear canal.

> Battery
> Zinc air battery
> 1.3 - 1.4 volts
> Button cell

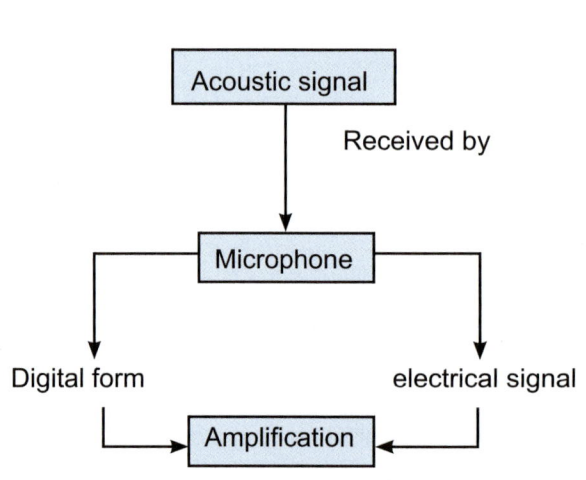

5. COCHLEAR IMPLANTS

Dr. Kashmira P. Chavan

A cochlear implant is a surgically implanted electronic device in individuals with severe to profound sensorineural hearing loss, who get no significant benefit with optimally fitted hearing aids. A cochlear implant performs the function of the damaged portion of the inner ear (cochlea)and delivers electrical signals to the ganglion cells close to the auditory (hearing) nerve. The auditory nerve relays these signals to the brain, which interprets them, and sound is perceived.

PARTS OF A COCHLEAR IMPLANT

External components .

- Speech processor with microphone.
- Transmission coil.

Internal components (surgically implanted) .

- Receiver-Stimulator.
- Electrode array.

The microphone picks up sounds, and the speech processor converts them into electrical signals. These signals are carried via the transmitter coil to the internal receiver-stimulator, from where the coded signals travel via the electrode array and stimulate the cochlear nerve endings in the cochlea. The cochlear nerve then relays these signals to the brain, which interprets them, and sound is perceived.

CANDIDACY CRITERIA

General Audiological Criteria

- Bilateral severe to profound hearing loss with inadequate benefit from optimally fitted hearing aids,

Expanded Candidacy Criteria

- Bilateral moderate-profound sensorineural hearing loss with inadequate benefit from optimally fitted hearing aids,
- Unilateral hearing loss or Single Sided Deafness (SSD).

Aided Testing

- 40% sentence speech perception in the worse ear.
- Up to 70% sentence speech perception in the better ear.

AGE

Adults

- No upper age limit
- Post-lingual hearing loss (Acquired or progressive).
- Bilateral moderate to severe hearing loss or worse.
- 75% or worse phenome score in better hearing ear.
- 55% or worse phenome score in better hearing ear.

Children

- Congenital or post-lingual (acquired or progressive) sensorineural hearing loss.
- To be ideally implanted within the first two years of life in case of a congenital hearing loss, as early implantation associated with better outcomes. Older the age of implantation in cases of congenital hearing loss, poorer the outcomes.
- Unaided PTA is 65 dBHL or worse in the better hearing ear.
- Unaided PTA is 75 dBHL or worse in the worse hearing ear,
- Best aided open set speech perception scores 70% or worse.
- No minimum age for referral for CI evaluation.
- FDA approval for CI in children ≥12 months old since 2000.

Older Children

- Congenital hearing loss history of regular hearing aid usage and following an aural communication mode
- Progressive or acquired hearing loss with good spoken language and consistent hearing aid usage

Medical / Surgical Criteria

- Absence of any medical / surgical contraindications for surgery
- Appropriate expectations and commitment from the patient / family

Radiological Criteria:

- Presence of cochlea and cochlear nerve

CONTRAINDICATIONS

- Patients not fitting into audiological criteria
- Hearing loss of neural or central origin
- Absence of cochlear nerve/ cochlea
- Active middle ear infections
- Other medical / surgical contraindications to surgery
- Psychological contraindications

PRE-IMPLANT EVALUATION

- Complete audiological evaluation (Unaided / Aided)
- Hearing Aid Trial
- Habilitation to begin prior to implantation (in children)
- Commitment to undergo habilitation (for a minimum period of 2-3 years or as may be required). And mapping post-implantation
- Radiological evaluation
    - HRCT Temporal Bone
    - MRI Brain (Limited) with cochlea and 7th 8th nerve complexes
- Vaccination
- Evaluation by a pediatrician / pediatric neurologist for fitness for cochlear implant surgery
- Physician / Anesthesia fitness
- Appropriate expectations counseling

STEPS OF SURGERY

- Postaural Lazy S incision.
- Connective tissue harvesting.
- Elevation of posterosuperiorly based musculoperiosteal flap.
- Creation of an adequately sized subperiosteal pocket underneath the musculo periosteal flap.
- Creation of a tunnel anteriorly below the muscle for the extracochlear electrode (for Nucleus Cochlear implants).
- Cortical mastoidectomy.
- Posterior Tympanotomy (Landmarks - Chorda tympani, Facial nerve, short process of the Incus).
- Drilling the well for the receiver-stimulator, and a channel for the electrode array.
- Identification of the round window.
- Drilling of any bony overhang over the round window for greater exposure.
- Creating a cochleostomy antero-inferior to the round window (for electrode insertions via a cochleostomy approach) / Incision in round window membrane (for electrode insertions via a round window approach) / Creating a cochleostomy flush with the antero-inferior margin of the round window (for electrode insertions via an extended round window approach).
- Implant placement and electrode insertion.
- Sealing of round window / cochleostomy with connective tissue.
- Closure in layers.
- Intra-operative neural response and impedance testing, and C-arm imaging to confirm functioning and appropriate implant placement.

COMPLICATIONS

- Intra-operative .
    - Bleeding
    - Damage to surrounding structures
    - Cerebrospinal fluid leakage
    - Damage to implant
    - Inappropriate implant placement
- Post-operative .
    - Wound infections
    - Facial paralysis: Temporary / Permanent
    - Implant Migration
    - Meningitis
    - Device failure

Diagrams by
Dr. Murallichand Nallamothu

External Portion: Outside the skin   Internal portion: Under the skin

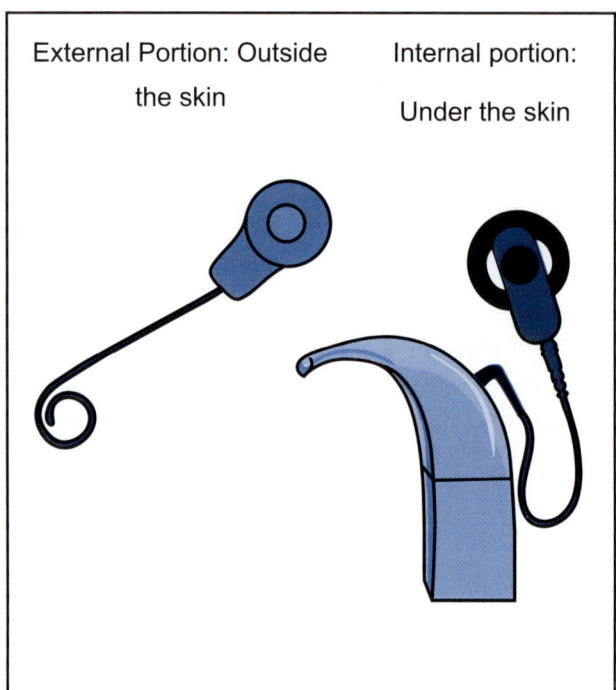

OW, RW and H forms 90 degree triangle

OW= Oval Window, **RW**= Round Window, **H**= Helicotrema

OW & RW & H forms 90° triangle.

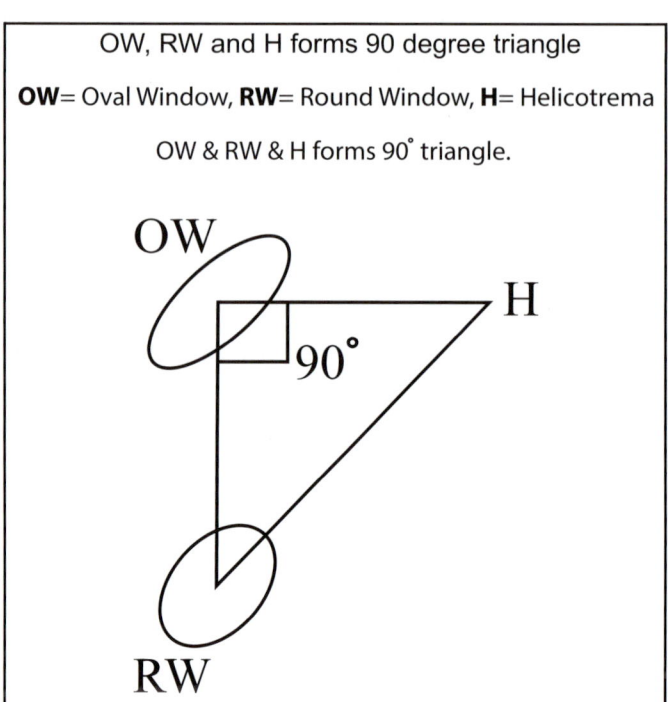

OW= Oval Window, **RW**= Round Window, **H**= Helicotrema

Centre of OW roughly corresponds to Groove of Tensor Tympani.

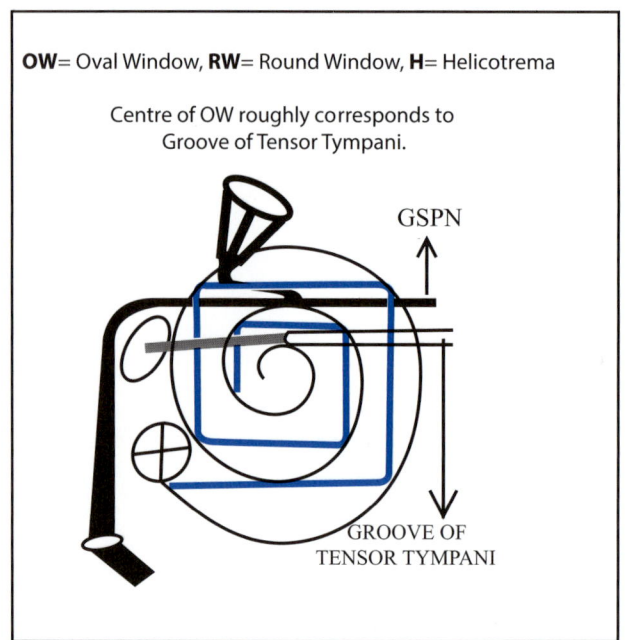

Below RW is divided into four quadrants.

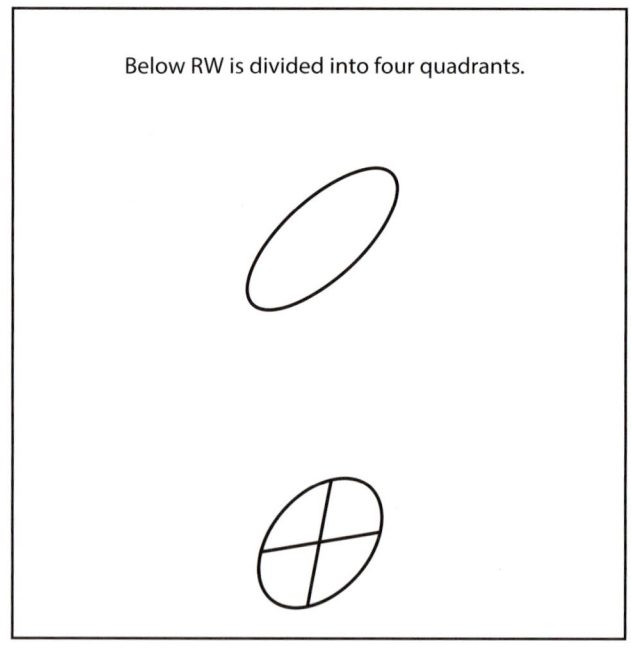

If we drill between OW & RW it is
SCALA VESTIBULAR COCHLEOSTOMY

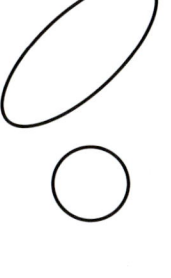
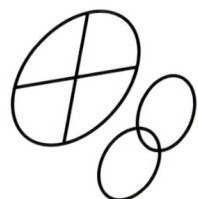

The round inferior to Antero - Inferior Cochleostomy is
INFERIOR COCHLEOSTOMY, which is direct trajectory
to Scala Tympani.

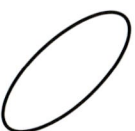
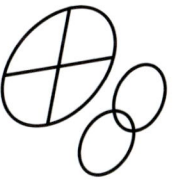

Osseus spiral laminae is seen through SUPERIOR
COCHLEOSTOMY. The space above osseus spiral
laminae is SCALA VESTIBULI and space below osseus
spiral laminae is SCALA TYMPANI

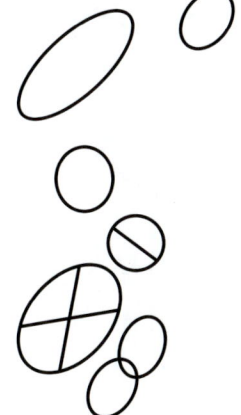

Overview of suggested surgical approaches in obliterated
cochlea.

- Partial drill-out of the basal turn.
  - Round window and beginning of basal turn
  - Half of the scala tympani of the basal turn

- Scala vestibuli insertion

- Complete drill-out of basal turn

- Complete drill-out of basal turn with middle turn cochleostomy
  with double array insertion

  - Anterograde insertion
  - Retrograde insertion

- Complete drill-out of the basal turn with middle turn drill-out
  with incomplete double array insertion

  - Anterograde insertion
  - Retrograde insertion

- No lumen found : Indication for ABI

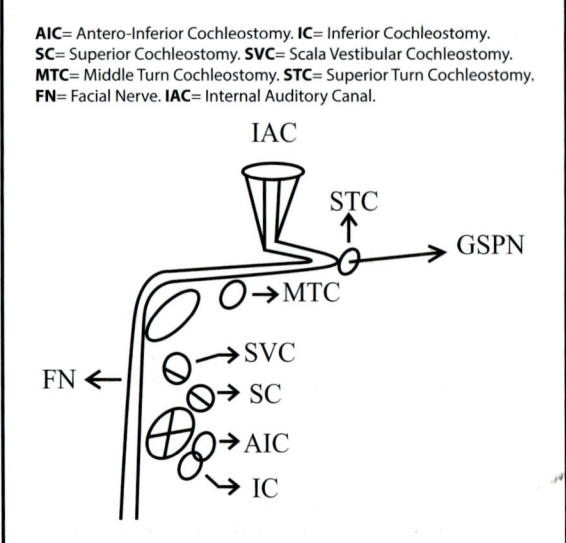

AIC= Antero-Inferior Cochleostomy. IC= Inferior Cochleostomy.
SC= Superior Cochleostomy. SVC= Scala Vestibular Cochleostomy.
MTC= Middle Turn Cochleostomy. STC= Superior Turn Cochleostomy.
FN= Facial Nerve. IAC= Internal Auditory Canal.

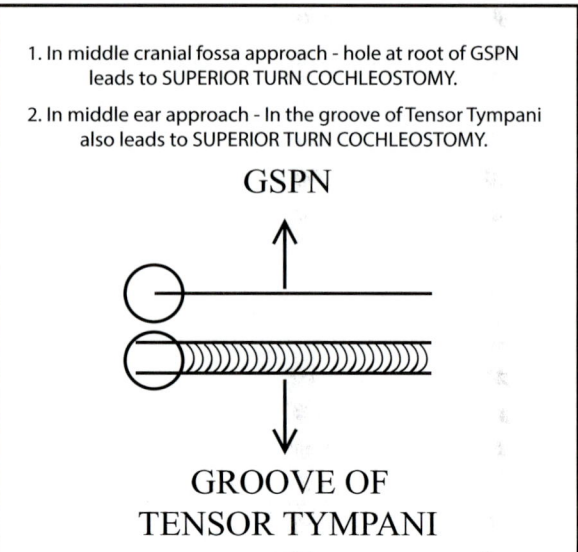

1. In middle cranial fossa approach - hole at root of GSPN leads to SUPERIOR TURN COCHLEOSTOMY.

2. In middle ear approach - In the groove of Tensor Tympani also leads to SUPERIOR TURN COCHLEOSTOMY.

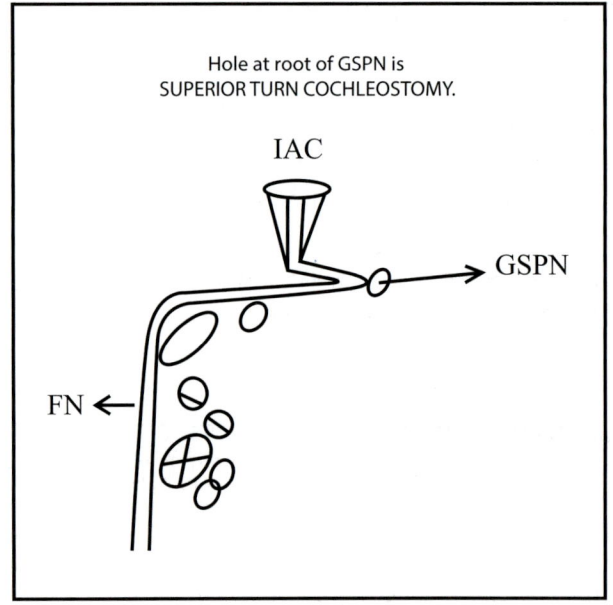

Hole at root of GSPN is
SUPERIOR TURN COCHLEOSTOMY.

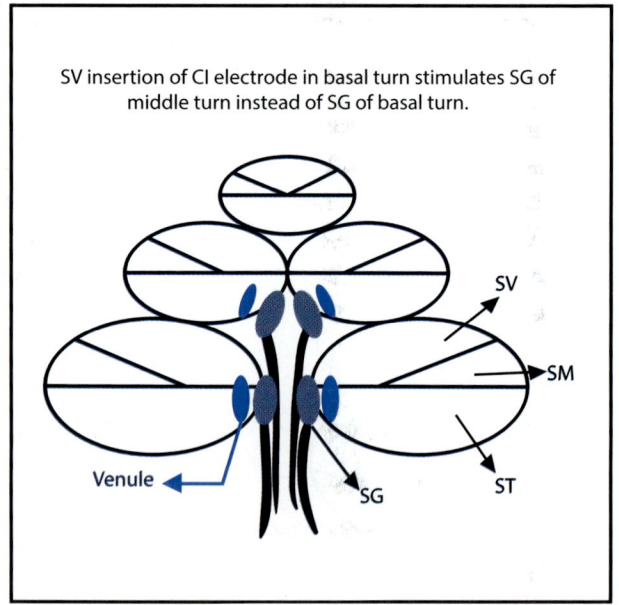

SV insertion of CI electrode in basal turn stimulates SG of middle turn instead of SG of basal turn.

INCISIONS FOR COCHLEAR IMPLANT

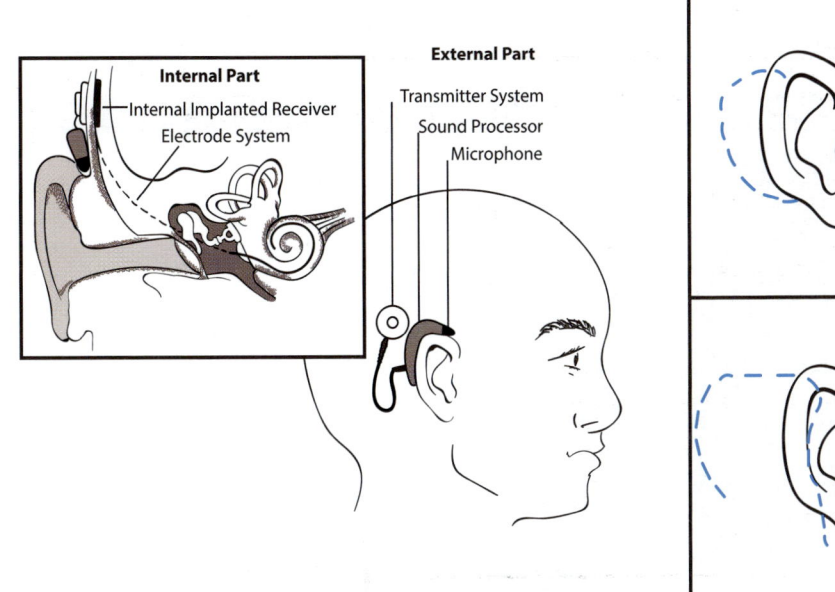

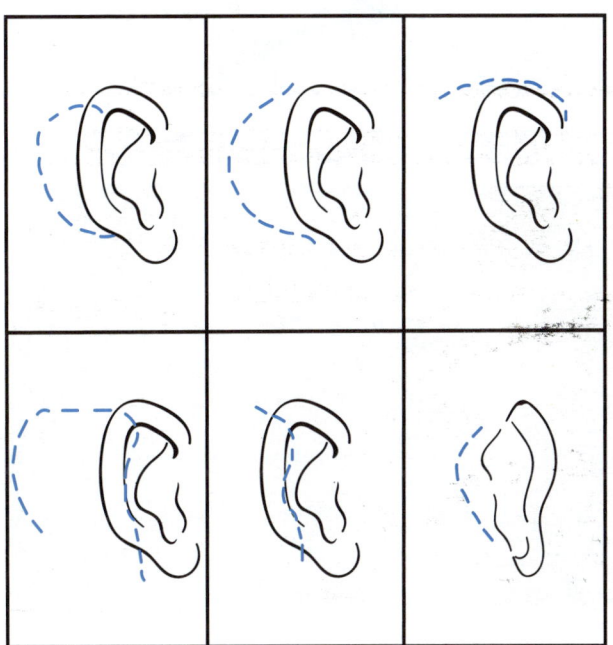

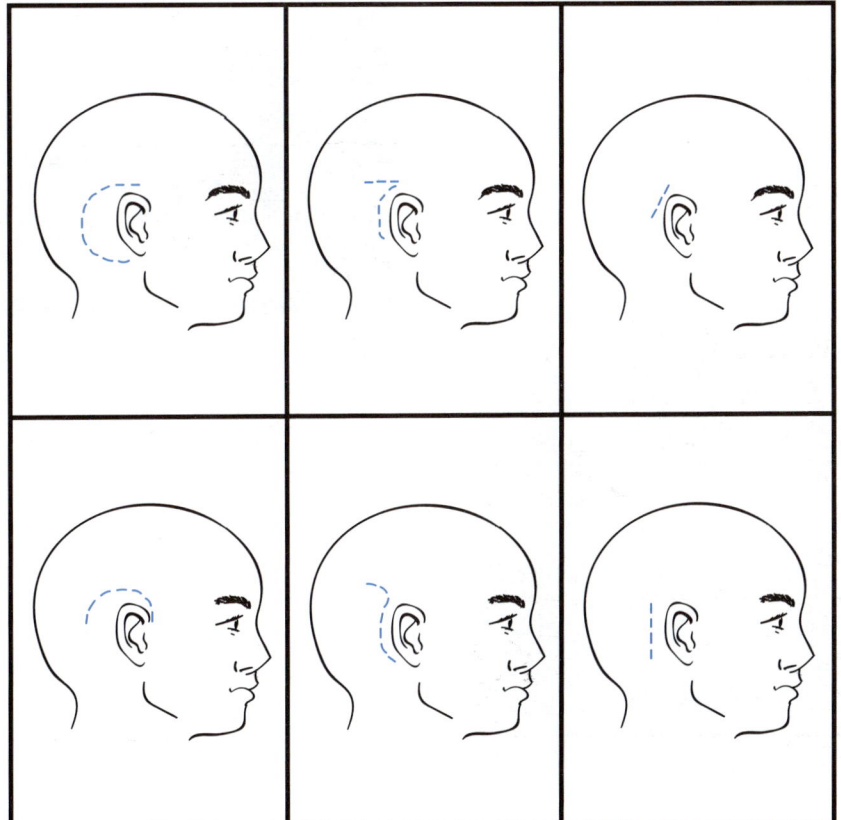

6. HOW TO READ A NORMAL HRCT TEMPORAL BONE

Dr. Kashmira P. Chavan

AXIAL SECTIONS (SERIAL CUTS – SUPERIOR TO INFERIOR)

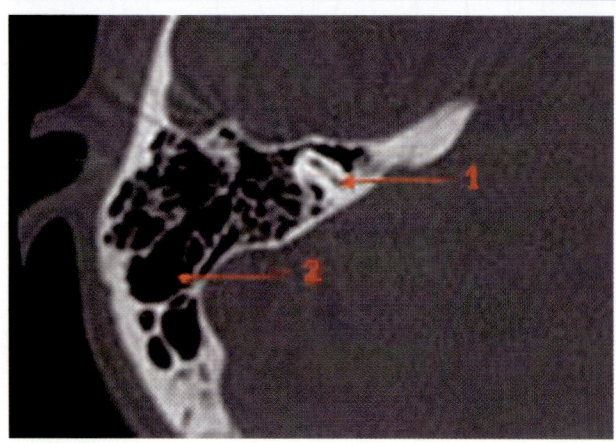

1. Superior Semicircular canal
2. Mastoid

1. Superior Semicircular canal
2. Mastoid

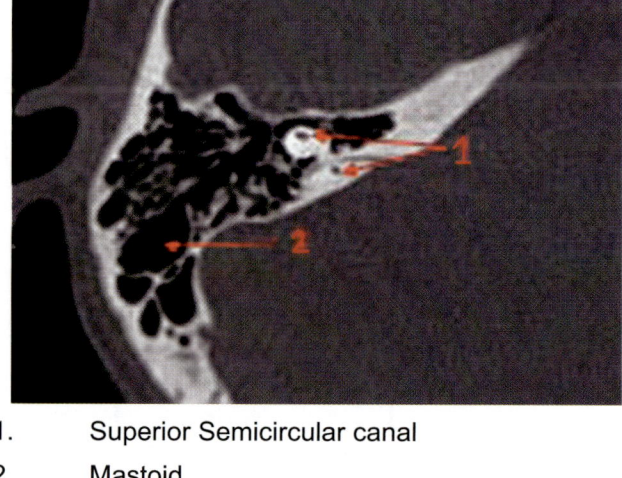

1. Superior Semicircular canal
2. Mastoid
3. Common crus
4. Posterior semicircular canal

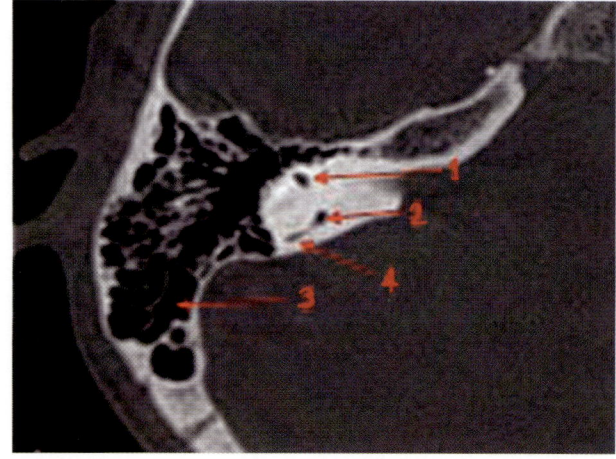

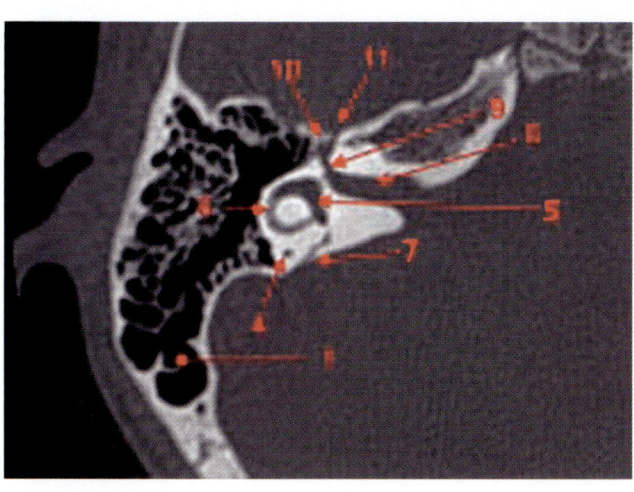

4. Posterior semicircular canal
5. Vestibule
6. Lateral SCC
7. Vestibular Aqueduct
8. Internal Auditory canal
9. Facial nerve (Labyrinthine segment)
10. Geniculate ganglion
11. Greater superficial petrosal nerve

1. Mastoid
4. Posterior Semicurcular canal
5. Vestibule
6. Lateral SCC
7. Vestibular Aqueduct
8. Internal Auditory canal
9. Facial Nerve
10. Geniculate ganglion
11. Greater superficial petrosal nerve
12. Cochlea labyrinthine
13. Facial nerve (Tympanic segment)
14. Ossicles segment
15. Sigmoid sinus

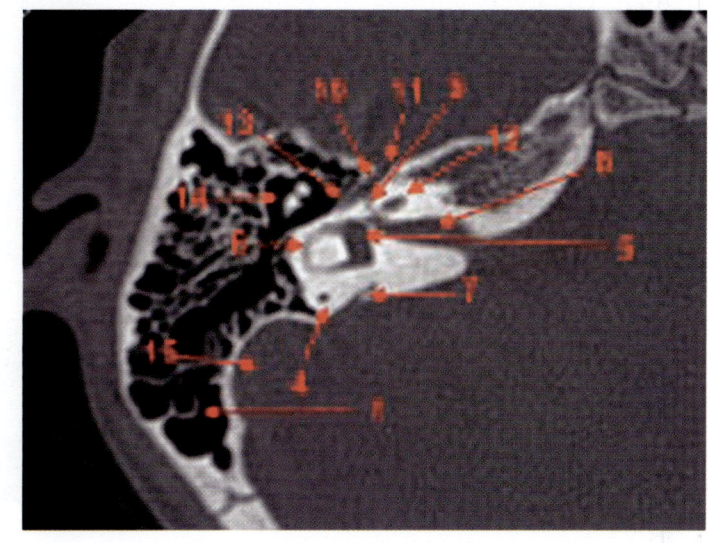

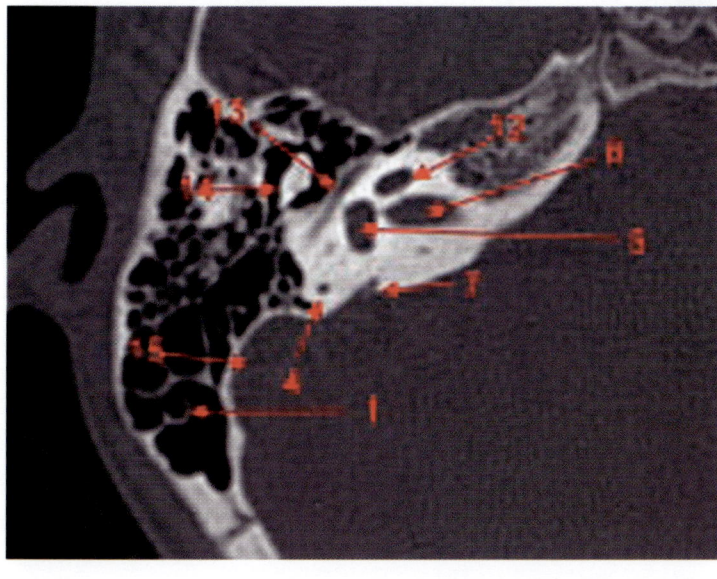

1. Mastoid
4. Posterior Semicircular canal
5. Vestibule
7. Vestibular Aqueduct
8. Internal Auditory canal
12. Cochlea
13. Facial nerve (Tympanic segment)
14. Ossicles
15. Sigmoid sinus

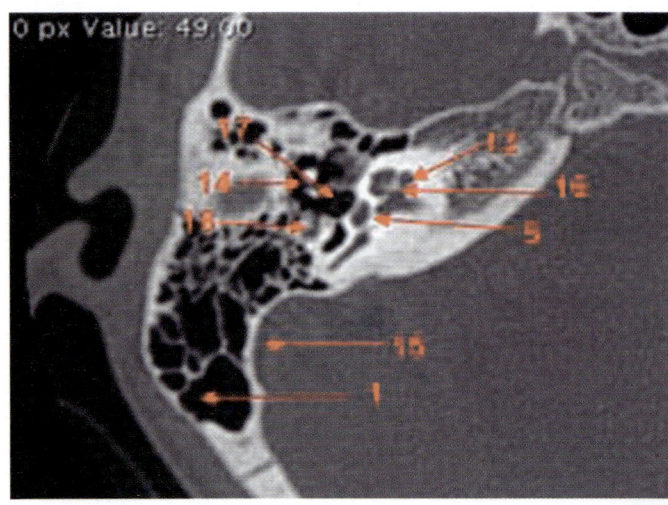

1.   Mastoid
5.   Vestibule
12. Cochlea
14. Ossicles
15. Sigmoid sinus
16. Modiolus
17. Stapes
18. Facial nerve (Vertical / Mastoid segment)

1.   Mastoid
12. Cochlea
14. Ossicles
15. Sigmoid sinus
18. Facial nerve (verticle / mastoid segment)
19. Round window niche
20. Cochlear aqueduct
21. Jugular bulb
22. Canal for tensor tympani

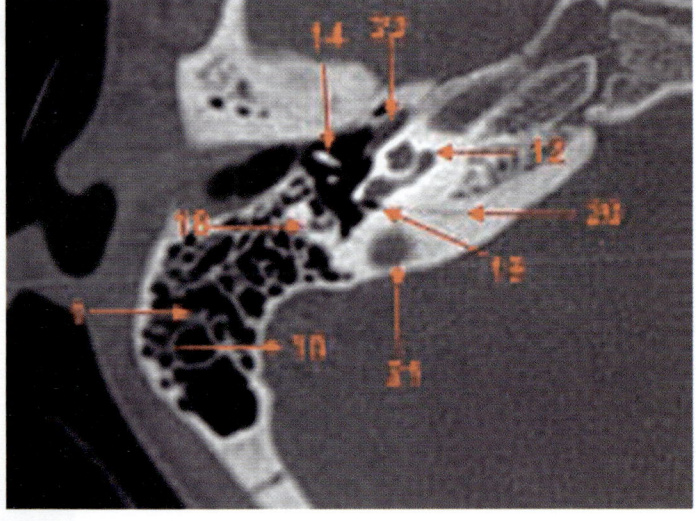

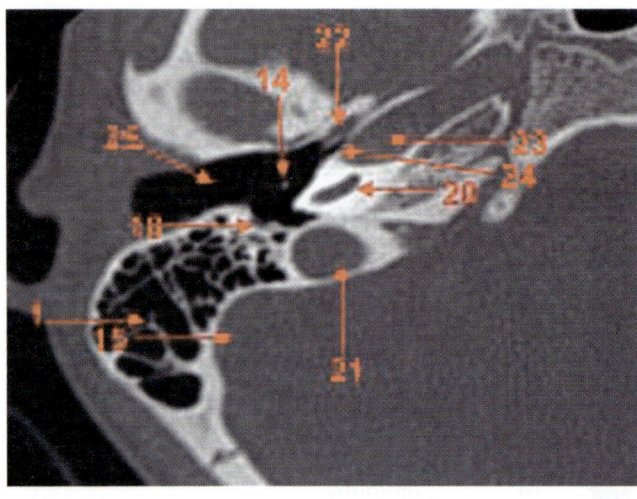

1.   Mastoid
12. Cochlea
14. Ossicle (Umbo)
15. Sigmoid Sinus
18. Facial nerve (vertical/mastoid segment)
21. Jugular bulb
22. Canal for tensor tympani
23. Carotid artery
24. Eustachian tube
25. External Canal

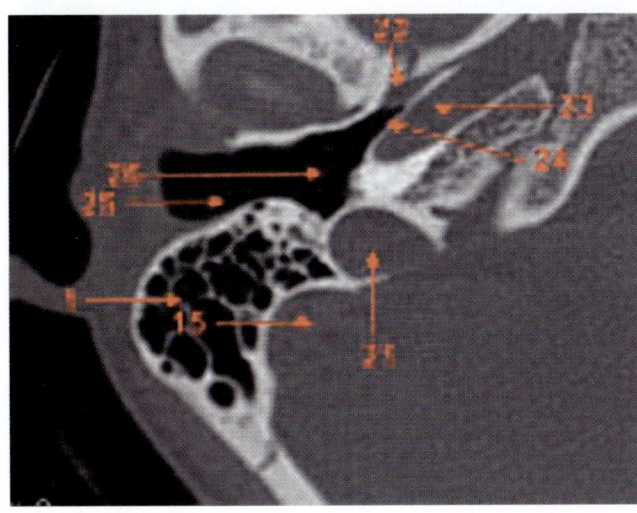

1. Mastoid
15. Sigmoid sinus
21. Jugular bulb
22. Canal for tensor tympani
23. Carotid artery
24. Eustachian tube
25. External auditory canal
26. Tympanic membrane

7. DENTISTRY IN ENT

Oral ulcer not healed in 3 weeks warrants Biopsy.

Facial pain:

- Tooth pathology
- Sinusitis
- TM joint dysfunction
- Salivary pathology
- Migraine
- Trigeminal neuralgia
- Cluster Headache
- Trauma
- Angina
- ENT tumours
- Osteomyelitis facial bones
- Atypical

Trismus:

- Dental Infections
- Neoplasia
- Tetanus

Dental caries - 3's'
• Streptococcus mutans
• Substrate - Sugar
• Susceptible tooth

Periodontal disease:
Gingivitis at the tooth-gingival interface by bacterial and polysaccharide complexes.

Vincent's angina:

- Ulcerative gingivitis
- Anaerobes
- Spirochetes

Oromandibular Devices:
• Mandibular Advancement Device
• Pushes / Pulls tongue forward
• Snoring / OSA

Gingival Swelling:
• Phenytoin
• Ciclosporin
• Nifedipine
• Scurvy
• Pregnancy
• Leukaemia
• Congenital

Dry mouth / Xerostomia
• Hypnotics
• Tricyclics
• Beta-blockers, diuretics
• Dehydration
• Sjogren's syndrome
• SLE, Scleroderma
• HIV/AIDS
• Sarcoidosis
• Salivary gland Sialoliths

8. OESOPHAGUS

Oesophageal tumours

- Most are malignant
- Less then 1% are benign
- Common benign: Leiomyoma
- Common malignant
  - Squamous Cell Carcinoma
  - Adenocarcinoma
  - Middle and lower third affected

Major Risk Factors

- Smoking
- Alcohol
- Barrett's oesophagus

Lesser factors

- Radiation
- Obesity
- Chronic oesophagitis
- Achalasia
- Tylosis
- Plummer Vinson syndrome
- Coeliac disease
- Caustic burns
- Chemicals
- HPV

Tylosis

- Non-epidermolytic palmoplantar keratoderma
- Rare autosomal disease
- Hyperkeratosis of palms
- More chance of developing (SCC) Squamous Cell Carcinoma
- 17q 25 chromosome abnormal

Plummer Vinson syndrome

- Dysphagia due to degeneration of oesophagus musculature
- Microcytic hypochromic anaemia
- Splenomegaly
- Achlorhydria
- Angular stomatitis
- Women > men

Imaging in oesophagus

- XRC
- BA swallow
- Oesophagoscopy
- Brush cytology
- Biopsy
- EUS
- C.T. Scan
- MRI
- PET scan

X-ray findings in oesophageal tumours

- Tumour seen
- Lymph nodes seen in mediastinum
- Displacement of normal mediastinal structures
- Aspiration pneumonitis
- Air fluid levels in oesophagus
- Pulmonary metastasis
- Pleural effusions

Ba Swallow findings in Oesophageal tumours

- Stricture
- Ulceration
- Irregular ulcerated mucosa
- Dilatation proximal to mass
- Shelf like luminal narrowing
- Apple - core lesion
- Tracheo-oesophageal fistula
- Metastatic lymph node
- Stenosis and overt obstruction

EUS

- Valuable diagnostic tool
- Correctly determines tumour depth and nodal stage
- Mediastinal, perigastric, coeliac nodes

C.T. Chest - Abdomen

- Reveals invasion of mediastinal structures
- Nodal metastases
- Distant metastasis in liver, lungs, pleura, adrenals
- C.T. may miss nodes in mediastinum and retro peritoneum
- MRI not considered superior to C.T. in these cases

PET Scan

- For screening metastases to liver, lung, adrenal, skeleton
- Superior for distant metastasis
- Limited use in local staging due to its resolution

Oesophageal carcinoma

- Squamous Cell Carcinoma
- Adenocarcinoma
- Fast spread
- Lack of serosal layer

Palliation

- Chemoradiation +/- Surgery in combination
- Oesophageal stent
- Newer self expanding metal stents
- Endoscopic laser debulking
- Intraluminal brachytherapy
- Photodynamic therapy
- External beam irradiation
- Surgical bypass
- Tracheostomy
- Gastrostomy
- Jejunostomy
- Pain control
- Family counselling

Chemotherapy

- 5Fu

- Cisplatin

- Anti growth factor antibodies

- Squamous cell carcinoma of oesophagus-moderately radioresponsive

Surgeries to treat oesophageal carcinoma

Cervical Oesophagus - Complete laryngo - pharyngectomy with bilateral neck dissection with gastric pull-up, colon interposition, Jejunal free flap, other flaps for reconstruction

All other Oesophageal carcinomas -

- Three - hole technique

- Cervical approach

- Laparotomy

- Right Thoracotomy to remove all tumour and regional nodes

9. TRACHEOSTOMY CARE

Dr. KK Ezzy (Valiullah)
Dr. Anjoo Choudhary
Prince Aly Khan Hospital

TRACHEOSTOMY CARE

- Keep your neck clean and dry.
- Change the dressing daily and if soiled.
- Change neck straps weekly and if soiled.
- In case of granulations, apply antibiotic and steroid ointment like gentamicin-clobetasone on the stomal skin using sterile cotton swab.
- Keep your mouth clean. Brush your teeth at least two times a day. Salivary secretions have germs that cause infection if they get into your airway.
- Each person that comes into your home should wash their hands.

Cleaning the tube

- Check the air blast three times a day.
- Suction if increased secretions are present.
- In case of inner tube, remove and clean using brush and warm water.
- In case of children, clean the outer part of tube with sterile swab stick.

In case of blocked tube

- Pinch the catheter and insert upto the tip.
- Suction while withdrawing.
- Recheck the air blast.
- If no improvement then instill 0.5 cc soda bicarbonate and re-suction.
- Nebulise and retry.
- If no improvement then remove tube, extend the neck and stretch the stomal skin. Patient will breathe through the stoma.
- Replace the tube as soon as possible.

Humidification

- Keep wet gauze over stoma throughout the day and night to avoid secretions from getting dried.
- Or use humidifier and change once blocked.

Changing of tracheostomy tube

- Tube should be changed every 28 days.
- Under sterile conditions, open a new tube and attach straps.
- Lubricate with lignocaine jelly.
- Make the patient lie down, lift the chin to extend the cheek, remove the old tube.
- Insert the new tube directing it backwards then downwards towards the patient's feet.
- Confirm position with air blast and tie it around the neck

Communication with the tube

- Deflate cuff in case of cuffed tube, insert a smaller size.
- Use a speaking valve or fenestrated tube for speech.

Key Point to remember:

- Always keep a same sized tube and a smaller size tube ready near the patient.
- Always keep a mode of communication like alarm bell near the patient.
- In case the tube dislodges, DON'T PANIC, extend neck and breathe normally through the stoma and patiently insert a clean tube.

10. SALIENT POINTS

DYSPHAGIA

Growths which present with dysphagia:

- Base of tongue
- Posterior pharyngeal wall
- Supraglottis
- Posterior cricoid
- Pyriform fossa

Growth which present with change of voice

1. Base of tongue — Due to mass effect, problem with articulation and resonance
2. Post pharyngeal wall — Problems with articulation and resonance and mass effect.
3. Supraglottis — Muffled speech due to articulaton and resonance problem.
4. Post – Cricoid — Due to Cricoarytenoid fixation
5. Pyriform fossa — Because of invasion of cricoarytenoid joint Invasion and invasion of posterior Cricoarytenoid muscle and recurrent laryngeal nerve.

Dysphagia	Symptom
Oropharyngeal	– Difficulty initiating swallowing
	- Nasal regurgitation
Oesophageal	– food stuck in the throat
	- Pain retrosternal area

Muscles of Soft Palate:

- Tensor palatini
- Levator palatini
- Palatoglossus
- Palatopharyngeus
- Musculus uvulae

Muscles of mastication

- Medial pterygoid
- Lateral pterygoid
- Temporalis
- Masseter
- Buccinator

Structures passing through sinus of morgagni
Eustachian tube
Tensor palatini muscle
Levator Veli palatini muscle
Ascending pharyngeal artery.

Sinus of Morgagni

Space between superior constrictor and base of skull

OSA

Friedman Classification

The Friedman classification is used to assess: palatine tonsil, modified mallampati score, BMI (Body mass index)

Friedman tongue position (FTP)

a) FTP I visualizes the uvula and tonsils / pillars.

b) FTP IIa visualizes most of the uvula but not the tonsils / pillars

c) FTP IIb visualizes the entire soft palate to the uvular base.

d) FTP III shows some of the soft palate with the distal end absent.

e) FTP IV visualizes only the hard palate.

Tonsil Grading System

a) size 0 absence of tonsillar tissue

b) size 1 within the pillars

c) size 2 extended to the pillars

d) size 3 extended past the pillars

e) size 4 extended to the midline.

The Mallampati Score

Class I	Complete visualization of soft palate
Class II	Complete visualization of the uvula
Class III	Visualization of only the base of uvula
Class IV	Soft palate is not visible at all.

Apnoea-Hypopnoea Index - AHI (Adults)

- Normal: AHI: < 5
- Mild: AHI: 5-15
- Moderate: AHI: 15-30
- Severe: AHI: > 30

EAR

Exostoses

- Smooth, multiple, bilateral
- Swellings of bony canal
- Localised bony hypertrophy
- Response to cold exposure / aquatic sports

Main Complication of grommets
• Infections
• Tympanosclerosis

11. OSTEOLOGY POINTS

Embryology

Calvarium (Roof) - Frontal, Parietal, Occipital

Base - Sphenoid, Ethmoid, Occipital, Temporal, Anterior and posterior fontanelle.

Calvarium (Roof)

Frontal Bone part

- Orbital plate
- Glabella
- Supraorbital notch

Parietal Bone

- Sagittal Suture
- Galea aponeurotica
- Superior and Inferior temporal line

Occipital Bone Part

- Lambdoidal Suture
- External Occipital Protuberances
- Hypoglossal canal
- Clivus

Bones of Base of Skull

- Part of frontal bone
- Part of occipital bone
- Temporal Bone
- Sphenoid Bone
- Ethmoid Bone

Frontal Bone parts

- Orbital Plate of frontal bone

Occipital Bone parts

- Part of Occipital bone forms base
- Clivus
- Foramen magnum

Temporal Bone

Squamous

- Fish scale
- Temporal fossa

Petrous

- Wedge
- Dense
- IAM

Tympanic

- Curved plate
- Separate bone
- Contains EAC

Mastoid

- Mastoid and styloid process
- Mastoid air cells
- Mandibular fossa - TMJ

Zygomatic process

- Zygomatic arch
- Articular tubercle

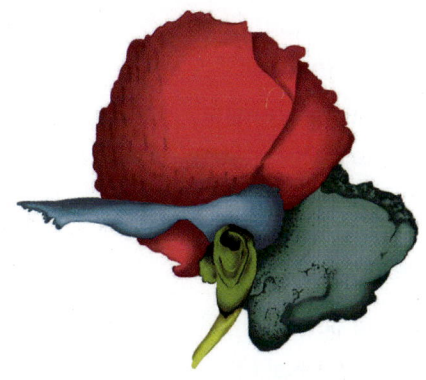

Muscles
- **Temporalis**
- **Masseter**
- **Posterior belly digastric**
- **Splenius capitis**

Sphenoid bone

- Butterfly shape body
  - Chiasmatic groove
- Greater wings
- Lesser wings
- Anterior & Posterior clinoid process
- Sella Turcica
  - Tuberculum sellae
  - Hypophyseal fossa
  - Dorsum sellae
- Orbital Surface
- Optic foramen / canal
- Foramen rotundum
- Superior orbital fissure
- Pterygoid process (Medial and lateral pterygoid plates)
- Foramen spinosum
- Foramen ovale

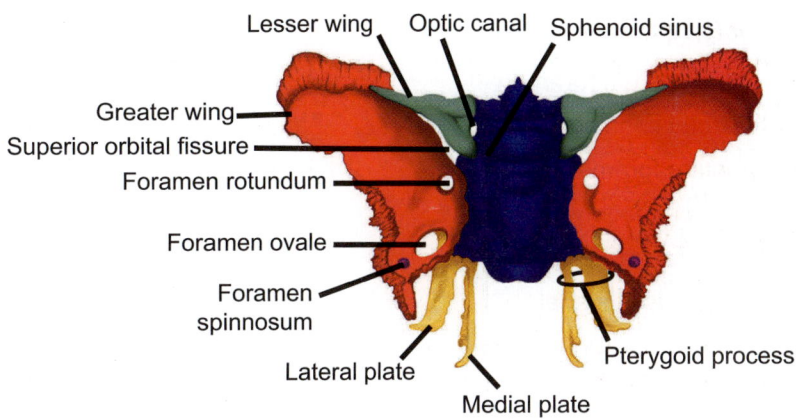

Lesser wing   Optic canal   Sphenoid sinus
Greater wing
Superior orbital fissure
Foramen rotundum
Foramen ovale
Foramen spinosum
Lateral plate
Medial plate
Pterygoid process

Ethmoid Bone

- Perpendicular Plate
- Cribriform plate
- Olfactory foramina
- Crista galli
- Nasal turbinates concha

Bones of the face

- Nasal bone
- Inferior nasal conchae
- Maxillae
- Lacrimal Bones
- Zygomatic Bone
- Palatine bones
- Vomer
- Mandible

Foramina of the Skull

- Olfactory
- Optic canal
- Superior orbital fissure
- Foramen rotundum
- Foramen ovale
- Foramen spinosun
- Internal acoustic meatus
- Stylomastoid foramen
- Carotid canal
- Jugular foramen
- Foramen lacerum
- Foramen magnum
- Hypoglossal canal

Skull Sutures

- Frontal metopic suture
- Coronal suture
- Sagittal suture
- Lambdoidal suture
- Squamosal suture

Maxillary bones

- Body-maxillary sinus
- Infra-orbital foramen
- Alveolar Process
- Palatine process
  (Zygomatic and frontal process)

Landmarks

Anterior surface

- Infra-orbital foramen
- Anterior nasal spine - junction
- Alveolar process
- Zygomatic process
- Frontal process
- Nasal notch
- Incisive fossa

Inferior surface / palatine surface

- Alveolar sockets
- Incisive canal
- Greater palatine foramen
- Median palatine suture

Nasal bones   .

- Forms bridge at the junction
  - Superior border
  - Medial border
  - Lateral border
  - Inferior border

Zygomatic Bones

(Cheek bone / Malar bone)

Landmarks

- Frontal (in frontal process)
  - Zygomatico-orbital foramen
  - Infra orbital process
  - Zygomatico - facial foramen
- Lateral
  - Orbital process
  - Zygomatico facial foramen

- Temporal process
- Zygomatico - temporal foramen

- Body
- Rami
- Angle of Mandible
- Condylar process
- Coronoid process
- Alveolar process
- Mental foramen

Landmarks

Inner Surface

- Genial tubercle
- Mylohyoid line and groove
- Mandibular foramen
- Mandibular notch
- Genial angle
- Ascending ramus
- Digastric fossa
- Submandibular fossa
- Lingula
- Sphenomandibular ligament
- Sublingual fossa
  (Head, neck, body, ramus, condylar, coronoid process)

Outer surface

- Mandibular notch
- Head
- Condylar process
- Body
- Alveolar process
- Coronoid process
- Mental tubercle
- Mental foramen
- Mental protruberance (Symphysis mentii in centre / medially)
- Base
- Oblique line
- Angle
- Ramus
- Neck

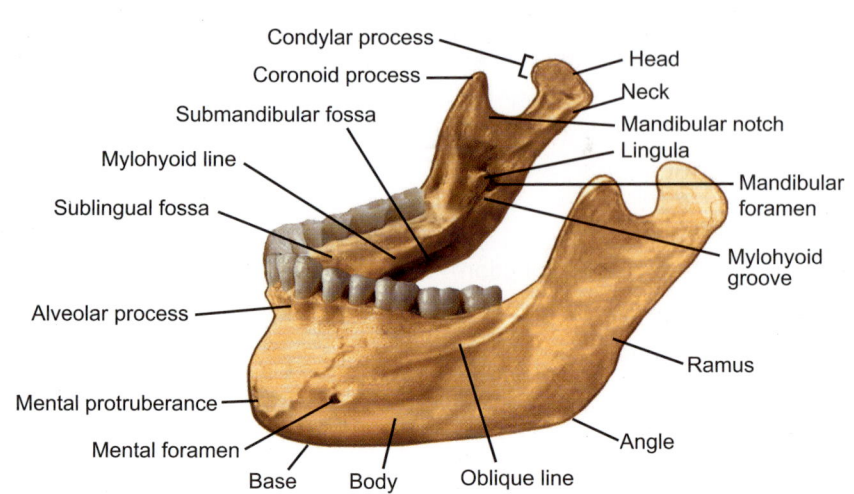

MUSCLES, BLOOD VESSELS, NERVES IN RELATION

- Temporalis
- Masseter
- Lateral pterygoid
- Medial pterygoid
- Mylohyoid
- Masseteric nerves and vessels
- Buccinator
- Facial vessels
- Platysma
- Depressor anguli oris
- Orbicularis Oris
- Mentalis
- Depressor labii inferioris
- Superior constrictor
- Auriculotemporal nerve
- Superficial temporal artery
- External carotid artery
- Mental foramen with mental nerves and vessels
- Mylohyoid groove with nerve and artery to mylohyoid
- Maxillary artery
- Geniohyoid
- Digastric anterior belly
- Genioglossus
- Pterygomandibular raphe
- Lingual nerve
- Inferior alveolar artery and nerve

Lacrimal Bone

- Small fragile bone
- Lacrimal sac
- Nasolacrimal duct

Palatine Bone

- Horizontal portion
- Perpendicular portion
- Floor of nasal cavity
- Roof of mouth
- Floor of orbit

12. MCQs

Q.1   The tonsils lie on which muscle:

A.   Musculus uvulae
B.   Superior constrictor
C.   Palatoglossus
D.   Palatopharyngeus

Ans. B)

Q.2   Which of it is not part of adenoid facies?

A.   Open mouth
B.   High arched palate
C.   Cleft palate
D.   Open anterior bite

Ans. C)

Q.3   Simonart's band is

A.   Thin tissue in floor of nasal vestibule in cleft lip patients
B.   Associated with incomplete cleft
C.   Associated with Vincents Angina
D.   Not related to Simonart, a Belgian Doctor

Ans. A)

Q.4   The primary and secondary palate are separated by

A.   Foramen lacerum
B.   Incisive foramen
C.   Foramen ovale
D.   Nasal placodes

Ans. B)

Q.5   The primary palate consists of not one of the following:

A.   Lip
B.   Alveolar arch
C.   Pre maxilla (palate anterior to incisive foramen)
D.   Hard palate

Ans. D)

Q.6   Cleft lip/palate is mainly associated with the following syndromes but

A.   Apert's syndrome
B.   Plummer-Vinson syndrome
C.   Treacher Collins syndrome
D.   Stickler's syndrome

Ans. B)

Q.7   Submucous cleft includes all but

A.   Bifid uvula
B.   Zona pellucida
C.   Notch in posterior hard palate
D.   Immunotherapy

Ans. D)

Q.8   Allergic salute is all but one

A.   Allergic shiners
B.   Horizontal crease on skin of nose
C.   Muscle relaxant
D.   Allergic gape

Ans. C)

Q.9   Septal perforations from Syphilis are usually

A.   Anterior
B.   Posterior
C.   None of the above

Ans. B)

Q.10   State true or false

Salicylates ototoxicity is

A.   Flat bilateral hearing loss
B.   Tinnitus
C.   Reversible HL within 72 hours of discontinuation

Ans. All true

Q.11   The following disease are associated with myoclonus:

A.   Syphilis
B.   Psychogenic illness
C.   Multiple sclerosis
D.   Intracranial neoplasm

Ans. All true

Q.12   Drugs causing tinnitus are:

A.   Chloroquine
B.   Gentamycin
C.   Enalapril
D.   B-blocker timolol

Ans. All true

Q.13   Trail sign is

A.   Of crusting or keratin leading from the margin of a TM perforation
B.   Seen in cholesteatoma
C.   Both of the above

Ans. C)

Q.14   Carhart's notch is characteristically seen at

A.   500 Hz
B.   1000 Hz
C.   2000 Hz
D.   4000 Hz

Ans. C)

Q.15   Organ of corti is in

A.   Scala media
B.   Scala vestibuli
C.   Scala tympanum
D.   Saccule

Ans. A)

Q.16   Caloric test has

A.   Slow component only
B.   Fast component only
C.   Slow and fast components
D.   None of the above

Ans. C)

Q.17   Features of cholesteatoma include all but

A.   Deafness
B.   Keratinized stratified squamous epithelium
C.   Bone erosions
D.   Lymphatic permeation

Ans. D)

Q.18   Acoustic neuroma is common in

A.   Facial nerve
B.   Cochlear nerve
C.   Superior vestibular nerve
D.   Inferior vestibular nerve

Ans. C)

Q.19   Kobrak test is used for

A.   Eliciting nystagmus
B.   Check for deafness
C.   Check for cochlear nerve affection
D.   Minimal caloric stimulation

Ans. D)

Q.20   For coalescent mastoiditis ideal is

A.   Cortical mastoidectomy
B.   MRM
C.   Radical mastoidectomy
D.   Stapedotomy

Ans. A)

Q.21 Basal turn dysplasia of cochlea is

A. Mondini dysplasia
B. Bing Schiebenman dysplasia
C. Scheibe dysplasia
D. Alexander dysplaisa

Ans. D)

Q.22 Ramsay Hunt Syndrome involves:

A. Stellate ganglion
B. Geniculate ganglion
C. Scarpa ganglion
D. Spiral ganglion

Ans. B)

Q.23 Fistula test causes vertigo and nystagmus towards

A. Non-affected ear
B. Affected ear
C. Both ears
D. None of the above

Ans. B)

Q.24 Hennebert's sign is

A. Positive fistula test without middle ear / mastoid disease
B. Seen in Meniere's disease
C. Seen in Congenital Syphilis
D. All of the above

Ans. D)

Q.25 The following pass through superior orbital fissure but one:

A) Oculomotor nerve
B) Trochlear nerve
C) Ophthalmic branch of trigeminal nerve
D) Mandibular nerve

Ans. D)

Q.26 Hypoglossal nerve is motor to muscles of the tongue except:

A) Palatoglossus
B) Genioglossus
C) Hyoglossus
D) Styloglossus

Ans. A)

Q.27 Vagus nerve branchial motor is motor to all except:

A) Motor to constrictor muscles of pharynx
B) Muscles of larynx
C) Tensor veli palatini
D) Intrinsic muscles of larynx

Ans. C)

Q.28 Maxillary division of trigeminal nerve

A)   Passes through foramen rotundum
B)   Supplies skin of face, over maxilla, upper lip,maxillary teeth.
C)   Supplies mucosa of nose, maxillary sinuses, palate.
D)   All of the above

Ans. D)

Q.29 Olfactory hallucinations

A)   False perceptions of smell
B)   Lesions in temporal bone
C)   Accompany deep to uncus lesion
D)   All of the above

Ans. D)

Q.30 Irritating lesions of lateral olfactory area are:

A)   Temporal lobe epilepsy
B)   Uncinate fits
C)   Disagreeable odours
D)   Involuntary movements of lips/tongue
E)   All of the above

Ans. E)

Q.31 State true or false

A)   Section of right Optic nerve results in blindness in the temporal and nasal visual fields area right eye
B)   Section of optic chiasm reduces peripheral vision - bitemporal hemianopia.
C)   Section of right Optic tract eliminates vision from left temporal and right nasal - contralateral homonymous hemianopsia
D)   All of above true

Ans. D)

Q.32 Stage 1 sleep

A)   Transition b/w wakefullness and sleep.
B)   Low-voltage EEG.
C)   Slow rolling eye movements.
D)   All of the above

Ans. D)

Q.33 Stage 2 sleep

A)   Lack of eye movements
B)   Sleep spindles
C)   K. Complexes
D)   All of the above

Ans. D)

Q.34 Stage 3 and 4

A)   Deeper sleep
B)   Delta waves in stage 4
C)   Slow delta waves in stage 3
D)   All of the above

And. D)

Q.35 Dreams are during

A)   REM sleep
B)   Non-REM sleep

Ans . A)

Q.36 REM sleep

A)   Paradoxical sleep
B)   20-25% of sleep cycle
C)   Saw tooth waves on EEG
D)   Mixed frequency and low voltage activity on EEG.
E)   All of the above

Ans. E)

Q.37 Obstructive events occur most in:

A)   stage II sleep
B)   stage III sleep
C)   stage IV sleep
D)   B) + C)

Ans. D)

Q.38 Blow-out fracture

A)   Blunt non penetrating object
B)   Increased intra-orbital pressure
C)   Out-fracture of orbital wall
D)   All of the above

Ans. D)

Q.39 Signs of disruption of medial canthal tendon

A)   Telecanthus
B)   Epiphora
C)   Narrow palpebral fissure
D)   All of the above

Ans. D)

Q.40 Forced duction test examines for extraocular muscle entrapment in blow out fractures

Ans. True

Q.41 Battle's sign is periorbital ecchymosis

Ans. False

Q.42 Raccoon sign is post auricular ecchymosis due to fracture mastoid cortex.

Ans. False

Q.43 Laryngopharyngeal reflux is

A.   Hoarseness
B.   Dry cough
C.   Cervical dysphagia
D.   Globus sensation
E.   All of the above

Ans. E)

Q.44   Sulzberger's Powder

A.   Antiseptic
B.   2 gm Iodine and Boric acid
C.   Powder blown in radical mastoid cavity
D.   All of the above

Ans. D)

STATE TRUE OR FALSE

Q.45   Botulinum toxin irreversibly blocks the presynaptic release of acetylcholine:- localised muscle paralysis

Ans. True

Q.46   Rhinitis medicamentosa is the medical name for "Hooked-on-Afrin nose."

Ans. True

Q.47   Digital endoscopic photography offers numerous advantages over analog photography in clinical practice.

Ans. True

Q.48   Botox is used in facial plastic surgery for treatment of cervicofacial rhytids as in - around the eyes and forehead.

Ans. True

Q.49   Most common organism for septal crusting is

A.   Staphylococcus aureus
B.   Streptococcus
C.   Anaerobes
D.   None of the above

Ans.   A)

Q.50   Most common malignant tumour of the thyroid gland is papillary carcinoma

Ans. True

Q.51   Papillary carcinoma accounts for

A.   Best prognosis
B.   Women more affected
C.   "Orphan-annie's eye" nuclei
D.   Psammoma bodies
E.   All of the above

Ans. E)

Q.52   Most common tumour of the thyroid is follicular adenoma.

Ans. True

Q.53 ^{131}I ablation complications are

A.   Acute radiation thyroiditis
B.   Acute Sialoadenitis
C.   Hypoparathyroidism
D.   Increase risk of bladder carcinoma
E.   All of the above

Ans. E)

Q.54   MEN1 is also known as Wermer Syndrome

Ans. True

Q.55   MEN IIA is also known as Sipple's Syndrome

Ans. True

Q.56   Of all paraganglionamas, paraganglionic tissue at carotid body bifurcation is the most common location.

Ans.   True

Q.57   Schirmer's test is a method used to assess <u>parasympathetic</u> / <u>sympathetic</u> **innervation to the lacrimal gland via the Greater superficial petrosal nerve.**

Ans. Parasympathetic

Q.58   Facial myokimia is a worm-like motion in the mid facial muscles associated with multiple sclerosis or malignant neoplasms.

Ans.   True

Q.59   Trench mouth presents with crater like punched out depressions along the gingival margins.

Ans. True

Q.60   Sjogren's syndrome

A. Buccal biopsy with histological grading is the diagnostic investigation

B. Small percentage can develop lymphoma in parotid gland, hence long-term follow-up is essential.

C. Parotid enlargement and also lacrimal gland involvement is due to lymphocytic infiltration.

D. All of the above

Ans.   D)